I0982968

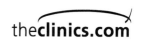

GASTROINTESTINAL ENDOSCOPY CLINICS OF NORTH AMERICA

Eosinophilic Esophagitis

GUEST EDITOR
Glenn T. Furuta, MD

CONSULTING EDITOR
Charles J. Lightdale, MD

January 2008 • Volume 18 • Number 1

SAUNDERS

An Imprint of Elsevier, Inc.
PHILADELPHIA   LONDON   TORONTO   MONTREAL   SYDNEY   TOKYO

W.B. SAUNDERS COMPANY
A Division of Elsevier Inc.

Elsevier Inc. • 1600 John F. Kennedy Blvd. • Philadelphia, Pennsylvania 19103-2899

http://www.giendo.theclinics.com

GASTROINTESTINAL ENDOSCOPY CLINICS	Volume 18, Number 1
OF NORTH AMERICA	ISSN 1052-5157
January 2008	ISBN-13: 978-1-4160-5841-0
Editor: Kerry Holland	ISBN-10: 1-4160-5841-9

The ideas and opinions expressed in *Gastrointestinal Endoscopy Clinics of North America* do not necessarily reflect those of the Publisher. The Publisher does not assume any responsibility for any injury and/or damage to persons or property arising out of or related to any use of the material contained in this periodical. The reader is advised to check the appropriate medical literature and the product information currently provided by the manufacturer of each drug to be administered to verify the dosage, the method and duration of administration, or contraindications. It is the responsibility of the treating physician or other health care professional, relying on independent experience and knowledge of the patient, to determine drug dosages and the best treatment for the patient. Mention of any product in this issue should not be construed as endorsement by the contributors or editors, or the Publisher of the product or manufacturers' claims.

Gastrointestinal Endoscopy Clinics of North America (ISSN 1052-5157) is published quarterly by Elsevier Inc., 360 Park Avenue South, New York, NY 10010-1710. Months of issue are January, April, July, and October. Business and Editorial Offices: 1600 John F. Kennedy Blvd., Suite 1800, Philadelphia, PA, 19103-2899. Customer Service Office: 6277 Sea Harbor Drive, Orlando, FL 32887-4800. Periodicals postage paid at New York, NY and additional mailing offices. Subscription prices are $240.00 per year of US individuals $357.00 per year for US institutions, $123.00 per year for US students and residents, $265.00 per year for Canadian individuals, $426.00 per year for Canadian institutions, $315.00 per year for international individuals, $426.00 per year for international institutions, and $161.00 per year for Canadian and foreign students/residents. To receive student/resident rate, orders must be accompanied by name of affiliated institution, date of term, and the *signature* of program/residency coordinator on institution letterhead. Orders will be billed at individual rate until proof of status is received. Foreign air speed delivery is included in all *Clinics* subscription prices. All prices are subject to change without notice. POSTMASTER: Send address change to *Gastrointestinal Endoscopy Clinics of North America*, Elsevier Periodicals Customer Service, 6277 Sea Harbor Drive, Orlando, FL 32887-4800. **Customer Service: 1-800-654-2452 (US). From outside of the US, call 1-407-345-4000. E-mail: hhspcs@harcourt.com.**

Gastrointestinal Endoscopy Clinics of North America is covered in *Excerpta Medica, Index Medicus, and MEDLINE/MEDLARS*.

Printed in the United States of America.

CONSULTING EDITOR

CHARLES J. LIGHTDALE, MD, Professor, Department of Medicine, Columbia University Medical Center, New York, New York

GUEST EDITOR

GLENN T. FURUTA, MD, Section of Pediatric Gastroenterology, Hepatology and Nutrition, The Children's Hospital; Associate Professor of Pediatrics, University of Colorado Denver, School of Medicine, Aurora, Colorado

CONTRIBUTORS

SEEMA S. ACEVES, MD, PhD, Division of Allergy, Immunology, Rady Children's Hospital; Assistant Adjunct Professor of Pediatrics, University of California, San Diego, California

AMAL ASSA'AD, MD, Professor of Pediatrics, Division of Allergy and Immunology, Cincinnati Children's Hospital Medical Center, Cincinnati, Ohio

CARINE BLANCHARD, PhD, Research Fellow, Division of Allergy and Immunology, Cincinnati Children's Hospital Medical Center; Department of Pediatrics, University of Cincinnati College of Medicine, Cincinnati, Ohio

MIRNA CHEHADE, MD, Assistant Professor of Pediatrics, Pediatric Gastroenterology and Nutrition, Pediatric Allergy and Immunology, Mount Sinai School of Medicine, New York, New York

MARGARET H. COLLINS, MD, Professor of Pathology, University of Cincinnati; and Division of Pathology and Laboratory Medicine, Cincinnati Center for Eosinophilic Disorders, Cincinnati Children's Hospital Medical Center, Cincinnati, Ohio

VICTOR L. FOX, MD, Assistant Professor of Pediatrics, and Director, GI Procedure Unit and Endoscopy Program, Harvard Medical School, Division of Gastroenterology and Nutrition, Children's Hospital Boston, Boston, Massachusetts

GLENN T. FURUTA, MD, Section of Pediatric Gastroenterology, Hepatology and Nutrition, The Children's Hospital; Associate Professor of Pediatrics, University of Colorado Denver, School of Medicine, Aurora, Colorado

NIRMALA GONSALVES, MD, Assistant Professor of Medicine, Division of Gastroenterology, Northwestern University, Feinberg School of Medicine, Chicago, Illinois

SANDEEP K. GUPTA, MD, Associate Professor of Clinical Pediatrics, Indiana University School of Medicine, James Whitcomb Riley Hospital for Children, Indianapolis, Indiana

DAVID A. KATZKA, MD, Professor of Medicine, University of Pennsylvania School of Medicine, Philadelphia, Pennsylvania

CHRIS A. LIACOURAS, MD, Professor of Pediatrics, University of Pennsylvania School of Medicine; Attending Pediatric Gastroenterologist, The Children's Hospital of Philadelphia, Division of Gastroenterology, Hepatology and Nutrition, Philadelphia, Pennsylvania

SAMUEL NURKO, MD, MPH, Director, Center for Motility and Functional Gastrointestinal Disorders, Children's Hospital Boston; Associate Professor in Pediatrics, Harvard Medical School, Boston, Massachusetts

LAURA J. ORVIDAS, MD, Associate Professor of Otolaryngology, Division of Pediatric Otolaryngology, Mayo Clinic; Mayo Eugenio Litta Children's Hospital; Mayo Clinic College of Medicine, Rochester, Minnesota

PHILIP E. PUTNAM, MD, FAAP, Associate Professor of Pediatrics, Director of Endoscopy Services, and Medical Director, Cincinnati Center for Eosinophilic Disorders, Division of Gastroenterology, Hepatology, and Nutrition, Cincinnati Children's Hospital Medical, Cincinnati, Ohio

RACHEL ROSEN, MD, MPH, Center for Motility and Functional Gastrointestinal Disorders, Children's Hospital Boston; Instructor in Pediatrics, Harvard Medical School, Boston, Massachusetts

MARC E. ROTHENBERG, MD, PhD, Professor of Pediatrics, Director, Division of Allergy and Immunology, and Director, Cincinnati Center for Eosinophilic Disorders, Cincinnati Children's Hospital Medical Center; Department of Pediatrics, University of Cincinnati College of Medicine, Cincinnati, Ohio

HUGH A. SAMPSON, MD, Professor of Pediatrics, Pediatric Allergy and Immunology, Mount Sinai School of Medicine, New York, New York

MICHELE SHUKER, MS, RD, CSP, LDN, Program Coordinator, Center for Pediatric Eosinophilic Disorders, The Children's Hospital of Philadelphia, Philadelphia, Pennsylvania

STUART JON SPECHLER, MD, Professor of Medicine, Department of Medicine, Dallas Department of Veterans Affairs Medical Center, The University of Texas Southwestern Medical Center at Dallas, Dallas, Texas

JONATHAN M. SPERGEL, MD, PhD, Associate Professor of Pediatrics, Allergy Section Chief, Division of Allergy and Immunology and Director of the Center for Pediatric Eosinophilic Disorders, The Children's Hospital of Philadelphia; Department of Pediatrics, University of Pennsylvania School of Medicine, Philadelphia, Pennsylvania

ALEX STRAUMANN, MD, Associate Professor of Medicine, Department of Gastroenterology, Kantonsspital Olten, Olten, Switzerland

DANA M. THOMPSON, MD, Associate Professor of Otolaryngology, Division of Pediatric Otolaryngology, Cincinnati Children's Hospital Medical Center; University of Cincinnati College of Medicine, Cincinnati, Ohio

CONTENTS

Previously believed a rare condition, there has been a rising number of cases of eosinophilic esophagitis in adult and pediatric populations over the past several years. Because of this increase, it is important for clinicians to be able to recognize, diagnose, and manage this disease. This article focuses on the history and nomenclature of eosinophilic esophagitis and its evolution as a separate entity from gastroesophageal reflux disease. It also outlines currently accepted diagnostic criteria for this increasingly common condition.

During the past decade, the increasing number of recognized cases of eosinophilic esophagitis in children and adults has resulted in a dramatic expansion of the medical literature surrounding it. Clinical and basic research has contributed to a better, but still incomplete, body of knowledge regarding its clinical and histologic manifestations, as well as its immunologic and genetic pathogenesis. This article provides a broad framework for recognizing the remarkable variety of clinical manifestations of eosinophilic esophagitis in children, which must be considered as part of the differential diagnosis in many different clinical situations.

EE, and the correct diagnosis can be made only if the histology is correlated with clinical findings. The histology of the normal esophagus is reviewed and contrasted with the findings in EE. The characteristic findings in EE are illustrated. Selected research in humans and animal models pertinent to EE are briefly reviewed.

The understanding of esophageal motility alterations in patients who have eosinophilic esophagitis (EE) is in its infancy despite the common presenting complaint of dysphagia. A diversity of motility disorders has been reported in patients who have EE including achalasia, diffuse esophageal spasm, nutcracker esophagus, and nonspecific motility alterations including high-amplitude esophageal body contractions, tertiary contractions, abnormalities in lower esophageal sphincter pressure, and other peristaltic problems. Some evidence suggests that treatment of EE will improve motility. Technological advances such as high-resolution manometry and combined manometry with impedance may provide new insight into more subtle motility abnormalities.

Similar to gastrointestinal symptoms of eosinophilic esophagitis (EE), symptoms of otorhinolaryngologic disease associated with EE often are refractory to traditional treatment of gastroesophageal reflux disease. Patient demographics and characteristics often are similar. Clinicians must maintain a high index of suspicion to accurately diagnose and manage airway findings related to esophagitis. Team collaboration between otolaryngologists, allergists, and gastroenterologists will assure the best treatment in this select group of predisposed patients.

Eosinophilic esophagitis is a chronic disease limited to the esophagus and has a persistent or spontaneously fluctuating course. So far it does not seem to limit life expectancy, but it often substantially impairs the quality of life. To date, there has been no association with malignant conditions, but there is concern that the chronic, uncontrolled inflammation will evoke irreversible structural alterations of the esophagus, leading to tissue fibrosis, stricture formation, and impaired function. This esophageal remodeling may result in several disease-inherent and procedure-related complications.

FORTHCOMING ISSUES

RECENT ISSUES

THE CLINICS ARE NOW AVAILABLE ONLINE!

Access your subscription at:
http://www.theclinics.com

Gastrointest Endoscopy Clin N Am
18 (2008) xiii–xiv

GASTROINTESTINAL
ENDOSCOPY CLINICS
OF NORTH AMERICA

Foreword

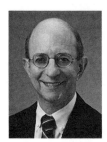

Charles J. Lightdale, MD
Consulting Editor

One of the joys of reading is the discovery of a word not previously encountered. Before long, you see it with increasing frequency and start using it yourself. Could it have been there all the time, or for some reason is it just being used more frequently? In any case, it is your word now. In the professional life of a physician, a similar thing can happen with a disease. What brings it to attention might be an article or a lecture. Suddenly, you see a patient who seems to have all the diagnostic hallmarks of the disease. Additional patients are encountered in short order. The patients respond to a specific treatment. In gastrointestinal endoscopy, this happened in recent years with eosinophilic esophagitis. Earlier, there were descriptive case reports of "ringed esophagus" in young patients, but it was the pediatric specialists who first described the additional characteristics of vertical furrows and white exudates, and who made the critical associations with extensive eosinophilic infiltrates in the esophageal mucosa and allergy. Eosinophilic esophagitis may be the paradigm for a disease that begins in childhood and that evolves and extends into adult life.

Eosinophilic esophagitis is complex and may have more than one pathogenesis in its varying presentations in children and adults. One thing is certain: eosinophilic esophagitis is an important disease that causes considerable morbidity in those afflicted. It is a major cause of esophageal symptoms, particularly dysphagia. Eosinophilic esophagitis seems to be increasing in frequency like bronchial asthma, to which it has been compared. The relationship of eosinophilic esophagitis to gastroesophageal reflux disease remains poorly defined in some cases. Chronic eosinophilic

doi:10.1016/j.giec.2007.11.001   *giendo.theclinics.com*

esophagitis seems to lead to fibrosis in some patients, and eosinophilic esophagitis has been linked to the Schatzki ring long associated with hiatal hernia and GERD.

There is much to be learned about eosinophilic esophagitis, and major lines of clinical and laboratory research have been established. Dr. Glenn Furuta, Children's Hospital of Denver, has pioneered in clinical and basic research and has a tremendous grasp of the field. As Guest Editor, he is like a *maestro* conducting a major orchestra. He has assembled an extraordinary group of highly accomplished individual players—pediatric and adult gastroenterologists, endoscopists, surgeons, pathologists, immunologists, and allergists–to produce a symphonic, magnificent state-of-the-art issue on eosinophilic esophagitis, including current approaches to diagnosis and therapy.

The word is out. Read this issue of the *Gastrointestinal Endoscopy Clinics of North America* and make eosinophilic esophagitis part of your vocabulary.

Charles J. Lightdale, MD
Department of Medicine
Columbia University Medical Center
161 Fort Washington Avenue, Room 812
New York, NY 10032, USA

E-mail address: CJL18@columbia.edu

Gastrointest Endoscopy Clin N Am
18 (2008) xv–xix

GASTROINTESTINAL
ENDOSCOPY CLINICS
OF NORTH AMERICA

Preface

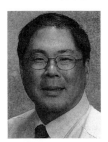

Glenn T. Furuta, MD
Guest Editor

Seven years ago, we published an article in the *Gastrointestinal Endoscopy Clinics of North America* and a review article in *Gastrointestinal Endoscopy* to bring features of an emerging disease, eosinophilic esophagitis (EE), to a new audience, the gastrointestinal endoscopist. Since that time, clinical experience has demanded and research studies have supported that EE is no longer an emerging disease but one that must be "swallowed" without any degree of dysphagia. In fact, its importance sparked the formation of two international conferences focusing on clinical, histologic, and pathogenic aspects of EE (the First and Second International Gastrointestinal Eosinophil Research Symposia). Now, Dr. Lightdale has afforded us with another opportunity to provide the latest update on this disease in this issue of *Gastrointestinal Endoscopy Clinics of North America*.

What makes this disease so interesting, and complicated, is its multidisciplinary nature. This edition of *Gastrointestinal Endoscopy Clinics of North America* emphasizes this point in a dramatic fashion; its authorship consists of 4 adult and 15 pediatric specialists, 1 pathologist, 5 allergists, 3 basic scientists, 9 clinical scientists, 2 surgeons, a dietician and 11 gastroenterologists. In the true academic spirit, each of these authors found the mental space and physical energy, somewhere between their clinical duties, educational responsibilities, and research projects, to provide an outstanding, unique contribution herein. In this introduction I will not elaborate extensively on the specific topic of each author's contribution but rather provide a bit of biographic information that puts their work in context, especially because many are neither gastroenterologists nor endoscopists.

1052-5157/08/$ - see front matter © 2008 Elsevier Inc. All rights reserved.
doi:10.1016/j.giec.2007.10.001   *giendo.theclinics.com*

Nirmala Gonsalves, MD, is an adult gastroenterologist whose enthusiasm and insights bring new approaches to evaluating and treating patients who have EE. Her work taught us how many biopsies (five) are required to make the diagnosis of EE and now she is investigating whether dietary management may provide a therapeutic option for affected adults. Dr. Gonsalves fosters interactions between adult and pediatric gastroenterologists and is active in advocacy work. She represents one of the young movers and shakers in this field.

Hugh Sampson, MD, is the internationally recognized expert in mechanisms of IgE-mediated food allergic diseases. In 1995, Dr. Sampson published the seminal work that was the first to identify EE in children and to show that elemental diets could serve as primary treatment for the disease. Since then, he has continued to lead the charge in understanding this disease. His longitudinal experiences and unique insights are critical to future advances in this field.

Mirna Chehade, MD, is a pediatric gastroenterologist who is one of the leaders in performing translational research in children who have food allergic diseases. This work provides us with important insights into a still-murky area of allergic gastroenteropathy especially as it relates to long-term follow-up and natural history of these diseases. In her article, she dissects translational and epidemiologic works to forecast the future of the field.

The English language–centric medical community could have been light years ahead in its identification of this disease if it had recognized one of the first descriptions published by a private practice gastroenterologist from Olten County, Switzerland in 1994. The original publication by Alex Straumann, MD, described many of the now well-recognized features of EE. Since then, he has taken his passionate interest in this disease to new levels with clinical descriptions, translational studies, and therapeutic trials. He has documented the longest natural history of EE in adults, thus making his article in this issue priceless. When, in whom, and how rapidly these observations will arise can be the focus of his next study.

Phil Putnam, MD, is a master endoscopist of children. His tireless efforts in the endoscopy suite and hospital have trained a cadre of pediatric gastroenterologists and brought extraordinary care to children who have EE. The complete nature of his care is emphasized by his regular visits to the pathologist's microscope where he reviews all of his biopsy specimens. The described experiences with hundreds of complicated patients make his chapter not a collection of anecdotes but a virtual textbook of clinical features of pediatric EE.

David Katzka, MD, is an expert esophagologist who took on the early mission of being an adult gastroenterologist who believed that EE represented a distinct disease. Throughout the 1990s he cared for patients who had eosinophilic gastrointestinal diseases, and now he speaks frequently on his clinical experiences, serves on abstract review committees, and performs clinical research and writes about his clinical insights to a broad audience with the goal of improving care and expanding knowledge.

Victor Fox, MD, is the master endoscopist at the Children's Hospital Boston. His meticulous attention to detail brought early insights to the white exudates, full-thickness inflammation, furrowing, and shearing associated with EE. But Dr. Fox's scientific nature emphasized that these findings were not unique to EE, and in fact that the squamous epithelium represents a target organ for newly recognized inflammatory responses. His chapter builds on this fascinating hypothesis and as this field continues to mature we will likely see this thinking endoscopist's tenets gain further support.

Samuel Nurko, MD, is the master of motility at the Children's Hospital Boston. He represents the rare breed of master clinician and funded translational researcher whose insights and data bring new diagnostic and therapeutic modalities to affected patients. His early observations emphasized that many of the symptom complexes associated with EE represented intermittent dysmotility and studies presented in his chapter provide support for his claim.

Rachel Rosen, MD, is an outstanding physician-scientist who possesses clinical insights and investigational rigor that provide us with new mechanisms for observed symptoms related to dysmotility in EE. Her work on this disease examines not only the esophagus but also its potential connection with the aerodigestive tract and the impact of non-acid refluxate in esophageal injury. We look forward to more unique contributions from this dedicated professional.

Sandeep Gupta, MD, is a dedicated multitalented pediatric gastroenterologist who has a longstanding clinical and research expertise in EE. His early work identified vertical furrows, the now well-known endoscopic feature that is highly suggestive of EE, and his recent trendsetting translational studies seek to determine potential noninvasive markers of disease activity and inflammation. Dr. Gupta is a nationally recognized speaker on this topic and a well-known advocate for patients who have EE.

Dana Thompson, MD, and Laura Orvidas, MD, are unique pediatric otolaryngologists who focus on EE. Dr. Thompson was the first to study the link between the upper tract and EE. This is particularly interesting because both are lined by squamous epithelium and basic studies suggest the intimate relationship between these two organs. We await her discovery, as a surgeon, of novel markers of inflammation associated with the upper tract that gastroenterologists have not yet recognized.

Margaret Collins, MD, is a master pathologist who has a longstanding expertise in histologic patterns of mucosal eosinophilia. With her calm demeanor, Dr. Collins consistently emphasizes the importance of viewing the intestinal mucosa in the context of the clinical parameters in which it was obtained, a rule that makes her contributions to this field particularly important. She is always engaged and very interested in discussing the clinical features of the diseases. Her tremendous dedication to patient care is manifest by her advocacy in speaking and writing about this disease to a vast array of audiences, including patient groups.

Amaal Assad, MD, is an expert pediatric allergist who has broad and deep experience in eosinophilic gastrointestinal diseases and food allergies. She is a noted researcher, enthusiastic speaker, and interesting writer whose efforts are focused on improving care for patients. Always poised to give her valuable opinion, Dr. Assad's rigorous approach emphasizes that although EE is often viewed as a food allergic disease, the present-day tools and treatments for patients are still in need of refinement.

The visionary, tireless efforts of Marc Rothenberg, MD, PhD, have led the way in determining clinical features, identifying pathogenic mechanisms, advocating for patients and families, and establishing novel therapeutic techniques. In his dual role as pediatric allergist and funded physician-scientist, he has developed a unique, multidisciplinary team whose contributions to the field have been broad and deep, ranging from the identification of the genetic EE signature to the use of anti–IL-5 antibody as a potential treatment modality.

Carine Blanchard, PhD, is a bright young investigator whose novel basic and translational work with in vitro, ex vivo, and in vivo models of EE have brought us a wealth of understanding. Her innovative work identified the role of proinflammatory cytokines, including eotaxin-3 and IL-13, in the pathogenesis of squamous inflammation. We look forward to many more intriguing studies from this enthusiastic investigator.

Chris Liacouras, MD, is the master of pediatric gastrointestinal eosinophilia. His influence has touched every aspect of this disease, including patient care, clinical research, education, and advocacy. From the early days of this field, Dr. Liacouras recognized that patients who had EE did not respond to acid blockade. Since then he has documented the world's largest and longest experience with EE in his patient population. He was the first to recognize the vital importance of multidisciplinary care and his current program is the model that others strive to emulate. His selfless dedication to advocating for patients is unparalleled; it is not unusual for him to travel by train, plane, and automobile to give a 1-hour talk and then jet back home.

Jonathan Spergel, MD, PhD, is a forward-thinking pediatric allergist whose collaboration with Dr. Liacouras has brought novel approaches to patient testing and treatment. Realizing that EE may not be solely an IgE-mediated disease, he was the first to introduce atopy patch testing as an alternative method of identifying food allergens. His published work documents the validity of this concept and its use has brought new relief for his patients. In addition, he is a staunch advocate for patients, having hosted patient education seminars. He travels often for speaking engagements promoting the importance of disease recognition to new audiences.

Michele Shuker, RD, is a unique pediatric dietician whose groundbreaking work and commitment have improved the lives of countless patients who have EE. As the coordinator of the multidisciplinary EE program at Children's Hospital of Philadelphia, she performs the Herculean task of overseeing the work of the all the care providers. Most important, her nutritional expertise assures that children who receive dietary management are provided with a comprehensive plan allowing them to grow and develop normally.

Seema Aceves, MD, PhD, is a trend-setting pediatric allergist who recently entered the EE field with a large splash. In addition to her work identifying a novel method for the administration of topical corticosteroids with viscous sucralose, she has published an intriguing study determining potential mechanisms for esophageal fibrosis. Her enthusiasm and dynamic nature in combination with her scientific prowess make her a welcome addition to the field. Like others contributing to this issue, she is a staunch patient advocate, speaking and hosting educational symposia for patients who have EE.

Dr. Spechler is a world-recognized leader in esophagology with a focus on mechanisms of chronic squamous epithelial injury. With his vast and lengthy experience and visionary foresight, Dr. Spechler reminds his pediatric colleagues that although eosinophilic inflammation may be attributable to allergic causes, other causes are possible and therapeutic approaches should be individually tailored. His wisdom will continue to influence this evolving field.

As the editor of this issue of *Gastrointestinal Endoscopy Clinics of North America*, I feel particularly privileged to be associated with such an observant, selfless group of outstanding authors. Throughout my professional experiences with patients and research I have been fortunate to encounter so many dedicated people who have, in various ways, helped grow this field. In addition to these authors, a number of others, including Alan Leichtner, MD; Donald Antonioli, MD; Charles Lightdale, MD; Frank Twarog, MD; Christopher Duggan, MD, MPH; Allan Walker, MD; Barry Wershil, MD; Steve Ackermann, PhD; Jamie Lee, PhD; Jerry Gleich, MD; Peter Bonis, MD; Beth Mays; Sean Colgan, PhD; Ron Sokol, MD; and Dan Atkins, MD, provided me with invaluable insights and timely support that allowed me to continue in this quest. It is my hope that this edition of *Gastrointestinal Endoscopy Clinics of North America* will "degranulate" into the hands of neophyte eosinophilophiles who will bring new ideas, innovative approaches, and unbridled enthusiasm to this fascinating field. Finally, I am grateful to my parents, sister, wife Lauren, and children Henry and Ellie for keeping me grounded during this intriguing professional adventure.

Glenn T. Furuta, MD
Section of Pediatric Gastroenterology, Hepatology and Nutrition
The Children's Hospital, 13123 East 16th Avenue
B290 Aurora, CO 80045, USA

E-mail address: furuta.glenn@tchden.org

ELSEVIER
SAUNDERS

Gastrointest Endoscopy Clin N Am
18 (2008) 1–9

GASTROINTESTINAL
ENDOSCOPY CLINICS
OF NORTH AMERICA

Eosinophilic Esophagitis: History, Nomenclature, and Diagnostic Guidelines

Nirmala Gonsalves, MD

*Division of Gastroenterology, Northwestern University,
Feinberg School of Medicine, 676 North St. Claire Street, Suite 1400,
Chicago, IL 60611, USA*

History of eosinophils in the esophagus: the evolution from eosinophilic esophagitis to gastroesophageal reflux disease and back to eosinophilic esophagitis

In 1879, Paul Ehrlich named the eosinophil from "Eos," the Greek word for goddess of the dawn because its cytoplasmic granules stained red with eosin, similar to the colors of dawn. Since that time, considerable research has been devoted to the eosinophil and its role as lord of the esophageal rings. Eosinophils normally are present in the gastrointestinal tract, spleen, lymph nodes, and thymus. Within the gastrointestinal tract, eosinophils are located in the lamina propria of the stomach, small intestine, cecum, and colon and usually are not found in the esophagus. They likely serve a protective role in defending the host against infections. Eosinophilic gastrointestinal disorders (EGID) are characterized by eosinophilic infiltration and inflammation of the gastrointestinal tract in the absence of previously identified causes of eosinophilia, such as parasitic infections, malignancy, collagen vascular diseases, drug sensitivities, and inflammatory bowel disease [1]. These disorders include eosinophilic esophagitis (EE), eosinophilic gastritis, eosinophilic gastroenteritis (EG), eosinophilic enteritis, and eosinophilic colitis. This article focuses on EE.

Previously believed a rare condition, over the past several years, esophageal eosinophilia increasingly has been recognized in adult and pediatric populations. This condition may occur in isolation and under proper circumstances is termed EE or as a part of the spectrum of EG [1]. Although EE was described first as a distinct entity in 1978, there was a shift in belief

---

E-mail address: n-gonsalves@md.northwestern.edu

1052-5157/08/$ - see front matter © 2008 Elsevier Inc. All rights reserved.
doi:10.1016/j.giec.2007.09.010

over the next several years implicating gastroesophageal reflux disease (GERD) as the underlying cause of eosinophilic infiltration in the esophagus. Over the past 10 years, however, the tide has shifted back toward EE as a primary entity and the cause of significant esophageal eosinophilia.

One of the first cases describing eosinophilic infiltration of the esophagus was by Dobbins and colleagues [2] in 1977. This case report described a 51-year-old man who had symptoms of dysphagia, substernal pain, esophageal spasm on manometry, negative pH testing, peripheral eosinophilia, and eosinophilic infiltration of the small intestine and esophagus. Isolated EE then was described in an adult patient by Landres and coworkers [3] in 1978. This case report describes a 44-year-old man who had symptoms of epigastric and substernal pain, dysphagia, peripheral eosinophilia, vigorous achalasia, and eosinophilic infiltration of the esophagus. After these early reports, however, much of the research that followed pointed to GERD as the primary cause of eosinophils in the esophagus.

One of the first studies to suggest this affiliation was by Winter and colleagues [4] in the pediatric literature in 1982. This group correlated the presence of esophageal eosinophilia with markers of reflux esophagitis. They studied 46 children who had a diagnosis of reflux esophagitis and who had completed pH studies, manometry, and endoscopy. Eighteen of their patients had intraepithelial eosinophils (>1/high-power field [HPF]) present in the proximal, distal, and midesophagus. They reported that the presence of intraepithelial eosinophils correlated with abnormal pH monitoring studies and histologic features consistent with reflux.

This association was further supported by Lee [5] in 1985. Lee's group reviewed esophageal mucosal biopsies in their pathology files for findings of marked eosinophilia (defined as more than 10 intraepithelial eosinophils in two HPFs of each biopsy). They found 11 patients who met these criteria and that 91% had evidence of reflux esophagitis and concluded that marked eosinophilia may indicate prolonged or severe GERD.

The association of esophageal eosinophilia and GERD finally changed in 1993 with a pivotal study by Attwood and colleagues [6] that suggested esophageal eosinophilia may not represent solely a reflux phenomenon. They performed a retrospective review of 12 adult patients who had esophageal eosinophilia from 1988 to 1990. All these patients had undergone an esophagram, manometry, and 24-hour pH monitoring study. The histologic specimens from these patients were reviewed and characterized as low-grade infiltration (less than 20 eosinophils [eos]/HPF) or high-grade (greater than 20 eos/HPF). Hyperplastic mucosal changes also were assessed. Eleven of 12 patients who had high-grade esophageal eosinophilia had normal 24-hour pH monitoring. These patients all were labeled as having a "normal" endoscopy and barium swallow. The majority of patients suffered from intermittent dysphagia and frequent food impactions. Seven of 12 were found to have allergic diseases, such as asthma or sinusitis. Their mean eosinophil count (MEC) per HPF was 56 with a range of 21 to 100. Attwood and colleagues noted a tendency for eosinophil location to be near the epithelial surface and that the patients had marked hyperplastic changes (mean papillary height was 75% of the epithelial thickness and mean basal zone thickness was 40%). They compared this group to a reference population of 90 patients who had proved acid reflux on 24-hour pH monitoring. The majority of patient symptoms in this group included heartburn, regurgitation, and dysphagia. Only 43 of 90 patients had eosinophilia on esophageal biopsies. Unlike the previous subset of patients, however, there was no dense infiltrate. The mean eosinophils per HPF in this group was 3.3 with a range of 1 to 19. The investigators concluded that in patients who had symptoms of dysphagia, the presence of high esophageal eosinophilia, normal endoscopy, and normal 24-hour pH studies represents a distinct clinical syndrome. Since the initial description of EE by Landres and colleagues [3] in 1978, this was the first study to suggest that the presence of eosinophils in the esophagus may be attributed to disease states other than GERD.

Several studies followed, supporting the notion that esophageal eosinophilia may be related to factors other than GERD. Kelly and colleagues [7] in 1995 investigated 75 pediatric patients who had longstanding reflux who were unresponsive to medical therapy. They found that 23 patients had persistent esophageal eosinophilia despite medical treatment for reflux. They hypothesized that there may be an allergic component to this entity and placed the patients on an elemental diet for a period of 6 weeks. Of the 17 patients who began the trial, 12 completed the trial and 10 underwent repeat endoscopy. If patients had improvement in their symptoms, a repeat endoscopy with biopsy then was performed followed by food challenges. On completion of the elemental diet, 80% patients became free of long-term complaints and all others reported substantial improvement in their symptoms. The median time for improvement of symptoms was 3 weeks. Seventy percent of patients had asthma or eczema. On repeat endoscopy, 60% showed complete resolution of endoscopic findings. There was a significant reduction of esophageal eosinophilia in all patients and complete resolution seen in 50%. The mean eosinophils per HPF before and after therapy was 41 and 0.5, respectively. The investigators also showed a decrease in basal zone hyperplasia and papillary height in biopsy specimens. During a controlled reintroduction of foods, symptoms were recreated in 9 of 10 patients a median of 1 hour after the reintroduction of the offending food. The most common agents were cow milk, soy protein, wheat, peanut, and egg. With this evidence, Kelly and colleagues [7] suggested an association between EE and an allergic predisposition.

Another landmark study that further supports the finding that causes other than GERD contribute to esophageal eosinophilia was performed by Ruchelli and colleagues [8] in 1999. Their goal was to determine whether or not the degree of esophageal eosinophilia predicted symptomatic improvement after antireflux therapy. The investigators identified pediatric patients who had GERD and who had esophageal eosinophilia. After

3 months of antireflux therapy, they repeated the endoscopy and evaluated symptoms and the degree of esophageal eosinophilia. Treatment response was classified as improvement, relapse, or failure. They identified significant differences in the eosinophil counts in patients who improved versus patients who failed antireflux treatment (1.1 versus 24.5 eos/HPF, respectively). In addition, they determined that a threshold MEC value greater than 7 provided sensitivity of 61.3%, specificity of 95.7%, and predictive value of treatment failure of 86.1%, and that a MEC less than 7 provided an 85% predictive value of successful therapy. Finally, they determined that the history of allergic phenomena (wheezing, atopy, and rhinitis) was significantly higher in the failed group (56%) versus the improvement group (6%) or relapsed group (7%). Of the 16 patients in the failure group, eight patients had complete resolution with corticosteroids, four had marked improvement with elimination diet, and four were lost to follow-up. The investigators concluded that the finding of severe eosinophilia predicted failure of conventional therapy and suggested, therefore, a cause other than GERD.

The association of EE and food allergens was supported further in a study by Markowitz and colleagues [9] in 2003. They treated 51 pediatric patients who had EE with an elemental diet for 4 weeks. Forty-nine of 51 patients experienced significant improvement in symptoms of vomiting, abdominal pain, and dysphagia after the diet. The median number of esophageal eosinophils per HPF decreased from 33.7 to 1.0 after the diet, with an average time to clinical improvement of 8.5 days.

Together, these early studies provided the groundwork to establish EE as a distinct clinicopathologic entity separate from GERD. Although investigation of EE was active among pediatric researchers, and there was some early evidence that this condition also existed in adults, there was a delay in acceptance of EE as a distinct entity by some adult gastroenterologists and pathologists. This ongoing association of eosinophils in the esophagus with GERD may have contributed to delayed recognition of EE in many adult patients and the dearth of studies in adults until recent years.

Previously considered a rare condition, over the past several years, there has been a dramatic increase in reports of EE in the adult and pediatric literature from North and South America, Europe, Asia, Australia, and the Middle East [10–19]. The cause for this increase likely is a combination of increasing incidence of EE and growing awareness of the condition among gastroenterologists, allergists, and pathologists. Noel and coworkers [20] calculated an incidence of EE in a population of children in Ohio to be 1 in 10,000 per year and a prevalence of 4 in 10,000 in 2003. Portmann and colleagues estimated an incidence of 0.17 cases per 10,000 adult inhabitants with a prevalence of 3.3 per 10,000 inhabitants of their catchment area in Switzerland [21]. These numbers likely underestimate the true prevalence, because these data include only patients who had symptoms sufficient to warrant endoscopy. A recent population-based study in Sweden randomly surveyed 3000 adults; more than 50% (1563 adults) were invited to have endoscopy and 1000 agreed and underwent esophageal biopsies. This study found that eosinophilia was present in 5% of the population, and histologic criteria for EE was met in 1% of the population [22]. These numbers suggest that EE is becoming as common as other immunologically influenced diseases, such as inflammatory bowel disease [23]. In addition, the many publications about EE in the past several years have contributed to increasing the awareness of this condition in the gastroenterology and pathology communities [17].

Nomenclature

Since its description in 1879, the interest in the eosinophil and its role in EE has grown tremendously and resulted in the formation of a collaborative group termed, The International Gastrointestinal Eosinophil Researchers (TIGERS). Given the rising number of cases of this condition seen in the community and academic settings and the plethora of publications, it is important to define this condition properly and to establish a common language when reporting this condition. Many terms and acronyms previously have been used in the literature to describe this entity, including allergic esophagitis, idiopathic EE, primary EE, and ringed esophagus. The term, "eosinophilic esophagitis," is accepted as the unifying term. Accepted abbreviations for this condition include EE and EoE (which, when spoken, is pronounced "EE").

Diagnostic guidelines

The diagnostic guidelines regarding this condition are evolving continuously as more is learned about this disease from ongoing research. The guidelines reviewed in this section are many that have been adapted from the First International Gastrointestinal Eosinophilic Research Symposium (FIGERS). The consensus statement developed from this meeting was based on the collaboration of 32 researchers in the field of EGID. The guidelines presented by the group comprise the latest literature review in combination with expert opinion when literature was lacking [24].

The diagnosis of EE depends on many factors, including clinicians recognizing its features and obtaining adequate biopsies and pathologists performing appropriate evaluations. In years past, this diagnosis often was overlooked, as many patients who had EE had prior endoscopic evaluations with alternative diagnoses, such as Schatzki's rings or GERD [25,26]. In many cases, misdiagnoses lead to repeat endoscopies, esophageal dilations, and a delay in the institution of appropriate medical therapy. Also, because of the previous overlap of histologic features of EE and GERD, many biopsy specimens were misread as GERD. Therefore, if considering a diagnosis of EE, gastroenterologists should perform esophageal biopsies and request that a pathologist perform eosinophil counts on the tissue (see the article by Collins, elsewhere in this issue).

EE is a clinicopathologic disease; therefore, symptoms and histologic findings must be present to diagnose this condition. The currently accepted histologic criteria include a peak eosinophil count per HPF of greater than or equal to 15 in the esophagus with normal gastric and duodenal biopsies (Table 1) [24]. Although GERD may be a cofactor in some patients, this needs to be treated effectively or ruled out. It previously was believed that GERD would cause only a moderate degree of esophageal eosinophilia rather than the markedly elevated numbers seen in EE. A recent case report, however, describes three pediatric cases of EE with markedly elevated eosinophilia, which responded to acid suppression [27]. Therefore, despite the degree of histologic eosinophilia, biopsies must be taken after at least 6 to 8 weeks of acid suppression with twice-daily proton pump inhibitors. Alternatively, a pH monitoring study of the distal esophagus may be performed and demonstrate negative acid exposure. A reliable diagnosis of EE can be made only under these circumstances and in patients who are symptomatic [24]. Patients who have asymptomatic esophageal eosinophilia by definition do not have EE. The significance of asymptomatic esophageal eosinophilia has yet to be determined.

To obtain adequate histologic material to maximize sensitivity for EE, endoscopists must know where to biopsy and how many biopsies to take. As discussed later, the eosinophilic infiltration in the esophagus observed in EE can be heterogeneous and patchy [28,29]. Taking too few biopsies in the esophagus may result in the diagnosis being overlooked. Previous studies have demonstrated this heterogeneity and have shown that the degree of eosinophilia is slightly higher in the distal than proximal esophagus [26]. A recent study in adults shows that using a diagnostic threshold of greater than or equal to 15 eosinophils per HPF, taking one biopsy has a sensitivity of only 55%. This sensitivity increases to 100% after five biopsies are procured (Fig. 1) [25]. The investigators also showed that although there

Table 1
Diagnostic criteria for eosinophilic esophagitis

Histology	Esophageal biopsies ≥15 eos/HPF	
	Normal gastric and duodenal biopsies	
	Patients must have biopsies after 6–8 weeks of	
	twice daily acid suppression with proton pump	
	inhibitors or have a documented negative pH study	
Presence of	Adults	Children
symptoms	Dysphagia	Abdominal pain
	Food impaction	Heartburn
	Heartburn	Regurgitation
	Regurgitation	Nausea/vomiting
	Chest pain	Dysphagia
	Odynophagia	Failure to thrive

was no significant difference in eosinophilia between biopsies taken in the proximal or distal esophagus, if biopsies were taken in only the proximal esophagus, the diagnosis could not have been made in 20% of cases. The investigators concluded that at least five biopsies should be obtained in the proximal and distal esophagus to help maximize diagnostic yield. A recent study in the pediatric literature also demonstrates this. Using a diagnostic threshold of greater than or equal to 15 eosinophils per HPF, one biopsy has a sensitivity of 73% whereas four biopsies are needed to obtain a sensitivity of 100% [30]. Using this information, a reasonable approach is to obtain four quadrant biopsies in the proximal and distal esophagus. The proximal and distal landmarks may vary slightly by center, but accepted definitions include defining "distal" as 5 cm above the squamocolumnar junction and "proximal" as 10 cm above the distal mark.

Gastroenterologists also should be aware of endoscopic features of EE that should prompt tissue sampling. Features, such as concentric mucosal rings, linear furrowing, and white plaques, are characteristic of this condition and should alert endoscopists to obtain biopsies [15]. The esophagus may be visually normal however, in as many as 30% of children and 9% of adults [18,31]. Therefore, appropriate biopsies to evaluate for EE should be obtained during an endoscopy for evaluation of unexplained dysphagia, refractory heartburn, odynophagia, and chest pain despite a normal-appearing esophagus [24]. (See the article by Fox, elsewhere in this issue.)

Other major requirements for diagnosis are based on clinical symptoms and are discussed in greater detail in the articles by Putnam and Katzka, elsewhere in this issue. Common presenting symptoms in adults include dysphagia, food impaction, reflux symptoms, and chest pain [32]. Common presenting symptoms in children include heartburn, regurgitation, vomiting,

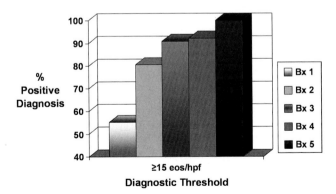

Fig. 1. Number of biopsy specimens needed to make the diagnosis of EE by using a diagnostic threshold of ≥15 eos/HPF. A single biopsy specimen had a sensitivity of 55%, which increased to 100% with five biopsy specimens. (*Data from* Gonsalves N, Policarpio-Nicolas M, Zhang Q, et al. Histopathologic variability and endoscopic correlates in adults with eosinophilic esophagitis. Gastrointest endosc 2006;64(3):313–9.)

abdominal pain, and dysphagia [31]. Patients must have symptoms related to EE to be diagnosed with this condition. Also, other causes of eosinophilia need to be ruled out, such as EG, parasitic infections, malignancy, collagen vascular diseases, drug sensitivities, and inflammatory bowel disease. Biopsies of the stomach and duodenum always should be obtained to rule out EG adequately.

Summary

The diagnostic guidelines of EE are evolving continuously as more is learned about this disease. With ongoing collaborative efforts, clinical and basic science research over the next several years will be critical to improving understanding of the pathophysiology, treatment, and natural history of this condition. Improved recognition and diagnosis of this condition hopefully will lead to earlier medical treatment of EE and prevent complications of untreated disease, such as esophageal strictures and food impaction. In this new dawn of the eosinophil era, results of forthcoming research eagerly are anticipated and promise to shed new light on this once elusive condition.

References

[1] Rothenberg M. Eosinophilic gastrointestinal disorders (EGID). J Allergy Clin Immunol 2004;113:11–28.
[2] Dobbins J, Sheahan D, Behar J. Eosinophilic gastroenteritis with esophageal involvement. Gastroenterology 1977;72:1312–6.
[3] Landres RT, Kuster GG, Strum WB. Eosinophilic esophagitis in a patient with vigorous achalasia. Gastroenterology 1978;74:1298.
[4] Winter HS, Madara JL, Stafford RJ, et al. Intraepithelial eosinophils: a new diagnostic criterion for reflux esophagitis. Gastroenterology 1982;83:818–23.
[5] Lee R. Marked eosinophilia in esophageal mucosal biopsies. Am J Surg Pathol 1985;7:475–9.
[6] Attwood S, Smyrk T, Demeester T, et al. Esophageal eosinophilia with dysphagia. A distinct clinicopathologic syndrome. Dig Dis Sci 1993;38:109–16.
[7] Kelly K, Lazenby A, Rowe P, et al. Eosinophilic esophagitis attributed to gastroesophageal reflux: improvement with an amino-acid based formula. Gastroenterology 1995;109: 1503–12.
[8] Ruchelli E, Wenner W, Voytek T, et al. Severity of esophageal eosinophilia predicts response to conventional gastroesophageal reflux therapy. Pediatr Dev Pathol 1999;2:15–8.
[9] Markowitz J, Spergel J, Ruchelli E, et al. Elemental diet is an effective treatment for eosinophilic esophagitis in children and adolescents. Am J Gastroenterol 2003;98(4):777–82.
[10] Croese J, Fairley S, Masson J, et al. Clinical and endoscopic features of eosinophilic esophagitis in adults. Gastrointest Endosc 2003;58(4):516–22.
[11] Straumann A, Spichtin H, Grize L, et al. Natural history of primary eosinophilic esophagitis: a follow-up of 30 adult patients for up to 11.5 years. Gastroenterology 2003;125:1660–9.
[12] Lucendo A, Carrion G, Navarro M, et al. Eosinophilic esophagitis in adults: an emerging disease. Dig Dis Sci 2004;49(11):1884–8.
[13] Esposito S, Marinello D, Paracchini R, et al. Long-term follow-up of symptoms and peripheral eosinophil counts in seven children with eosinophilic esophagitis. J Pediatr Gastroenterol Nutr 2004;38:452–6.

[14] Khan S, Orenstein S, Di Lorenzo C, et al. Eosinophilic esophagitis: strictures, impactions, dysphagia. Dig Dis Sci 2003;48(1):22–9.

[15] Fox V, Nurko S, Furuta G. Eosinophilic esophagitis: it's not just kid's stuff. Gastrointest Endosc 2002;56(2):260–70.

[16] Zimmerman S, Levine M, Rubesin S, et al. Idiopathic eosinophilic esophagitis in adults: the ringed esophagus. Radiology 2005;236(1):159–65.

[17] Arora A, Yamazaki K. Eosinophilic esophagitis: asthma of the esophagus? Clin Gastroenterol Hepatol 2004;2:523–30.

[18] Potter J, Saeian K, Staff D, et al. Eosinophilic esophagitis in adults: an emerging problem with unique esophageal features. Gastrointest Endosc 2004;59(3):355–61.

[19] Cheung KM, Oliver MR, Cameron DJ, et al. Esophageal eosinophilia in children with dysphagia. J Pediatr Gastroenterol Nutr 2003;37(4):498–503.

[20] Noel R, Putnam P, Rothenberg M. Eosinophilic esophagitis. N Engl J Med 2004;351(9): 940–1.

[21] Portmann S, Heer P, Bussman C, et al. Epidemiology of eosinophilic Esophagitis: data from a community-based longitudinal study work carried out by the Swiss EE study group [abstract]. Gastroenterology 2007;132:A609.

[22] Ronkainen J, Talley N, Aro P, et al. Prevalence of oesophageal eosinophils and eosinophilic oesophagitis in adults: the population-based Kalixanda study. Gut 2007;56(5):615–20.

[23] Kugathasan S, Judd R, Hoffman R, et al. Epidemiologic and clinical characteristics of children with newly diagnosed inflammatory bowel disease in Wisconsin: a statewide population-based study. J Pediatr 2003;143:525–31.

[24] Furuta GT, Liacouras CA, Collins MH, et al. First International Gastrointestinal Eosinophil Research Symposium (FIGERS) Subcommittees. Related Articles, Links Eosinophilic esophagitis in children and adults: a systematic review and consensus recommendations for diagnosis and treatment. Gastroenterology 2007;133(4):1342–63.

[25] Gonsalves N, Policarpio-Nicolas M, Zhang Q, et al. Histopathologic variability and endoscopic correlates in adults with eosinophilic esophagitis. Gastrointest endosc 2006;64(3): 313–9.

[26] Remedios M, Campbell C, Jones D, et al. Eosinophilic esophagitis in adults: clinical, endoscopic, histologic findings, and response to treatment with fluticasone propionate. Gastrointest Endosc 2006;63(1):3–12.

[27] Ngo P, Furuta GT, Antonioli D. Eosinophils in the esophagus—peptic or allergic eosinophilic esophagitis? Case series of three patients with esophageal eosinophilia. Am J Gastroenterol 2006;101(7):1666–70.

[28] Noel R, Putnam P, Collins M, et al. Clinical and immunopathologic effects of swallowed fluticasone for eosinophilic esophagitis. Clin Gastroenterol Hepatol 2004;2:568–75.

[29] Attwood S, Lewis C, Bronder C, et al. Eosinophilic esophagitis: a novel treatment using Montelukast. Gut 2003;52:181–5.

[30] Shah A, Gonsalves N, Aldana-Melina H, et al. Histologic variability and clinical findings in children with eosinophilic esophagitis [abstract]. Gastroenterology 2007.

[31] Liacouras C, Spergel J, Ruchelli E, et al. Eosinophilic esophagitis: a 10-year experience in 381 children. Clin Gastroenterol Hepatol 2005;3:L1198–206.

[32] Sgouros S, Bergele C, Mantides A. Eosinophilic esophagitis in adults: a systematic review. Eur J Gastroenterol Hepatol 2006;18:211–7.

ELSEVIER
SAUNDERS

Gastrointest Endoscopy Clin N Am
18 (2008) 11–23

GASTROINTESTINAL
ENDOSCOPY CLINICS
OF NORTH AMERICA

Eosinophilic Esophagitis in Children: Clinical Manifestations

Philip E. Putnam, MD, FAAP

*Cincinnati Center for Eosinophilic Disorders, Division of Gastroenterology, Hepatology,
and Nutrition, Cincinnati Children's Hospital Medical Center, 3333 Burnet Avenue,
ML 2010, Cincinnati, OH 45229, USA*

During the past decade, the increasing number of recognized cases of eosinophilic esophagitis in children and adults has resulted in a dramatic expansion of the medical literature surrounding it. Clinical and basic research has contributed to a better, but still incomplete, body of knowledge regarding its clinical and histologic manifestations, as well as its immunologic and genetic pathogenesis.

This article provides a broad framework for recognizing the remarkable variety of clinical manifestations of eosinophilic esophagitis in children. There is not a convenient "one size fits all" description of the presentation of eosinophilic esophagitis, and therefore physicians must consider it as part of the differential diagnosis in many different clinical situations. Prompt, accurate diagnosis is required for timely management, symptom control, and prevention of untoward sequelae from the disorder.

Much of the medical literature related to eosinophilic esophagitis exists as case reports, case series, and reviews from centers in North America. The larger case series form the basis for the current understanding of the clinical manifestations of eosinophilic esophagitis in children and come from the tertiary referral centers that focus on diagnosis and management of pediatric eosinophilic esophagitis [1–6]. In addition, the recent publication of diagnostic guidelines will allow standardization for clinical care and future research studies [7].

Although most of these works were not designed primarily as epidemiologic studies, the demographics of the identified patients support several common findings. For reasons that remain unclear, approximately 70% of children who have eosinophilic esophagitis are males. A series in the United

---

E-mail address: phil.putnam@cchmc.org

1052-5157/08/$ - see front matter © 2008 Elsevier Inc. All rights reserved.
doi:10.1016/j.giec.2007.09.007

States also has confirmed the clinical impression that the majority (94.4%) of patients are white [2].

In southwest Ohio, the incidence of eosinophilic esophagitis in children has been estimated at 1.25 cases per 10,000 children per year [6]. Formal epidemiologic studies encompassing the broader population are needed to understand more precisely the risk for developing eosinophilic esophagitis in North America and abroad.

Symptoms of eosinophilic esophagitis

The most frequent symptoms of eosinophilic esophagitis are nonspecific and include dysphagia, pain, and vomiting. The age at which the symptoms develop varies considerably [6]. Feeding difficulty was the predominant reason for referral and evaluation of infants and toddlers ultimately diagnosed as having eosinophilic esophagitis. Preschool and school-aged children commonly complained of abdominal pain or vomiting, whereas dysphagia generally appeared as a primary complaint in the preadolescent years. In that analysis the chief complaint was recorded, but most patients had more than one symptom attributable to the disorder.

Dysphagia

Dysphagia caused by eosinophilic esophagitis is described variously by affected individuals and is notoriously intermittent. Age and ability to communicate effectively play influence how a child describes his or her own difficulty swallowing. Some note that food "goes down slowly," whereas others say that food gets stuck temporarily somewhere in the throat or chest before proceeding down. Some report difficulty initiating the swallow while the bolus is still in the mouth or recognize anxiety promoted by prior episodes of food impaction. Retrospective analyses note that dysphagia was present for more than 2 years before diagnosis in some patients [8,9]. As detailed in the article by Katzka, elsewhere in this issue, dysphagia has been the predominant presenting symptom in adults.

A careful history in patients who complain of dysphagia reveals that they have learned to compensate by eating slowly, drinking after each bite, taking small bites, chewing excessively, or avoiding specific food consistencies that are problematic such as meat or bread. This phenomenon may help to explain the intermittent experience of dysphagia, because the failure to compensate at a particular meal or even for a single bite may allow the symptom to manifest and "reset" the compensatory mechanisms.

Food impaction requiring endoscopic removal as the initial contact between an adolescent and the medical community is a fairly common presentation for eosinophilic esophagitis. Often the dysphagia has been long standing but mild and intermittent. Many individuals report years of symptoms that were ignored, compensated for, attributed to "taking too big a bite", or that were blamed on "not chewing food well enough."

The author and colleagues also have diagnosed eosinophilic esophagitis when called to remove from the esophagus impacted but nonobstructing foreign bodies that normally would have passed, such as coins. It is good practice to obtain mucosal biopsies from the esophagus, remote from the site of the impaction, after endoscopic removal of a foreign body, especially food impactions. Endoscopic evidence for eosinophilic esophagitis (thickening, furrowing, or pinpoint or diffuse white exudate) (Figs. 1 and 2) is frequently present in affected individuals at the time of the impaction, but because the endoscopic appearance may be influenced by the foreign body on the one hand, and because up to one third of patients who have eosinophilic esophagitis may have a normal-appearing esophagus at endoscopy on the other hand [4], mucosal biopsy is warranted after extracting a foreign body in children.

Less common but clearly problematic, gastroenterologic consultation has been requested for some individuals after long periods of psychiatric evaluation and treatment of chronic dysphagia without radiographic evidence for dysmotility or stricture. The authors have seen children ultimately proved to have eosinophilic esophagitis whose dysphagia has been attributed to underlying anxiety, obsessive-compulsive disorder, eating disorder, or pervasive developmental disorder. One boy was diagnosed with bulimia at age 10 years because he vomited after eating, although he had symptoms since infancy.

Dysphagia in patients who have eosinophilic esophagitis can be caused by mechanical obstruction of the esophagus and can manifest endoscopically and/or radiographically as a ring (Fig. 3) focal stricture, Schatzki ring, or long-segment narrowing (so-called "small-caliber esophagus") [10]. It is more common, however, for children to complain of dysphagia in the absence of radiographic narrowing of the esophagus [9]. Nurko and

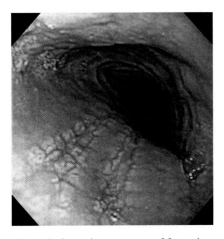

Fig. 1. Endoscopic appearance of furrowing.

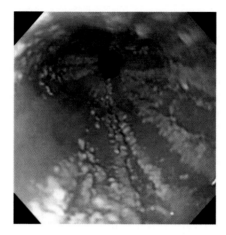

Fig. 2. Endoscopic appearance of exudate.

colleagues [8] examined the esophageal histology proximal to radiographically diagnosed Schatzki rings in 18 children and discovered that eosinophilic esophagitis was present in 8 of them. Notably, endoscopic evidence
for Schatzki ring was not present in the children who had histologic eosinophilic esophagitis, suggesting that focal transient spasm accounted for the
radiographic finding.

It is tempting to attribute dysphagia to the degree of inflammation, duration of disease, degree of lamina propria fibrosis, or the impact of chronic
inflammation on deeper layers of the esophagus. The deep layers of the
esophagus are affected, as evidenced by the thickening of the entire wall
of the esophagus demonstrated by endoscopic ultrasound [11]. Nonspecific
manometric abnormalities were observed in 60% of studied adult patients
who had eosinophilic esophagitis [12]. In that study, parallel improvement
in manometric and histologic findings was observed.

It is tempting to speculate that adolescents and adults who have had
long-standing untreated disease develop dysphagia as a consequence of persistent inflammation-induced damage including lamina propria fibrosis or
remodeling, but because the age of disease onset often is unknown in that
group, it has not been possible to associate dysphagia directly with the duration of inflammation in many individuals [13,14].

Stricture is a feared complication of eosinophilic esophagitis and has been
described as early as 7 months of age [9]. Although the strictures are ame-
nable to dilatation, esophageal mucosa with eosinophilic inflammation is
more prone to tear during dilatation than the mucosa overlying a peptic
stricture, and perforation of the esophagus has been described as a complication of attempted dilatation in adults [10,15,16]. Many clinicians managing adults who have eosinophilic esophagitis–associated dysphagia now
recommend aggressive medical management of the inflammation before

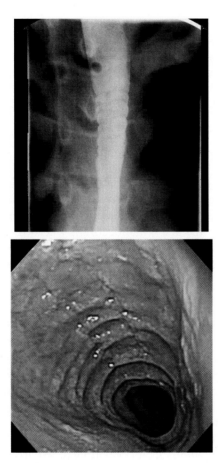

Fig. 3. (*Top*) Radiographic appearance and (*bottom*) endoscopic and radiographic appearance of the ringed proximal esophagus.

attempting dilatation unless clinical circumstances dictate more immediate relief of the obstruction [17]. Prospective study has not confirmed that this approach reduces the number of dilatations or the risk of perforation, but this approach is reasonable until refuted. Similarly, dogmatic historical concepts generated by experience in dilating peptic strictures should be abandoned and replaced by recommendations for gentle, gradual dilatation only when necessitated by failure of medical therapy for eosinophilic esophagitis.

Infants and preverbal toddlers who have eosinophilic esophagitis may present with feeding difficulties that manifest as gagging, choking, food refusal/aversion, or vomiting [18]. It is not well understood whether these problems are consequences of dysphagia, nausea, anorexia, pain, fear or anxiety after untoward experiences with eating, or a combination of these factors. Clinicians participating in the evaluation of young children who have feeding disorders must be knowledgeable in the evaluation and treatment options for eosinophilic esophagitis and have a low threshold for early evaluation and intervention. Because there are overlapping issues, concurrent therapy to account for all of the child's conditions (gastroesophageal reflux disease [GERD], behavioral feeding aversion, and eosinophilic esophagitis) may be necessary.

Vomiting

Vomiting as a primary complaint among pediatric patients who have eosinophilic esophagitis occurs most often in young children. It can mimic reflux, manifest as effortless regurgitation, but eosinophilic esophagitis is seldom diagnosed in the first 6 months of life when GERD is common. Accurate diagnosis of eosinophilic esophagitis in very young children who vomit is often delayed by months to years, during which time treatment for symptoms attributed to GERD is attempted. In the author's experience, parents describe vomiting more often than effortless regurgitation.

Circumstances surrounding episodes of vomiting vary. Vomiting can be part of an overt and immediate allergic response to a recently ingested food. In that case, the family generally recognizes that there is a consistent reaction to that food and chooses to avoid it. Immediate vomiting may be associated with other manifestations of an adverse immune response such as hives, diarrhea, pain, or even anaphylaxis. Some children who have eosinophilic esophagitis and multiple food allergies have a history of developing different constellations of symptoms in response to various foods, up to and including food protein–induced enterocolitis syndrome.

Chronic, episodic, unpredictable vomiting of variable severity also occurs in patients who have eosinophilic esophagitis, and it is not clinically distinguishable from other causes of emesis. This vomiting does not occur proximate to exposure to a particular food, which precludes devising an appropriate diet based solely on history.

In the first year of life, clues that eosinophilic esophagitis, rather than reflux, is the underlying culprit include early onset of vomiting (within days to weeks of birth) associated with eczema, vomiting associated with irritability that does not respond to acid suppression, and onset of vomiting in the second half of the first year of life during the introduction of solid foods.

After infancy, vomiting is more chronic, intermittent, and not readily associated with particular foods, although it is usually meal related. Vomiting to the point of excess calorie loss resulting in failure to gain weight or weight loss is possible but uncommon.

Rarely, nausea without vomiting is the sole presenting manifestation of eosinophilic esophagitis. Although usually present with other symptoms, it has been an isolated complaint in a few individuals. Nausea has been responsive to standard treatment of the esophagitis in most individuals, but the author and colleagues have seen other children who have remarkably re-calcitrant nausea as a persistent complaint after resolution of active eosino-philic inflammation.

Retching to remove a piece of food that is stuck may be called "vomit-ing" by some patients and needs to be distinguished from emesis of gastric contents. Retching can be recognized as such by careful history. The patient will report that something got stuck and he or she retched to remove or oth-erwise dislodge it.

Pain

Pain is a frequent but not universal complaint among individuals who have untreated eosinophilic esophagitis. Children who have pain associated with eosinophilic esophagitis report chest, epigastric, and/or abdominal pain. Overt odynophagia is not typical. Some individuals have been evalu-ated the emergency department for episodic crushing substernal pain con-cerning for heart disease. Those individuals have been remarkably free of symptoms between pain attacks, which have been unpredictable in fre-quency and which lack an obvious inciting event.

The pain may be described as heartburn and may respond to acid sup-pression. When histologic eosinophilic inflammation persists despite effec-tive therapy for GERD, a clinical diagnosis of eosinophilic esophagitis is established.

A remarkable number of children indicate that their pain is in the epigas-trium or the periumbilical area. They often have difficulty describing the pain in more sophisticated terms. It is imperative that these complaints pro-mote appropriate investigation, particularly when the broader clinical pic-ture is concerning, such as a boy who has asthma or eczema or a history of food allergy. The absence of complaints referable to the chest should not preclude consideration of esophageal disease.

Associated conditions

Communicative children who have eosinophilic esophagitis may present with a single symptom, but careful questioning often elicits additional symp-toms that are attributable to the inflammation. In addition, many children who have eosinophilic esophagitis have other medical conditions with symp-toms that may overlap, contribute to, or serve to confuse the issue at presen-tation. For example, chest pain may accompany episodes of bronchospasm in a child who has asthma, and that phenomenon may divert attention away from other potential causes of chest pain, such as esophagitis (reflux or otherwise).

The profile of individuals who have eosinophilic esophagitis is quite var-ied, but there are notable associations. Because definitions and rigor in es-tablishing a formal diagnosis vary, the precise frequency of associated conditions is subject to interpretation. Nevertheless, eosinophilic esophagitis coexists or is a parallel phenomenon associated with asthma, eczema, and environmental and food allergies in up to 75% of children [2,19].

The association of eosinophilic esophagitis with other conditions is becoming more apparent from experience. The epidemiology and immunobiology are as yet unexplored. For example, esophageal eosinophilia has been seen in the Cincinnati Center for Eosinophilic Disorders in a handful of children who have other gastrointestinal conditions such as *Helicobacter pylori* gastritis, Crohn's disease, or celiac disease.

Esophageal involvement can be seen in patients who have eosinophilic gastroenteritis. It is inappropriate to make a clinical diagnosis of eosinophilic esophagitis when substantial eosinophilic inflammation of stomach, small intestinal, or colon is present concurrently or sporadically in a patient who has had eosinophilic infiltration of the esophagus. Studies have examined the number of eosinophils in normal gastrointestinal mucosa, but formal histologic and clinical definitions of eosinophilic gastroenteritis are yet to be developed [20,21]. As such, separating patients who have eosinophilic esophagitis who happen to have mild and clinically irrelevant mucosal eosinophilia distal to the esophagus from cases of eosinophilic gastroenteritis with esophageal involvement can be challenging. Diarrhea, anemia, hypoalbuminemia, failure to thrive, and gastrointestinal bleeding are not typical features of isolated eosinophilic esophagitis, and individuals who display them should be evaluated appropriately, even if a provisional diagnosis of eosinophilic esophagitis has been made.

A number of children who have underlying neurologic or neurodevelopmental conditions have been diagnosed as having eosinophilic esophagitis. Eosinophilic esophagitis has been seen in children who also have intractable seizures, cerebral palsy, Chiari malformation, pervasive developmental disorder, sensory integration disorder, or migraine. Hypersensitivity to antiepileptic drugs has been implicated in the development of eosinophilic esophagitis, so it is important to account for medication use in this group [22]. Otherwise, no obvious, direct, cause-and-effect relationship between these neurologic conditions and eosinophilic esophagitis has been discerned to date.

The epidemiology of eosinophilic esophagitis in children who have concurrent neurodevelopmental conditions has not been explored formally. It is not clear whether the prevalence of eosinophilic esophagitis is indeed higher in that population of children or whether clinicians have become more thorough in evaluating them. GERD is said to occur frequently in this population as well, but it is no longer safe to assume that GERD is responsible for nonspecific upper gastrointestinal symptoms.

Similarly, eosinophilic esophagitis has been discovered in children who have other syndromes, without comment on the epidemiology. A case report notes the association of eosinophilic esophagitis in Rubenstein-Taybi syndrome [23]. The author and colleagues have seen eosinophilic esophagitis in children who have coloboma, heart anomalies, choanal atresia, retardation of growth and development, and genital and ear anomalies (CHARGE syndrome), vertebral, anal, tracheo-esophageal, and radial limb or renal anomalies (VATER syndrome), Pierre-Robin syndrome, Klinefelter's syndrome, Moebius syndrome, and Pfeiffer syndrome.

Eosinophilic esophagitis and disease of the respiratory tract

Eosinophilic esophagitis has been discovered in children presenting with airway and respiratory complaints, who may or may not have concomitant gastrointestinal symptoms [24,25]. Although the prevalence of eosinophilic esophagitis in children presenting with primary airway disease is unknown, it must be considered in children who present with stridor, adenoidal hypertrophy, recurrent croup, recurrent pneumonia, or aspiration. The diagnosis has been made in children who have airway anomalies such as subglottic stenosis or laryngeal cleft [26].

No criteria yet exist on which to base recommendations for formal diagnostic evaluation for eosinophilic esophagitis in patients who have these presenting symptoms. At the Cincinnati Center for Eosinophilic Disorders, more than 50 children who have eosinophilic esophagitis have been seen in the tertiary, multidisciplinary clinic dedicated to the evaluation and treatment of significant airway problems resulting in tracheostomy tube dependence. Most have had subglottic stenosis caused by prolonged intubation after premature birth, and none were suspected of having or diagnosed as having eosinophilic esophagitis before evaluation in this institution. Many had failed prior attempts at surgical laryngotracheoplasty. Because the mechanisms involved are not established, it is not clear whether there is any direct relationship between the esophagitis and the recurrent stenosis, but the association and concern has been sufficient for the author and colleagues to consider evaluation for and treatment of eosinophilic esophagitis in this population warranted before committing to elective airway surgery until prospective studies further examine the pathogenesis.

Do different phenotypes of eosinophilic esophagitis exist?

Studies that describe the symptom complex in children who have eosinophilic esophagitis have generally lumped all individuals with defined histology together, and the disorder is considered as a single entity. Those who have followed a large number of children with eosinophilic esophagitis, however, suspect that clinically distinct patterns occur. Whether these presentations are simply at opposite ends of a continuum or deserve a separate diagnosis or classification scheme is not established. A particular single nucleotide polymorphism in the eotaxin-3 gene is present in some individuals with eosinophilic esophagitis, but it is not clear how that information can or should be used in clinical practice at this time [27].

In clinical practice, it is possible to categorize children loosely into clinical subtypes or phenotypes. For example, there is a group of children in which the individuals are extraordinarily atopic and exhibit a constellation of eosinophilic esophagitis, eczema, chronic rhinitis, asthma, repeated respiratory infections, and multiple food allergies. These children often present in early infancy with vomiting and irritability. Eczema, chronic nasal congestion, recurrent bronchospasm, and repeated upper respiratory infection become apparent in the first 2 years of life. In some, the eczema has been severe. Although the gastrointestinal symptoms respond to dietary restriction (most often requiring an elemental diet with an amino acid-based formula), the asthma is generally an independent phenomenon requiring standard therapy and does not resolve as a result of diet change alone. In this group, a clinical diagnosis of GERD has been made almost universally, but the children do not respond completely to antireflux therapy. Some of these children have been extraordinarily sensitive to food and exhibit recurrent eosinophilic esophagitis with virtually any food added to the diet.

At the other end of the spectrum is group of children who have eosinophilic esophagitis in the absence of atopy, eczema, or asthma. Evidence for food allergies is lacking by formal allergy testing, and the children do not respond to dietary therapy even with an elemental diet. This group of patients generally responds well to topical (swallowed) steroids (usually fluticasone or budesonide) as mainstay of chronic therapy. Recurrence after discontinuation of steroids is nearly universal, although follow-up of these patients is still relatively brief (< 10 years for children).

If these presentations are considered as a spectrum, the middle of the spectrum is populated by children who have eosinophilic esophagitis and food allergies, often with asthma, and/or mild eczema. They develop eosinophilic esophagitis with several foods but can be maintained on an elimination diet, avoiding those foods that trigger the inflammation. This group seems to be large and to incorporate the majority of children who have eosinophilic esophagitis who have been evaluated in the Cincinnati Center for Eosinophilic Disorders.

Familial eosinophilic esophagitis

Eosinophilic esophagitis has been demonstrated in more than one individual within many families [28]. The occurrence across generations suggests a genetic rather than environmental pathogenesis, but only now are the details being explored. Careful assessment of the family history may identify other individuals who already have been diagnosed, but the author and colleagues frequently hear about adults with longstanding dysphagia, perhaps requiring dilatation, attributed to reflux or Schatzki ring. Siblings who exhibit symptoms deserve early endoscopic evaluation to establish a diagnosis.

Response to therapy

Much of what has been learned about children who have eosinophilic esophagitis has come directly from studies designed to observe the response of the inflammatory process to therapy, be it dietary antigen elimination or steroids [4,19,29–33]. By convention, eosinophilic esophagitis is distinguished from reflux by the failure to respond to aggressive antireflux therapy. In the landmark description of eosinophilic esophagitis in children, the complete response of otherwise recalcitrant eosinophilic esophagitis to an elemental diet was a defining feature [34]. Now, the same parameters are used to make a formal diagnosis (ie, failure to respond to antireflux therapy) and to distinguish the food allergic variant (ie, response to diet). Specifically, complete clinical and histologic resolution of active eosinophilic esophagitis in response to diet therapy either with specific antigen avoidance or total antigen elimination (eg, diet replaced by an elemental formula) supports a diagnosis of the allergic variant of eosinophilic esophagitis. In theory, patients who do not respond to an elemental diet still may have an allergic variant, although the assumed nonfood environmental antigens involved remain unclear. Because up to 98% of children who have eosinophilic esophagitis respond to an elemental diet, the vast majority of affected children would seem to have the disease as a manifestation of adverse response to dietary antigens [32].

Controversies in eosinophilic esophagitis

One of the great difficulties in managing children who have eosinophilic esophagitis has been the absence of symptoms in treated individuals who nevertheless have active esophageal eosinophilia. Symptoms typically abate with therapy (diet or medication), but some patients still have unaltered or only minimally improved esophageal histology.

Another common scenario is for the esophagitis to return without overt symptoms during attempts at reintroducing food to the diet or upon withdrawal of steroid therapy [2,4]. This phenomenon has generated considerable debate as to whether the symptom(s) or the histology should be treated. Because only endoscopy with biopsy has been an adequate method for reassessment in the absence of symptoms, one of the concerns has been the risk and cost of the number of endoscopies that need to be performed during the lifetime of an individual undergoing food elimination/reintroduction. Early work that examined genetic, biochemical, and/or immunologic markers for the disease failed to discover factors with sufficient predictive value to be used routinely in place of endoscopy and histology [27,35,36]. The debate has not been resolved officially, although expert consensus now supports treating the histology irrespective of the absence of symptoms, because of the known longer-term risks of esophageal remodeling, fibrosis, and potential stricture formation [17].

References

[1] Orenstein SR, Shalaby TM, Di Lorenzo C, et al. The spectrum of pediatric eosinophilic esophagitis beyond infancy: a clinical series of 30 children. Am J Gastroenterol 2000; 95(6):1422–30.

[2] Assa'ad AH, Putnam PE, Collins MH, et al. Pediatric patients with eosinophilic esophagitis: an 8-year follow-up. J Allergy Clin Immunol 2007;119(3):731–8.

[3] Aceves SS, Newbury RO, Dohil R, et al. Distinguishing eosinophilic esophagitis in pediatric patients: clinical, endoscopic, and histologic features of an emerging disorder. J Clin Gastroenterol 2007;41(3):252–6.

[4] Liacouras CA, Spergel JM, Ruchelli E, et al. Eosinophilic esophagitis: a 10-year experience in 381 children. Clin Gastroenterol Hepatol 2005;3(12):1198–206.

[5] Fox VL, Nurko S, Furuta GT. Eosinophilic esophagitis: it's not just kid's stuff. Gastrointest Endosc 2002;56(2):260–70.

[6] Noel RJ, Putnam PE, Rothenberg ME. Eosinophilic esophagitis. N Engl J Med 2004;351(9): 940–1.

[7] Furuta GT, Liacouras CA, Collins MH, et al. Eosinophilic esophagitis in children and adults: a systematic review and consensus recommendations for diagnosis and treatment. Gastroenterology 2007;133(4):1342–63.

[8] Nurko S, Teitelbaum JE, Husain K, et al. Association of Schatzki ring with eosinophilic esophagitis in children. J Pediatr Gastroenterol Nutr 2004;38(4):436–41.

[9] Khan S, Orenstein SR, Di Lorenzo C, et al. Eosinophilic esophagitis: strictures, impactions, dysphagia. Dig Dis Sci 2003;48(1):22–9.

[10] Vasilopoulos S, Murphy P, Auerbach A, et al. The small-caliber esophagus: an unappreciated cause of dysphagia for solids in patients with eosinophilic esophagitis. Gastrointest Endosc 2002;55(1):99–106.

[11] Fox VL, Nurko S, Teitelbaum JE, et al. High-resolution EUS in children with eosinophilic "allergic" esophagitis. Gastrointest Endosc 2003;57(1):30–6.

[12] Lucendo AJ, Castillo P, Martín-Chávarri S, et al. Manometric findings in adult eosinophilic oesophagitis: a study of 12 cases. Eur J Gastroenterol Hepatol 2007;19(5):417–24.

[13] Aceves SS, Newbury RO, Dohil R, et al. Esophageal remodeling in pediatric eosinophilic esophagitis. J Allergy Clin Immunol 2007;119(1):206–12.

[14] Straumann A, Spichtin HP, Grize L, et al. Natural history of primary eosinophilic esophagitis: a follow-up of 30 adult patients for up to 11.5 years. Gastroenterology 2003;125(6):1660–9.

[15] Eisenbach C, Merle U, Schirmacher P, et al. Perforation of the esophagus after dilation treatment for dysphagia in a patient with eosinophilic esophagitis. Endoscopy 2006 [Epub ahead of print].

[16] Lucendo AJ, De Rezende L. Endoscopic dilation in eosinophilic esophagitis: a treatment strategy associated with a high risk of perforation. Endoscopy 2007;39(4):376.

[17] Liacouras CA, Bonis P, Putnam P, et al. FIGER summary. J Pediatr Gastro Nutr 2007;45: 370–91.

[18] Pentiuk SP, Miller CK, Kaul A. Eosinophilic esophagitis in infants and toddlers. Dysphagia 2007;22(1):44–8, Epub 2006 Oct 6.

[19] Spergel JM, Andrews T, Brown-Whitehorn TF, et al. Treatment of eosinophilic esophagitis with specific food elimination diet directed by a combination of skin prick and patch tests. Ann Allergy Asthma Immunol 2005;95(4):336–43.

[20] DeBrosse CW, Case JW, Putnam PE, et al. Quantity and distribution of eosinophils in the gastrointestinal tract of children. Pediatr Dev Pathol 2006;9(3):210–8.

[21] Lowichik A, Weinberg AG. A quantitative evaluation of mucosal eosinophils in the pediatric gastrointestinal tract. Mod Pathol 1996;9(2):110–4.

[22] Balatsinou C, Milano A, Caldarella MP, et al. Eosinophilic esophagitis is a component of the anticonvulsant hypersensitivity syndrome: description of two cases. Dig Liver Dis 2007 [Epub ahead of print].

[23] Noble A, Drouin E, Faure C. Eosinophilic esophagitis and gastritis in Rubinstein-Taybi syndrome. J Pediatr Gastroenterol Nutr 2007;44(4):498–500.

[24] Mandell DL, Yellon RF. Synchronous airway lesions and esophagitis in young patients undergoing adenoidectomy. Arch Otolaryngol Head Neck Surg 2007;133(4):375–8, 13.

[25] Dauer EH, Ponikau JU, Smyrk TC, et al. Airway manifestations of pediatric eosinophilic esophagitis: a clinical and histopathologic report of an emerging association. Ann Otol Rhinol Laryngol 2006;115(7):507–17.

[26] Goldstein NA, Putnam PE, Dohar JE. Laryngeal cleft and eosinophilic gastroenteritis: report of 2 cases. Arch Otolaryngol Head Neck Surg 2000;126(2):227–30.

[27] Blanchard C, Wang N, Stringer KF, et al. Eotaxin-3 and a uniquely conserved gene-expression profile in eosinophilic esophagitis. J Clin Invest 2006;116(2):536–47.

[28] Zink DA, Amin M, Gebara S, et al. Familial dysphagia and eosinophilia. Gastrointest Endosc 2007;65(2):330–4.

[29] Konikoff MR, Noel RJ, Blanchard C, et al. A randomized double-blind placebo-controlled trial of fluticasone propionate for pediatric eosinophilic esophagitis. Gastroenterology 2006; 131(5):1381–91.

[30] Noel RJ, Putnam PE, Collins MH, et al. Clinical and Immunopathologic effects of swallowed Fluticasone for eosinophilic esophagitis. Clin Gastroenterol Hepatol 2004;2(7): 568–75.

[31] Kagalwalla AF, Shah A, Ritz S, et al. Cow's milk protein-induced eosinophilic esophagitis in a child with gluten-sensitive enteropathy. J Pediatr Gastroenterol Nutr 2007;44(3):386–8.

[32] Markowitz JE, Spergel JM, Ruchelli E, et al. Elemental diet is an effective treatment for eosinophilic esophagitis in children and adolescents. Am J Gastroenterol 2003;98(4):777–82.

[33] Teitelbaum JE, Fox VL, Twarog FJ, et al. Eosinophilic esophagitis in children: immunopathological analysis and response to fluticasone propionate. Gastroenterology 2002; 122(5):1216–25.

[34] Kelly KJ, Lazenby AJ, Rowe PC, et al. Eosinophilic esophagitis attributed to gastroesophageal reflux: improvement with an amino acid-based formula. Gastroenterology 1995; 109(5):1503–12.

[35] Konikoff MR, Blanchard C, Kirby C, et al. Potential of blood eosinophils, eosinophil-derived neurotoxin, and eotaxin-3 as biomarkers of eosinophilic esophagitis. Clin Gastroenterol Hepatol 2006;4(11):1328–36, Epub 2006 Oct 23.

[36] Gupta SK, Fitzgerald JF, Kondratyuk T, et al. Cytokine expression in normal and inflamed esophageal mucosa: a study into the pathogenesis of allergic eosinophilic esophagitis. J Pediatr Gastroenterol Nutr 2006;42(1):22–6.

ELSEVIER
SAUNDERS

Gastrointest Endoscopy Clin N Am
18 (2008) 25–32

GASTROINTESTINAL
ENDOSCOPY CLINICS
OF NORTH AMERICA

Demographic Data and Symptoms of Eosinophilic Esophagitis in Adults

David A. Katzka, MD

University of Pennsylvania School of Medicine, 3 Ravdin Building,
3400 Spruce Street, Philadelphia, PA 19104, USA

Eosinophilic esophagitis (EE) is a disease that affects both adults and children. Although a majority of the studies in this disease have been based on the pediatric experience, in more recent years the understanding of EE in adults has increased because of the growing recognition of adult EE by gastroenterologists and pathologists and because of the overall increasing prevalence of this disease in the population. Data from recent adult studies, when compared with the pediatric literature, have been helpful in discerning the similarities and the differences between adults and children who have EE. More specifically, although demographic characteristics and symptoms may be similar in young and older patients who have EE, the severity, chronicity, and predominance of a specific symptom may differ markedly between children and adults. For example, younger children who have EE may present with a plethora of evident upper gastrointestinal symptoms such as nausea, vomiting, and dyspepsia, in stark contrast to the surreptitious or subclinical presentation of longstanding EE in many adults. As a result, when describing the different symptomatic presentations of EE in different age groups, one must wonder whether there is a shared pathophysiology with varied clinical presentation or distinctly different mechanisms that separate the groups and define distinct diseases with the same histologic end point. In adults there is a greater prevalence of gastroesophageal reflux and therefore there is more interest in its role of as a cause of EE. With this caveat in mind, this article discusses specific characteristics of the patterns of EE presentation in adults (Box 1) and notes how these patterns differ or resemble the presentation in children.

E-mail address: david.katzka@uphs.upenn.edu

1052-5157/08/$ - see front matter © 2008 Elsevier Inc. All rights reserved.
doi:10.1016/j.giec.2007.09.005
giendo.theclinics.com

Box 1. Symptoms and clues to diagnosis in adults who have eosinophilic esophagitis

Common symptoms
Dysphagia
Food Impaction
Heartburn

Less common symptoms
Chest pain
Dyspepsia
Nausea and/or vomiting
Odynophagia
Abdominal pain
Weight loss

Subtle symptomatic clues
Long duration of symptoms before diagnosis
Slow eating and prolonged chewing
Swallowing liquids consistently with solid food
Avoidance of some solid foods (eg, meats, breads, raw
　vegetables)

Extra-esophageal factors commonly identified in adults who have eosinophilic esophagitis
Male gender
White race
Personal and family history of other allergic disorders
　(eg, asthma, rhinitis, atopic dermatitis and food allergy)
Seasonal variation in occurrence of symptoms (ie, more common
　when aeroallergens prominent)

Demographic data

Several studies investigating EE in adults (Table 1) have addressed gender distribution in adult patients who have EE [1–9]. All studies indicate that EE predominates in men, with an average male:female ratio of approximately 2.4 to 1 in most studies. In the largest study of adults who had EE, which used a national pathology database of 363 patients [10], the ratio was 2.9. This ratio held across all age groups in this study, including patients past their eighth decade of life. Although one would like to think this ratio speaks for a preserved single pathophysiology throughout all age groups, it is important to remember that EE is increasing in the adult population [11], as is gastroesophageal reflux. The more serious complications of gastroesophageal reflux disease, such as Barrett's esophagus, are also increasing [12,13] and are more prevalent in men [14].

Table 1
Studies of adult eosinophilic esophagitis

Symptom	Study Number in study (%)								
	Croese, et al [1][a]	Arora, et al [2][b]	Straumann, et al [3][a]	Potter, et al [4][b]	Lucendo, et al [5][b]	Desai, et al [6][b]	Remedios, et al [7][b]	Gonsalves, et al [8][a]	Muller, et al [9][b,c]
Impaction	12 (39)	15 (74)	30 (100)	8 (33)	2 (40)	17 (100)	17 (65)	41(55)	15 (13)
Dysphagia	9 (29)	21 (100)	30 (100)	24 (83)	5 (100)	17 (100)	26 (100)	65 (90)	82 (70)
Heartburn	5 (16)	4 (19)	2 (7)	8 (28)		2 (12)	10 (39)	22 (31)	55 (47)
Chest pain	4 (13)						2 (8)	1 (1)	34 (29)
Abdominal pain	1 (3)							3 (4)	34 (29)
Weight loss		10 (49)							11 (9)
Male:female ratio	24:7	17:4	22:8	21:8	5:0	14:3	18:8	57:17	84:33
Age in years (age range in years)	34 (14–77)	39 (15–49)	33 (6–65)	35 (19–65)	25 (15–35)	42	34 (17–65)		42 (<10–>70)
Time until diagnosis in years (range in years)		11 (3–26)	4.6 (0–17)				6 (1–45)		4.2 (0–44)

[a] Primary symptoms.
[b] Any symptom.
[c] Included nine children.

The lower age range in most adult studies of EE is 18 years (the conventional cut-off between adults and children); the upper range includes patients in their nineties. As a "pediatric" disease, one might expect a linear drop off in disease incidence with increasing age; instead, in series of adult patients, the peak incidence may fall in the 30- to 50-year-old age group. Whether this incidence reflects sample bias or a marked delay in diagnosis is unclear. There is little published data available on the racial or ethnic distribution of EE. In a series of 94 adult patients at the University of Pennsylvania School of Medicine, 91 were white, 2 were Indian, and 1 was Asian; none were African American or Hispanic. In a recent pediatric study of 89 patients who had EE, 84 were white, 4 were African American, and 1 was classified as "other" [15]. Notably, both these patient populations are derived from urban populations, perhaps with some referral bias given that the studies were conducted at university medical centers. Thus, although it seems likely that EE may affect varied racial and ethnic groups, it seems to be much more prevalent in the white adult population.

There is a high prevalence of allergy in the family members of patients who have EE. Also, several reports have documented families in which several members had EE [16,17], including a recent report in which three siblings had EE [18]. Although one cannot dissect out and exclude similar environmental influences in these families, this lineage is in keeping with work by Rothenberg and colleagues [19] demonstrating the presence of an abnormal eotaxin gene in almost 50% of children who have EE. This genetic hypothesis may also explain the prevalence of this disease in a single racial group.

Symptoms as identifiers of eosinophilic esophagitis in adults

Non-esophageal symptoms

Because identification of patients who have EE may rely on a strong family history of EE or other allergic disorders, the diagnosis also may rely on the presence of symptoms attributable to a personal history of other allergic disorders. These disorders may include asthma, allergic rhinitis, and atopic dermatitis. In adult series, the incidence of a personal history of asthma, atopic dermatitis, or other extra-esophageal manifestations of allergies ranges from 29% [2] to 90% [1,3,7,8]. Of these diseases, asthma is the one most commonly associated with EE, accounting for approximately two thirds or atopic disorders. A family history of one of these allergic disorders is also present in approximately 20% of families of adult patients who have EE [3]. More specific data using radioallergosorbent testing (RAST) have demonstrated allergy to ragweed (18%), tree (75%), grass (81%), and mite (75%) in patients who have EE [8] Thus, elicitation of such symptoms as wheezing, rhinorrhea, and rash in addition to esophageal symptoms might be valuable in identifying patients who have EE.

The data on food allergy in adults who have EE are limited but are similar to those for children who have EE, in whom allergy is highly prevalent. In preliminary data from Gonsalves and colleagues [20], 61% of adults who had EE had positive RAST for foods. Preliminary data from the University of Pennsylvania School of Medicine [21] also demonstrate a prevalence of positive RAST in a majority of patients. In this series, 78% of the patients had RAST positive to one or more foods, ranging from 1 to 56 different foods and with a median of 6 foods. Notably, many of these food allergies are "silent" except for their role in EE. More specifically, adult patients who have EE commonly lack the typical manifestations of food allergies such as lip, throat, or tongue swelling, hives, or diarrhea, despite clear-skin or serologic identification of food antigen response. Nevertheless, more classic symptoms of food allergy may be elicited and may be helpful.

Esophageal symptoms

Adults who have EE present with a fascinating range of esophageal symptomatology. As in many chronic diseases that progress over long periods of time, symptoms can be silent, intermittent, and/or subtle in nature. It is assumed that many of the symptoms are silent because EE in adults is characterized pathologically by both an inflammatory mucosal component and by a submucosal and perhaps deeper-layer fibrosis (detected by endoscopic ultrasound) that is assumed to develop steadily over time [3] and presumably before overt symptoms may occur. On the other hand, the symptoms can be dramatic and/or persistent. For example, one of the common presentations of EE in adults is food impaction. In some case series up to 100% of adults who diagnosed as EE had food impaction [3], with a lower limit of at least 13% in one series of patients [9]. The authors of one recent series demonstrated that EE is the most common cause of food impaction in adults presenting to the emergency room in a community setting [6]. That patients with EE may present with such a potentially catastrophic symptom but be otherwise asymptomatic again suggests a silent progression of this disease until significant luminal and/or motility compromise allows bolus obstruction. Whether food impaction is attributable solely to a low, subclinical level of esophageal inflammation or is also caused by subclinical or a global esophageal hyposensitivity in these patients remains unclear.

The most common presentation of adults who have EE is, in essence, a lesser form of food impaction, chronic solid food dysphagia. Dysphagia occurred in up to 100% of patients in several reports [2,3,7] and is almost twice as common as all other symptoms combined. The next most common symptom in published series is heartburn, which occurs in approximately 34% of patients. Other, far less common presenting symptoms of EE are chest pain, abdominal pain, nausea, vomiting, and weight loss. The data summarizing these relatively small series have been corroborated by preliminary data from a national pathology database [10]. In this database series, dysphagia occurred in 70% of 363 patients who had EE, heartburn occurred in 28%, and abdominal pain and dyspepsia occurred in 14%. Data from this study demonstrate that this distribution of symptoms holds across all ages and across both sexes. This finding suggests that the data in this series are examining only one disease (ie, allergy based) and makes it less likely that reflux is contributing to and confounding the data.

Although dysphagia may be a prominent presenting symptom in patients who have EE when determined retrospectively, one cannot underestimate the often subtle nature of symptomatology given the pathologic subclinical progression of the disease. Indeed, one must take a careful history in patients who have EE to elicit their means of accommodating to and often circumventing dysphagia as their earliest and sometimes only symptom. Concordantly and not surprisingly, many patients who have EE have infrequent or even no symptoms because they have learned to chew their food carefully, eat slowly, cut food into small pieces, and wash down solid boluses with liquid to avoid experiencing dysphagia. Although these symptoms are not well reported, most investigators in the field of EE have noted them. Similarly, when patients who have EE are questioned about their symptoms in detail, one of the striking aspects is the long duration of symptomatology endured by these patients. As a result, series in adults typically report a 6- to 7-year average duration of symptoms before the diagnosis of EE was made [2,3,7,9]. Some studies report patients who have had 30 years of intermittent dysphagia before diagnosis. Granted, these symptoms started at a time when EE was not recognized; perhaps, with greater awareness, these long delays in diagnosis will shorten considerably. Nevertheless, as with any slowly progressive and potentially silent but benign disease, there will be a population of EE patients who have subclinical disease for years, for reasons discussed previously.

Some authors have reported the occurrence of dysphagia or other esophageal symptoms after exposure to specific foods. In some cases, the exposure did not involve consumption. For example, one patient, a baker, reported an increase in dysphagia when exposed to wheat while working [7], and another, a horse trainer, after exposure to hay. In another series, two patients reported symptoms after eating eggs; one of them also experienced symptoms after eating chicken, and the other also experienced symptoms after eating bananas and mushrooms. A third patient avoided kiwis and strawberries because of a burning sensation [4]. The ingestion of these foods might cause an allergic response of the esophagus, resulting in acute mucosal edema, although this supposition is speculative.

Furthermore, given the strong data from basic science linking aeroallergens with EE [22–25] and data demonstrating a decreased chance of diagnosing EE during the winter when fewer aeroallergens are present [25], patients may develop symptoms more often when exposed to aeroallergens. Thus, a careful history for a seasonal variation of esophageal symptoms or symptomatic expression of more typical rhino/respiratory symptoms along with esophageal symptoms may be an important clue to the presence of EE.

Some patients who have EE may present catastrophically with esophageal perforation [26–28]. Variations of the perforation may include a Boerhaave's syndrome, perforation of a diverticulum, or perforation of an area of stricture formation.

Finally, one of the attractive approaches to diagnosis of EE may be combining predictive factors into a scoring system for the presence of EE. For example, patients who present with food impaction associated with EE tend to do so at a younger age [6]. EE is seen most commonly in white men and often is associated with a personal and family history of allergy. Combining such data with other symptomatology may provide a very specific, if not sensitive, means of diagnosing allergy- based EE noninvasively. This work has yet to be done but is likely to become important in the future.

Summary

EE in adults is an emerging disease with a constellation of clinical presentations [29]. As more information has been gained, it has become possible to paint the profile of a patient who has EE: male, white, presenting with dysphagia and/or food impaction, and with a personal and/or family history of allergy. Still, as the disease becomes more widely recognized and more populations are studied, it may be found that many races and ethnic groups are affected and that patients may present with a variety of symptoms or symptoms of varying intensity as manifestations of EE. At present it can be difficult to exclude confounding gastroesophageal reflux as a contributor to, if not the sole cause of, EE in some patients. In the future, there will be better ways to isolate distinct pathophysiologies in these patients and to use symptoms more accurately to identify and understand this disease in adults.

References

[1] Croese J, Fairley SK, Masson JW, et al. Clinical and endoscopic features of eosinophilic esophagitis in adults. Gastrointest Endosc 2003;58:516–22.

[2] Arora AS, Perrault J, Smyrk TC. Topical corticosteroid treatment of dysphagia due to eosinophilic esophagitis in adults. Mayo Clin Proc 2003;78:830–5.

[3] Straumann A, Spichtin H-P, Grize L, et al. Natural history of primary eosinophilic esophagitis: a follow-up of 30 adult patients for up to 11.5 years. Gastroenterology 2003;125: 1660–9.

[4] Potter JW, Saeian K, Staff D, et al. Eosinophilic esophagitis in adults: an emerging problem with unique esophageal features. Gastrointest Endosc 2004;59:355–61.

[5] Lucendo AJ, Carrion G, Navarro M, et al. Eosinophilic esophagitis in adults: an emerging disease. Dig Dis Sci 2004;49:1884–8.

[6] Desai TK, Stecevic V, Chang C-H, et al. Association of eosinophilic inflammation with esophageal food impaction in adults. Gastrointest Endosc 2005;61:795–801.

[7] Remedios M, Campbell C, Jones DM, et al. Eosinophilic esophagitis in adults: clinical, endoscopic, histology findings, and response to treatment with fluticasone propionate. Gastrointest Endosc 2006;63:3–12.

[8] Gonsalves N, Policarpio-Nicolas M, Zhang Q, et al. Histopathologic variability and endoscopic correlates in adults with eosinophilic esophagitis. Gastrointest Endosc 2006;64:313–9.

[9] Muller S, Puhl S, Vieth M, et al. Analysis of symptoms and endoscopic findings in 117 patients with histologic diagnosis of eosinophilic esophagitis. Endoscopy 2007;39:339–44.

[10] Kapel RC, Miller J, Torres C, et al. Eosinophilic esophagitis: a prevalent U.S. disease that affects all age groups. Am J Gastroenterol 2006;101(9):S67.

[11] El-Serag H. Time trends in gastroesophageal reflux: a systematic review. Clin Gastroenterol Hepatol 2007;5:17–26.

[12] Conio M, Cameron AJ, Romero Y, et al. Secular trends in the epidemiology and outcome of Barrett's esophagus in Olmsted County, Minnesota. Gut 2001;48:304–9.

[13] Pohl H, Welch HG. The role of overdiagnosis and reclassification in the marked increase of esophageal adenocarcinoma incidence. Journal of the National Cancer Institute 2005;97(2): 142–6.

[14] Sharma P, Sampliner R, editors. Barrett's esophagus and esophageal adenocarcinoma. 2nd edition. Malden, MA: Blackwell; 2006.

[15] Assa'ad AH, Putnam PE, Collins MH, et al. Pediatric patients with eosinophilic esophagitis: an 8 year follow-up. J Allergy Clin Immunol 2007;119:731–8.

[16] Zink DA, Amin M, Gebara S, et al. Familial dysphagia and eosinophilia. Gastrointest Endosc 2007;65:330–4.

[17] Meyer GW. Eosinophilic esophagitis in a father and a daughter. Gastrointest Endosc 2005; 61(7):932.

[18] Patel SM, Falchuk KR. Three brothers with dysphagia caused by eosinophilic esophagitis. Gastrointest Endosc 2005;61(1):165–7.

[19] Blanchard C, Wang N, Stringer KF, et al. Eotaxin-3 and a uniquely conserved gene-expression profile in eosinophilic esophagitis. J Clin Invest 2006;116:536–47.

[20] Gonsalves N, Anh T, Zhang Q, et al. Distinct allergic predisposition of children and adults with eosinophilic esophagitis. Gastroenterology 2006;130(Suppl 2):579.

[21] Ann Allergy Asthma Immunol 2007;98(Suppl 1):1–123.

[22] Mishra A, Hogan SP, Brandt EB, et al. An etiological role for aeroallergens and eosinophils in experimental esophagitis. J Clin Invest 2001;107(1):83–90.

[23] Mishra A, Rothenberg ME. Intratracheal IL-13 induces eosinophilic esophagitis by an IL-5, eotaxin-1, and STAT6-dependent mechanism. Gastroenterology 2003;125(5):1419–27.

[24] Akei HS, Mishra A, Blanchard C, et al. Epicutaneous antigen exposure primes for experimental eosinophilic esophagitis in mice. Gastroenterology 2005;129(3):985–9.

[25] Wang FY, Gupta SK, Fitzgerald JF. Is there a seasonal variation in the incidence or intensity of allergic eosinophilic esophagitis in newly diagnosed children? J Clin Gastroenterol 2007; 41(5):451–3.

[26] Cohen MS, Kaufman A, DiMarino AJ Jr, et al. Eosinophilic esophagitis presenting as spontaneous esophageal rupture (Boerhaave's syndome). Clin Gastroenterol Hepatol 2007;5: A24.

[27] Mecklenburg I, Weber C, Folwaczny C. Spontaneous recovery of dysphagia by rupture of an esophageal diverticulum in eosinophilic esophagitis. Dig Dis Sci 2006;51:1241–2.

[28] Prasad GA, Arora AS. Spontaneous perforation in the ringed esophagus. Dis Esophagus 2005;18(6):406–9.

[29] Furuta GT, Liacouras CA, Collins MH, et al. Eosinophilic esophagitis in children and adults: a systematic review and consensus recommendations for diagnosis and treatment. Gastroenterology 2007;133:1342–63.

ELSEVIER
SAUNDERS

Gastrointest Endoscopy Clin N Am
18 (2008) 33–44

GASTROINTESTINAL
ENDOSCOPY CLINICS
OF NORTH AMERICA

Epidemiology and Etiology of Eosinophilic Esophagitis

Mirna Chehade, MD[a,b,*], Hugh A. Sampson, MD[b]

[a]Pediatric Gastroenterology and Nutrition, Mount Sinai School of Medicine,
New York, NY, USA
[b]Pediatric Allergy and Immunology, Mount Sinai School of Medicine,
New York, NY, USA

Eosinophilic esophagitis (EE) is an inflammatory disease of the esophagus characterized by eosinophilic infiltration of the esophageal mucosa, the latter serving as its histologic hallmark. Symptoms of EE are variable, and include gastroesophageal reflux symptoms, abdominal pain, growth failure, and dysphagia [1]. Dysphagia is a more common presentation in adults and older children. Serious complications of EE consisting of esophageal food impactions necessitating urgent endoscopic removal of the food [2,3] and esophageal strictures requiring endoscopic balloon dilatations [4] are also seen. The potential severity of these symptoms points to the importance of proper recognition and management of the disease, especially given that EE has become more prevalent over the past decade. In this article, available evidence on the epidemiology and etiology of EE is discussed.

Epidemiology

EE is being increasingly reported in the medical literature, both in children and in adults. It is a relatively new disease from clinical and research standpoints, however. A simple search of articles published in the literature on EE in PubMed, a service of the National Library of Medicine and the National Institutes of Health, using the search term "eosinophilic esophagitis" resulted in 269 publications between 2000 and April 2007; half of these articles appeared during the past 3 years. In contrast, only 38 publications were retrieved from all the previous 23 years (1976–1999). Table 1

---

* Corresponding author. Pediatrics, Box 1198, Mount Sinai School of Medicine, One Gustave L. Levy Place, New York, NY 10029.
E-mail address: mirna.chehade@mssm.edu (M. Chehade).

1052-5157/08/$ - see front matter © 2008 Elsevier Inc. All rights reserved.
doi:10.1016/j.giec.2007.09.002
giendo.theclinics.com

Table 1
Epidemiology of eosinophilic esophagitis in different populations

Study	Type	Subjects/setting	Location	Population	Dates	Prevalence or percent of subjects examined
Noel, et al [7]	Retrospective	Outpatients/medical center	Hamilton, OH, USA	Children	2003	43.0/100,000
Straumann, et al [12,19]	Prospective	Outpatients/medical center	Olten County, Switzerland	Adults	2007	30.0/100,000
Ronkainen, et al [21]	Prospective	Symptomatic individuals/ general population	Northern Sweden	Adults	1998	0.4%
Cherian, et al [22]	Retrospective	Outpatients/medical center	Perth, Australia	Children	2004	8.9/100,000
Liacouras, et al [25]	Prospective	Patients who had reflux symptoms and esophagitis/medical center	Philadelphia, PA, USA	Children	1993–1995	9.3%
Fox, et al [26]	Retrospective	Patients who had esophagitis/medical center	Boston, MA, USA	Children	1997–2002	6.8%
Esposito, et al [11]	Retrospective	Patients who had esophagitis/medical center	Novara, Italy	Children	2000–2004	3.5%
Byrne, et al [27]	Retrospective	Patients who had esophageal food impaction/medical center	Salt Lake City, UT, USA	Adults	1999–2004	11%
Desai, et al [3]	Prospective	Patients who had esophageal food impaction/medical center	Detroit, MI, USA	Adults	2000–2003	54%
Kerlin, et al [28]	Prospective	Patients who had esophageal food impaction/medical center	Brisbane, Australia	Adults	2002–2004	48%

summarizes prevalence rates of EE from the studies discussed below among different groups of patients.

Eosinophilic esophagitis occurs worldwide

Cases of EE are being reported not only in various parts of the United States, including the Northeast, Central, Midwest, and South [5–10], but also in various parts of Europe, such as Italy, Switzerland, Spain, and England, among others [11–14]. In addition, several cases have been described from Canada, Brazil, Japan, and Australia [15–18]. Attempts at estimating the exact prevalence of the disease have been limited, however.

EE seems to be reported selectively in the Westernized, developed countries. The reason for this is unclear, although this selective prevalence mirrors that of atopic diseases, including asthma.

Incidence and prevalence of eosinophilic esophagitis in children and adults

Two studies have attempted to address the incidence and prevalence of EE by identifying cases of EE using medical center records and comparing the number of cases to the general population in the area surrounding the medical center. These studies were possible to perform because both centers serve as the sole medical providers for an area with few demographic changes. The first study was by Noel and colleagues [7], examining the incidence and prevalence of EE requiring medical care in children residing in Hamilton County, Ohio. Patients were defined by histologic examination as having EE based on finding a minimum of 24 distal esophageal eosinophils per high power field (HPF), epithelial basal zone hyperplasia, and absence of eosinophilia in any other gastrointestinal segment. The incidence seemed to have slightly increased from 9.1 cases/100,000 children in 2000 to 12.8 cases per 100,000 in 2003, and the prevalence has increased over those years from 9.9 per 100,000 in 2000 to 43 per 100,000 in 2003.

Straumann and colleagues found a similar trend in adults who had EE residing in Olten County, Switzerland [12,19]. Criteria for the diagnosis of EE consisted of typical history, consistent endoscopic abnormalities, and histologic infiltration of the esophageal epithelium by 24 or more eosinophils per HPF, after excluding gastroesophageal reflux disease clinically and endoscopically. Throughout an 18-year observation period, an annual incidence of 1.7 cases per 100,000 inhabitants was noted (range 0–8), with a marked increase in newly diagnosed cases in the past few years. Because EE is proving to be a chronic disease [4], the prevalence steadily increased from 2 per 100,000 in 1989 to 30 per 100,000 at the present time.

Figures obtained from both studies indicate that the disease is not as rare as previously believed. The incidence of EE is approaching that of other gastrointestinal diseases. For example, the incidence of inflammatory bowel disease in children was found to be 7.1 per 100,000 in the state of Wisconsin, comparable to that of EE [20]. Furthermore, the incidence rates obtained in both studies discussed above likely represent an underestimate of the true incidence of the disease, because the cases included only those who sought medical care for their symptoms that were severe enough to warrant an esophagogastroduodenoscopy with biopsies, hence establishing the diagnosis of EE. Our clinical experience and that of others suggests that children and adults who have EE present with a spectrum of manifestations, including discrete symptoms that require a detailed history to elucidate [12]. Although many of these patients may not seek medical attention as a result of the relatively infrequent or seemingly inconsequential nature of their symptoms, further questioning often reveals that they may eat more slowly than their peers or family, cut their food in smaller pieces, or avoid foods that could serve as allergens or those that are difficult to swallow (bagels, meats). These observations emphasize the importance of thorough history intake in suspected patients.

Epidemiology of eosinophilic esophagitis in the general population

Ronkainen and colleagues [21] conducted a population-based study in two communities in Northern Sweden (n = 28,988) with a similar age and gender distribution to that of Sweden as a whole. Of a random sample of 2860 adults surveyed for gastrointestinal symptoms, esophagogastroduodenoscopy with biopsies was performed in a representative sample of 1000 of the 2122 responders to the survey. On evaluation of esophageal biopsies, EE, defined as 20 or more esophageal eosinophils per HPF, was present in 4 cases (0.4%) of the population studied, which would be 13 times that reported by Straumann and colleagues in symptomatic adults. Three of the 4 cases found reported troublesome reflux symptoms without erosive esophagitis and had not consulted any physician or received any treatment of their symptoms. Probable EE, defined as 15 to 19 eosinophils per HPF, was present in 7 subjects (0.7%). The study is limited, however, by the absence of objective testing for gastroesophageal reflux disease, which could potentially account for the esophageal eosinophilia in some of these subjects.

Increased prevalence or recognition?

The above studies indicate that the prevalence of EE is increasing over time. Whether the increase is real or attributable to an increasing awareness about the disease among caregivers in the past few years has recently been the subject of debate among researchers in the field. To address this problem, Cherian and colleagues [22] in Perth retrospectively identified all pediatric cases of esophagitis following biopsy in children in their medical center, a state pediatric referral center and the site of practice of all pediatric gastroenterologists in Western Australia, in the years 1995, 1999, and 2004.

Esophageal specimens were blindly re-evaluated and reclassified into non-eosinophilic esophagitis or into EE when more than 24 eosinophils per HPF were found on esophageal biopsies. Although more patients were indeed reclassified as having EE on re-evaluation, based on the new counts, the prevalence of EE was still found to have increased by 18-fold over the past decade, from 0.5 cases per 100,000 in 1995 to 8.9 per 100,000 in 2004. The increase in prevalence in EE seems to be mirroring the increase in atopic diseases in Western countries, such as asthma and allergic rhinitis. This finding is not surprising because up to 50% to 70% of children and adults who have EE have concomitant atopic diseases [23,24].

Epidemiology of eosinophilic esophagitis among patients who have reflux symptoms

Of equal interest is the determination of the prevalence of EE in subsets of patients who have certain symptoms, such as gastroesophageal reflux or dysphagia, because knowing the prevalence of EE among patients who have these symptoms potentially influences diagnostic approaches for these patients.

In 1998, Liacouras and colleagues [25] evaluated 1809 children who had gastroesophageal reflux symptoms at their tertiary center in Philadelphia, Pennsylvania; 583 of those children underwent upper endoscopy with biopsies and 214 showed evidence of esophageal eosinophilia on biopsy. Twenty children ultimately proved to have EE, defined by lack of response to various antacids and the finding of more than 15 eosinophils per HPF on microscopic examination of the esophageal mucosa. These data indicate that 1.1% of the children who had reflux symptoms had EE, and 9.3% of the children who had evidence of eosinophils in the esophagus had EE. An almost similar proportion of children who had esophagitis proved to have EE in another tertiary center in Boston, Massachusetts, where the proportion was 6.8% [26].

In Europe, Esposito and colleagues [11] reported a prevalence of EE of 3.5% among children who had esophagitis evaluated in Novara, Italy. Finding greater than 20 eosinophils per HPF was used as the basis for the diagnosis of EE in that study. From these and other studies, it is apparent that EE occurs in a significant number of children who have gastroesophageal reflux symptoms severe enough to warrant esophagogastroduodenoscopy, and therefore needs to be considered in the differential diagnosis, especially with a history of lack of response to antacids.

Epidemiology of eosinophilic esophagitis among patients who have dysphagia and food impactions

A retrospective chart review conducted by Byrne and colleagues [27] of adult patients who had esophageal food impactions between 1999 and

2004 revealed that 11% of these cases were associated with EE. Among men in their study, EE was the second most common cause of esophageal food impactions after peptic strictures. The actual cases of EE may have even been more numerous because this retrospective study was limited by the lack of availability of esophageal biopsies on some of the patients, which may have resulted in an underestimate of the prevalence of EE among the patients. In fact, it is well known that EE can present with a normal-appearing esophagus on endoscopic examination [24].

A prospective study by Desai and colleagues [3] revealed a higher prevalence. The authors evaluated 31 consecutive adult patients presenting with food impaction to their gastroenterology practice between 2000 and 2003. Seventeen of these patients (54%), mostly younger men, had esophageal histologic features consistent with EE in biopsy specimens. Similarly, another prospective study of 43 adults presenting with esophageal food impaction in an Australian center found a high prevalence of EE among these patients. Fourteen of the 29 patients biopsied (48%) had histologic evidence of EE [28]. EE therefore seems to be highly prevalent among patients who have esophageal food impactions, particularly among young men. Unless medically contraindicated, obtaining esophageal biopsies needs to be considered in all cases of food impaction.

Demographic characteristics of patients with eosinophilic esophagitis

EE seems to have a male predilection in adults and children. In children, 60% to 80% of patients who had EE were males [24,29–31]. A similar trend was found in adults, with men forming approximately 75% of the population with EE [32]. The reasons for this gender predilection are still unclear.

With respect to age distribution, adults who have EE typically present in their third and fourth decades of life [10,32], although EE has been described in older patients, including 72- and 85 year-old patients [33,34]. In children, the diagnosis is more common after infancy, with no known recognized peak, although in the reported literature the diagnosis of EE seems to be slightly more common in the 5- to 10-year-old age group [6,24].

A familial pattern has been reported. In a case series of 381 children who had EE, 7% of patients had a parent who had either esophageal stricture or histologic evidence of EE, and 5% had siblings who had EE [24]. Case reports of EE spanning two generations or involving brothers were also reported [35]. An important feature of EE, however, is its strong association with atopic disorders (asthma, allergic rhinitis, and atopic dermatitis) in children and adults [23,24]. It is not known, therefore, whether the clustering of some cases in families is expected because atopy has a strong familial disposition. A single-nucleotide polymorphism in the gene encoding eotaxin-3, a key promoter of eosinophil recruitment into the esophagus, was associated with disease susceptibility [36], suggesting a genetic predisposition for EE.

Studies of family members of patients who have EE are not yet available to confirm these findings.

Etiology

The role of acid reflux disease in eosinophilic esophagitis

Historically, EE has been erroneously labeled as severe acid-induced gastroesophageal reflux disease, because of the overlapping histologic feature of extensive esophageal epithelial eosinophilia. This concept was prompted by a report by Winter and colleagues [37] associating the finding of esophageal eosinophilia with acid-induced reflux disease, although large numbers of esophageal eosinophils in those patients were not described. We now know that EE is a separate entity from acid-induced reflux disease, as demonstrated by negative pH probe findings in children who have EE [38] and lack of response to antacids [29,39]. (See the articles by Gonsalves, and Aceves and colleagues, elsewhere in this issue.)

The presence of EE does not preclude the coexistence of acid-induced gastroesophageal reflux in some patients [32]. These patients typically have only a partial response to antacid therapy.

The role of food allergens in eosinophilic esophagitis

Kelly and colleagues [29] first shed light on the role of food allergies as a causative factor in EE by studying a series of 10 children who had gastroesophageal reflux symptoms that were refractory to antacids and even fundoplication (see also the articles by Assa'ad, and Spergel and Shuker, elsewhere in this issue). These children had persistent esophageal eosinophilia on biopsy. A dietary trial consisting of an amino acid–based formula for a minimum of 6 weeks, in addition to corn and apples in those old enough to eat solid foods, resulted in symptom improvement and histologic resolution of the disease. Symptoms completely resolved in 80% of the children studied and improved in the remaining 20%. As for esophageal eosinophilia, the maximal intraepithelial counts dramatically decreased from a median of 41 per HPF (range, 15–100) to 0.5 per HPF (range, 0–22). Other reactive changes of the esophageal epithelium also significantly improved. Open challenge with various foods performed at a later stage resulted in re-creation of symptoms identical to those experienced before the dietary trial, confirming a link of the patients' disease to a possible immunologic reaction to foods. Patients showed symptomatic responses to a median of two foods for each patient (range, one to six foods). Foods mostly implicated in these children were cow's milk, soy, wheat, peanut, and egg. Avoidance of the offending foods allowed 8 of 10 subjects to remain asymptomatic without anti-reflux medications.

Similar findings were later demonstrated in various other studies addressing food allergies as a possible cause of EE. A study conducted by Markowitz and colleagues [38] in 2003 on 51 children who had EE demonstrated significant improvement in gastrointestinal symptoms and histologic findings following a dietary trial similar to that of Kelly and colleagues [29], using an amino acid–based formula and one food, grape or apple, for a month. All but two patients experienced clinical improvement on the dietary intervention. Distal esophageal eosinophils decreased from 33.7 ± 10.3 per HPF to 1.0 ± 0.6 per HPF.

Kagalwalla and colleagues [40] in 2006 empirically removed cow's milk, soy, wheat, egg, peanut, and seafood from the diet of 35 children who had EE for a duration of 6 weeks, and found significant histologic improvement, although not complete resolution of the disease, in 74% of the patients. Overall, esophageal intraepithelial eosinophils decreased from 80.2 ± 44 per HPF to 13.6 ± 23.8 per HPF. This study again points to the likely role of food antigens in the cause of EE.

The immunologic reaction underlying the role played by food antigens is believed to be a mix of IgE-mediated and non-IgE (cell-mediated) hypersensitivity responses. This phenomenon was first demonstrated by Kelly and colleagues [29] who found symptoms following introduction of certain foods despite negative skin prick tests to these foods, the latter reflecting IgE-mediated allergic reactions.

Spergel and colleagues [41] further demonstrated this phenomenon by performing a combination of skin prick tests and patch tests on children who had EE. Although skin prick tests reflect IgE-mediated allergic reactions, skin patch tests reflect delayed, cell-mediated allergic reactions. Twenty-six children who had EE were instructed to avoid foods identified by positive results of skin prick and patch tests, for a minimum of 6 weeks. Eighteen of those children (69%) had resolution of their symptoms. Overall, esophageal eosinophil counts improved from 55.8 ± 24.6 per HPF to 8.4 ± 8.4 per HPF following this dietary therapy. Although treatment of their coexisting atopic disease was concomitantly initiated, which may have potentially contributed to the response rate, the approach in dietary therapy demonstrates a role for immediate, IgE-mediated food reactions and delayed, cell-mediated reactions. Patients were positive to an average of 2.7 ± 3.3 foods (range, 0–13) by skin prick testing, and an average of 2.7 ± 1.8 foods (range, 0–7) by patch testing. Foods most commonly identified by skin prick testing were milk, egg, peanut, shellfish, peas, beef, fish, rye, tomato, and wheat. Foods most commonly identified on patch testing were wheat, corn, beef, milk, soy, rye, egg, chicken, oats, and potato.

A known limitation in atopy patch testing is the lack of its standardization of methods, food antigens used, and interpretation, which may limit its reliability. Identification of specific foods causing a cell-mediated allergic reaction in EE still needs to be optimized.

In adults, the role of food allergy remains controversial, partly because of the scarcity of studies on dietary modifications in adults who have EE. Simon and colleagues [42] prospectively examined six adult patients who had EE who had evidence of sensitization to grass pollen, wheat, and rye, but not to cow's milk, egg, or fish, as determined by skin prick testing or serum allergen-specific IgE antibody determinations. Elimination of wheat, rye, and barley from the diet of these patients for 6 weeks failed to reduce clinical disease activity. Although one patient noticed some improvement of symptoms, endoscopic and histologic findings remained unchanged. Whether the lack of response is due to lack of food sensitization in adult EE or to sensitization of the patients to foods other than those eliminated in the study, which could not be predicted by conventional allergy tests, remains unknown. As a result, the role of food allergens in the pathogenesis of EE in adults could not be confirmed based on this study.

More recently, Gonsalves and colleagues [43] used the same dietary elimination strategy used by Kagalwalla and colleagues [40], summarized above, in adult patients who had EE and found a much smaller response rate of 30%, compared with 70% in the pediatric study. It is not known whether the disease is less food-responsive in adults, whether different foods may be responsible for symptoms in adults, whether compliance with dietary therapy is more difficult in the adult population, or whether aeroallergens may play a more prominent role in adult EE, all of which could contribute to the lack of response to dietary therapy.

A major limitation in conducting further dietary elimination trials is the lack of acceptable methods of identifying the responsible food allergens, which limits the ability to test the effect of eliminating relevant food allergens from the diet, whether in children or adults.

The role of aeroallergens in eosinophilic esophagitis

Aeroallergen sensitization has been proposed as a potential cause of EE (see also the article by Blanchard and Rothenberg, elsewhere in this issue). This proposal stems from murine studies of EE in which intranasal instillation of antigen resulted in esophageal eosinophilia [44], and a report in 2003 of a woman who had EE with symptomatic and histologic exacerbations of her disease during pollen seasons while remaining on a constant diet [45].

In patients who had seasonal allergies without gastroesophageal reflux symptoms, eosinophilic infiltration of the esophagus was demonstrated by Onbasi and colleagues [46] to be present during the pollen season, although to a lower extent than that seen in patients who had EE. In their study, allergic patients had 5.5 ± 7.3 eosinophils per HPF in the proximal esophagus and 3.2 ± 3.7 eosinophils per HPF in the distal esophagus. These data implicate aeroallergens as potential triggers for esophageal eosinophilia, although the maximum number of esophageal eosinophils was 12.8 eosinophils per HPF, which is still lower than the threshold agreed on for the diagnosis of EE, that of at least 15 eosinophils per HPF [39].

The overwhelming beneficial response to dietary therapy with amino acid–based formula in children who have EE [29,38] despite many having other allergic diseases, including environmentally induced allergic rhinitis, raises considerable doubt about any major role for aeroallergens in the pathogenesis of EE. Clearly, more studies are needed to clarify this issue.

Summary

EE is an emerging disease with significant health impact in children and adults alike. Little is known regarding its epidemiology and etiology. The incidence and prevalence of EE continue to increase in many countries around the world. EE constitutes a significant proportion of patients who have reflux symptoms and dysphagia. Multiple food allergies are believed to play a role in its cause, mediated by IgE and non-IgE mechanisms. The role of aeroallergens in EE is still debated. Studies related to identification of the specific allergens causing the disease are eagerly awaited for further understanding of the mechanism of disease and tailoring specific, more efficient therapies.

References

[1] Sampson HA, Anderson JA. Summary and recommendations: classification of gastrointestinal manifestations due to immunologic reactions to foods in infants and young children. J Pediatr Gastroenterol Nutr 2000;30:S87–94.

[2] Khan S, Orenstein SR, Di Lorenzo C, et al. Eosinophilic esophagitis: strictures, impactions, dysphagia. Dig Dis Sci 2003;48:22–9.

[3] Desai TK, Stecevic V, Chang CH, et al. Association of eosinophilic inflammation with esophageal food impaction in adults. Gastrointest Endosc 2005;61:795–801.

[4] Straumann A, Spichtin HP, Grize L, et al. Natural history of primary eosinophilic esophagitis: a follow-up of 30 adult patients for up to 11.5 years. Gastroenterology 2003;125: 1660–9.

[5] Liacouras CA, Markowitz JE. Eosinophilic esophagitis: a subset of eosinophilic gastroenteritis. Curr Gastroenterol Rep 1999;1:253–8.

[6] Orenstein SR, Shalaby TM, Di Lorenzo C, et al. The spectrum of pediatric eosinophilic esophagitis beyond infancy: a clinical series of 30 children. Am J Gastroenterol 2000;95: 1422–30.

[7] Noel RJ, Putnam PE, Rothenberg ME. Eosinophilic esophagitis. N Engl J Med 2004;351: 940–1.

[8] Aceves SS, Newbury RO, Dohil R, et al. Esophageal remodeling in pediatric eosinophilic esophagitis. J Allergy Clin Immunol 2007;119:206–12.

[9] Gupta SK, Fitzgerald JF, Kondratyuk T, et al. Cytokine expression in normal and inflamed esophageal mucosa: a study into the pathogenesis of allergic eosinophilic esophagitis. J Pediatr Gastroenterol Nutr 2006;42:22–6.

[10] Gonsalves N, Policarpio-Nicolas M, Zhang Q, et al. Histopathologic variability and endoscopic correlates in adults with eosinophilic esophagitis. Gastrointest Endosc 2006;64:313–9.

[11] Esposito S, Marinello D, Paracchini R, et al. Long-term follow-up of symptoms and peripheral eosinophil counts in seven children with eosinophilic esophagitis. J Pediatr Gastroenterol Nutr 2004;38:452–6.

[12] Straumann A, Simon HU. Eosinophilic esophagitis: escalating epidemiology? J Allergy Clin Immunol 2005;115:418–9.

[13] Lucendo AJ, Carrion G, Navarro M, et al. Eosinophilic esophagitis in adults: an emerging disease. Dig Dis Sci 2004;49:1884–8.

[14] Attwood SE, Lewis CJ, Bronder CS, et al. Eosinophilic oesophagitis: a novel treatment using Montelukast. Gut 2003;52:181–5.

[15] Sant'Anna AM, Rolland S, Fournet JC, et al. Eosinophilic esophagitis in children: symptoms, histology and pH probe results. J Pediatr Gastroenterol Nutr 2004;39:373–7.

[16] Cury EK, Schraibman V, Faintuch S. Eosinophilic infiltration of the esophagus: gastro-esophageal reflux versus eosinophilic esophagitis in children-discussion on daily practice. J Pediatr Surg 2004;39:E4–7.

[17] Furuta K, Adachi K, Kowari K, et al. A Japanese case of eosinophilic esophagitis. J Gastroenterol 2006;41:706–10.

[18] Cheung KM, Oliver MR, Cameron DJ, et al. Esophageal eosinophilia in children with dysphagia. J Pediatr Gastroenterol Nutr 2003;37:498–503.

[19] Portmann S, Heer R, Bussmann C. Epidemiology of eosinophilic esophagitis: data from a community-based longitudinal study work carried out by the Swiss EE study group, Switzerland. Gastroenterology 2007;132:A609.

[20] Kugathasan S, Judd RH, Hoffmann RG, et al. Epidemiologic and clinical characteristics of children with newly diagnosed inflammatory bowel disease in Wisconsin: a statewide population-based study. J Pediatr 2003;143:525–31.

[21] Ronkainen J, Talley NJ, Aro P, et al. Prevalence of oesophageal eosinophils and eosinophilic oesophagitis in adults: the population-based Kalixanda study. Gut 2007;56:615–20.

[22] Cherian S, Smith NM, Forbes DA. Rapidly increasing prevalence of eosinophilic oesophagitis in Western Australia. Arch Dis Child 2006;91:1000–4.

[23] Simon D, Marti H, Heer P, et al. Eosinophilic esophagitis is frequently associated with IgE-mediated allergic airway diseases. J Allergy Clin Immunol 2005;115:1090–2.

[24] Liacouras CA, Spergel JM, Ruchelli E, et al. Eosinophilic esophagitis: a 10-year experience in 381 children. Clin Gastroenterol Hepatol 2005;3:1198–206.

[25] Liacouras CA, Wenner WJ, Brown K, et al. Primary eosinophilic esophagitis in children: successful treatment with oral corticosteroids. J Pediatr Gastroenterol Nutr 1998;26:380–5.

[26] Fox VL, Nurko S, Furuta GT. Eosinophilic esophagitis: it's not just kid's stuff. Gastrointest Endosc 2002;56:260–70.

[27] Byrne KR, Panagiotakis PH, Hilden K, et al. Retrospective analysis of esophageal food impaction: differences in etiology by age and gender. Dig Dis Sci 2007;52:717–21.

[28] Kerlin P, Jones D, Remedios M, et al. Prevalence of eosinophilic esophagitis in adults with food bolus obstruction of the esophagus. J Clin Gastroenterol 2007;41:356–61.

[29] Kelly KJ, Lazenby AJ, Rowe PC, et al. Eosinophilic esophagitis attributed to gastroesophageal reflux: improvement with an amino acid-based formula. Gastroenterology 1995;109:1503–12.

[30] Chehade M, Sampson HA, Morotti RA, et al. Esophageal subepithelial fibrosis in children with eosinophilic esophagitis. J Pediatr Gastroenterol Nutr 2007;45:319–28.

[31] Teitelbaum JE, Fox VL, Twarog FJ, et al. Eosinophilic esophagitis in children: immunopathological analysis and response to fluticasone propionate. Gastroenterology 2002;122:1216–25.

[32] Sgouros SN, Bergele C, Mantides A. Eosinophilic esophagitis in adults: a systematic review. Eur J Gastroenterol Hepatol 2006;18:211–7.

[33] Evrard S, Louis H, Kahaleh M, et al. Idiopathic eosinophilic oesophagitis: atypical presentation of a rare disease. Acta Gastroenterol Belg 2004;67:232–5.

[34] Stevoff C, Rao S, Parsons W, et al. EUS and histopathologic correlates in eosinophilic esophagitis. Gastrointest Endosc 2001;54:373–7.

[35] Zink DA, Amin M, Gebara S, et al. Familial dysphagia and eosinophilia. Gastrointest Endosc 2007;65:330–4.

[36] Blanchard C, Wang N, Stringer KF, et al. Eotaxin-3 and a uniquely conserved gene-expression profile in eosinophilic esophagitis. J Clin Invest 2006;116:536–47.

[37] Winter HS, Madara JL, Stafford RJ, et al. Intraepithelial eosinophils: a new diagnostic criterion for reflux esophagitis. Gastroenterology 1982;83:818–23.

[38] Markowitz JE, Spergel JM, Ruchelli E, et al. Elemental diet is an effective treatment for eosinophilic esophagitis in children and adolescents. Am J Gastroenterol 2003;98:777–82.

[39] Furuta GT, Liacouras CA, Collins MH, et al. Eosinophilic esophagitis in children and adults: a systematic review and consensus recommendations for diagnosis and treatment. Gastroenterology 2007;133:1342–63.

[40] Kagalwalla AF, Sentongo TA, Ritz S, et al. Effect of six-food elimination diet on clinical and histologic outcomes in eosinophilic esophagitis. Clin Gastroenterol Hepatol 2006;4: 1097–102.

[41] Spergel JM, Beausoleil JL, Mascarenhas M, et al. The use of skin prick tests and patch tests to identify causative foods in eosinophilic esophagitis. J Allergy Clin Immunol 2002;109: 363–8.

[42] Simon D, Straumann A, Wenk A, et al. Eosinophilic esophagitis in adults—no clinical relevance of wheat and rye sensitizations. Allergy 2006;61:1480–3.

[43] Gonsalves N, Ritz S, Yang G, et al. A prospective clinical trial of allergy testing and food elimination diet in adults with eosinophilic esophagitis (EE). Gastroenterology 2007;132:A6.

[44] Mishra A, Hogan SP, Brandt EB, et al. An etiological role for aeroallergens and eosinophils in experimental esophagitis. J Clin Invest 2001;107:83–90.

[45] Fogg MI, Ruchelli E, Spergel JM. Pollen and eosinophilic esophagitis. J Allergy Clin Immunol 2003;112:796–7.

[46] Onbasi K, Sin AZ, Doganavsargil B, et al. Eosinophil infiltration of the oesophageal mucosa in patients with pollen allergy during the season. Clin Exp Allergy 2005;35:1423–31.

ELSEVIER
SAUNDERS

Gastrointest Endoscopy Clin N Am
18 (2008) 45–57

GASTROINTESTINAL
ENDOSCOPY CLINICS
OF NORTH AMERICA

Eosinophilic Esophagitis: Endoscopic Findings

Victor L. Fox, MD

*Harvard Medical School, Division of Gastroenterology and Nutrition,
Children's Hospital Boston, 300 Longwood Avenue, Boston, MA 02115, USA*

Eosinophilic esophagitis (EE) is a condition characterized by a dense infiltration of eosinophils within the epithelium that may extend into the deeper layers of the esophagus associated with distinctive endoscopic changes [1,2]. It is frequently found in patients who have a background of allergic or atopic disease and is believed to result from immune-mediated hypersensitivity reactions to various foods and aeroallergens [3–5]. Excessive acid reflux, however, may trigger a similar histologic response and endoscopic appearance in susceptible individuals [6]. The terms "allergic esophagitis" or "allergic eosinophilic esophagitis" (AEE) may therefore be more appropriate when distinguishing between gastroesophageal reflux disease (GERD) and allergen-related disease. In contrast, the term EE is used here to denote the condition of esophageal tissue that is densely infiltrated with eosinophils, regardless of its etiology. This article identifies endoscopic findings that are characteristic for EE and also illustrates patterns that may help to further differentiate between AEE and GERD.

Endoscopists who perform meticulous inspection of the esophagus, obtain tissue samples to correlate histology with gross findings, and assimilate these features with clinical symptoms have facilitated worldwide recognition of this condition. It is therefore essential for all endoscopists to become familiar with the endoscopic findings associated with EE to avoid delays or errors in diagnosis and to optimally assess outcomes of treatment.

The normal esophagus

Eosinophilic esophagus has been under-recognized and therefore under-reported because of the subtlety of gross endoscopic findings when

---

E-mail address: victor.fox@childrens.harvard.edu

compared with those of erosive disease or tumors. A review of normal characteristics and endoscopic findings of the esophagus is useful to serve as a background for comparison. Recognizing subtle variance from normal requires more than a cursory inspection of the esophagus during advancement of the endoscope to the stomach. Rather, the endoscopist must pause within portions of the esophagus and actively interrogate the surface and wall.

Important attributes of the esophagus include color and vascularity, surface contours, contractility, wall compliance, lumen diameter, and echo layer patterns. The normal esophagus has a whitish-pink color, and the epithelium is opaque when inspected in a slightly contracted state. When the lumen is distended by insufflating air, however, the epithelium thins as it stretches, and the surface acquires a glistening translucency, revealing a delicate and well-defined network of subepithelial blood vessels (Fig. 1). Although this vascular pattern is generally well visualized with white light, it is accentuated by illuminating with filtered light restricted to the blue and green spectra, known as narrow-band imaging. This modified imaging has been used to highlight the microvascular architecture of columnar, dysplastic, and even eroded epithelia [7–9]. The surface of the esophagus has smooth contours with occasional scattered, raised, pale nodules representing epithelial aggregates of intracellular glycogen (glycogenic acanthosis) (Fig. 2). Transient longitudinal and circular ridging, representing normal fold patterns and activity of the longitudinal and circular muscle layers, may be seen during spontaneous contractions and smooths when the lumen is distended with air. These spontaneous physiologic changes in the esophagus are best seen in their natural state during capsule endoscopy, because no air is introduced into the lumen (Fig. 3). The normal esophagus is also compliant as noted while taking mucosal biopsies. The surface is easily

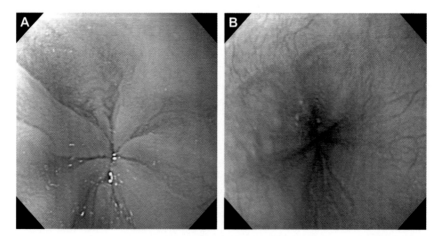

Fig. 1. (*A*) Normal esophagus showing whitish-pink color and opaque surface. (*B*) Slight air distension of the same normal esophagus reveals a distinct subepithelial vascular pattern.

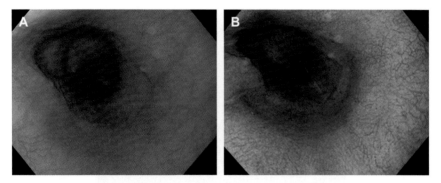

Fig. 2. Normal esophageal mucosa viewed with the Olympus GIF H180 high-definition gastro-scope (Olympus America, Center Valley, PA). Note few pale nodules caused by glycogenic acanthosis. (*A*) Conventional white light. (*B*) Narrow-band imaging mode.

grasped and the mucosa tents as the forceps are pulled away (Fig. 4). This normal esophageal compliance also allows easy passage of endoscopes with diameters in the range of 9 to 13 mm in a broad age range of children and adults without inducing surface trauma. High-resolution endosonography (EUS) of the normal esophagus and gastrointestinal wall using frequencies in the range of 15 to 30 MHz reveals seven to nine alternating hyperechoic and hypoechoic layers corresponding to the epithelial interface, mucosa (including muscularis mucosa), submucosa, circular and longitudinal muscle layers with an interface between muscle layers (muscularis propria), and adventitia (Fig. 5) [10,11]. Qualitative comparisons and quantitative measurements of layer thickness can be obtained using EUS [12,13].

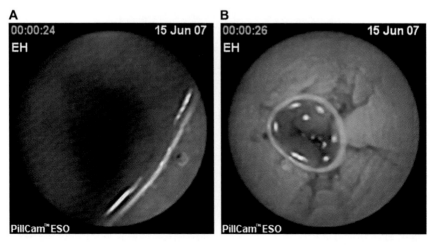

Fig. 3. Capsule endoscopy views of normal esophagus using the PillCam ESO capsule (Given Imaging, Yoqneam, Israel). (*A*) The surface appears smooth in the relaxed state. (*B*) Transient furrowing and circular ridging is seen during contractions.

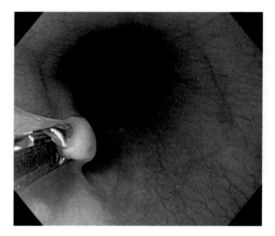

Fig. 4. Compliant mucosa of the normal esophagus, which tents while grasped with a biopsy forceps.

The inflamed esophagus

Although several published series have reported normal endoscopic findings in a substantial percentage of patients who have EE [14–18], less experienced observers may have failed to recognize subtle abnormalities [2]. Notably, when Croese and colleagues [17] reviewed archived images for their community-based retrospective case series, they reported that sentinel endoscopic features had been overlooked in 7 of 31 patients. In this author's

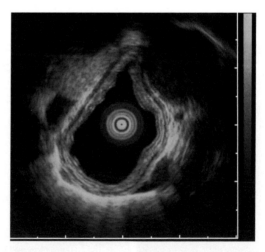

Fig. 5. High-resolution EUS image of the normal esophagus using a 20-MHz catheter probe (UM-3R, Olympus). Seven to nine alternating hyperechoic and hypoechoic sonographic layers can be seen representing the epithelial interface, mucosa and muscularis mucosa, submucosa, circular and longitudinal muscle (muscularis propria) and interface layers, and adventitia.

experience, an endoscopically normal appearing esophagus is incompatible with the diagnosis of active EE.

The only exception to this observation is the rare case of isolated submucosal or seromuscular disease, representing a form of eosinophilic gastroenteritis [19]. In this case, EUS may reveal the deeper wall abnormalities (Fig. 6). EUS findings in typical and atypical cases of EE have included total wall thickening, expansion of specific tissue layers such as submucosa and muscularis propria, disruption of the normal echo layer pattern, and extramural lymphadenopathy [13,20–23]. In most of these cases, surface or contour abnormalities were also endoscopically apparent.

Diminished vascular pattern

One of the most consistent abnormalities of a diffusely inflamed esophagus is attenuation or absence of the subepithelial vascular pattern, noted by Straumann and colleagues [24] in 93% of patients (Fig. 7). Extensive cellular infiltration correlates strongly with this avascular appearance, although minor degrees of histologic inflammation are not grossly detectable [25]. The attenuated vascular pattern presumably results from increased opacity of a thickened epithelium with expansion of the basal layer and edema and is not improved with distension of the lumen.

Furrowing

Linear furrowing, also called fissuring or vertical lines, has been reported in 25% to 100% of cases (Fig. 8) [16]. Thickening of the combined mucosal

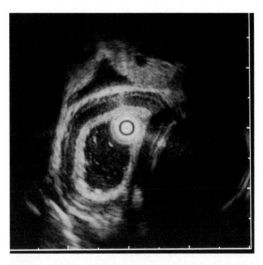

Fig. 6. Marked thickening of the muscularis propria revealed on EUS examination of the esophagus in a patient with eosinophilic gastroenteritis presenting with abdominal pain, dysphagia, and eosinophilic ascites.

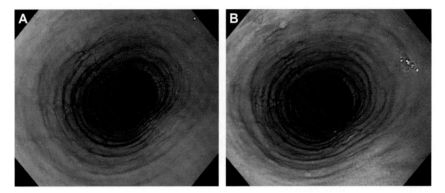

Fig. 7. (*A*) White-light and (*B*) narrow-band images showing absent vascular pattern, linear furrowing, and multiple concentric rings in a patient with eosinophilic esophagitis.

and submucosal layers revealed by EUS (Fig. 9) generates this topographic alteration [1]. Furrowing typically extends along the full length of the esophagus in cases of AEE. It may, however, also be limited to the mid and distal esophagus in patients who have GERD (Fig. 10) or found in a patchy distribution in patients who have mild or partially treated AEE.

Erosions, ulceration, and gastroesophageal reflux disease

Superficial erosions and deeper ulceration are not typically found in patients who have EE and imply peptic injury, which is a hallmark of GERD. Erosions, however, are occasionally seen in a background of other findings typical for AEE (Fig. 11). The two conditions may, therefore, coexist in a particular patient. In this case, although the erosive changes heal with adequate acid suppressive medication, the other background alterations

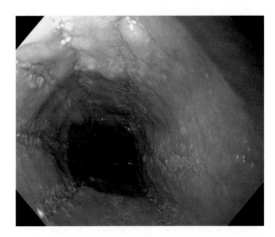

Fig. 8. Esophageal furrowing and mild surface exudate.

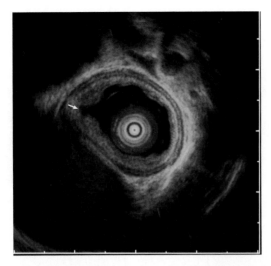

Fig. 9. Furrow (*arrow*) within thickened mucosa and submucosa layer revealed by high-resolution probe EUS. (*From* Fox VL, Nurko S, Furuta GT. Eosinophilic esophagitis: it's not just kid's stuff. Gastrointest Endosc 2002;56(2):260–70; with permission.)

remain unchanged, consistent with an allergen-induced process. When erosive and other changes are limited to the distal esophagus, GERD should be suspected as the primary disease process. In fact, overlapping clinical features of allergic and acid reflux esophagitis are common, particularly in the adult population [26–28].

Based on these and other observations, one might also speculate that there are at least two different phenotypic manifestations of GERD, one that is predominantly erosive and the other nonerosive. An individual patient may be genetically or immunologically primed to respond along one of these two pathways. Patients who have underlying atopy might be primed toward a nonerosive response seen with EE, even when the triggering agent is acid rather than a dietary allergen or aeroallergen.

Exudate

Another distinctive feature of EE is the finding of surface exudate consisting of clustered eosinophils or microabscesses breaking through the epithelium. The pattern may appear as pin-point white spots or broader, more amorphous plaques that resemble candidal infection (see Fig. 8; Figs. 12, 13, 15). See the articles by Putnam and Katzka, elsewhere in this issue. The sensitivity of this finding ranges from 30% to 50%, but the specificity may be as high as 95% [15,24,29].

Rings, strictures, and reduced compliance

Stacked circular rings appear and disappear during continuous inspection of an inflamed esophagus, suggesting intermittent contraction of the deep

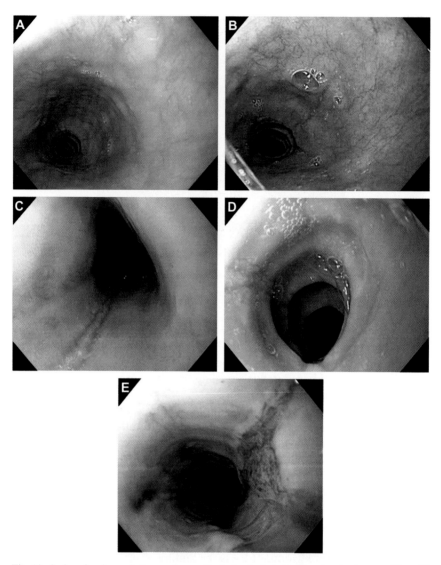

Fig. 10. Series of endoscopic images in a patient who had obstructive dysphagia caused by mid and distal esophageal stricturing inflammatory disease. Although severe distal involvement with sparing of the proximal esophagus is characteristic for GERD, the nonerosive morphology and histology are typical for EE. (*A*) White light examination showing normal epithelial surface in the proximal esophagus with ringed stricture arising more distally. (*B*) Narrow-band imaging view of proximal esophagus highlighting a normal vascular pattern. (*C, D*) Furrows and ringed fibrotic stricture beginning in the mid esophagus. (*E*) Deep linear tear after balloon dilation of stricture.

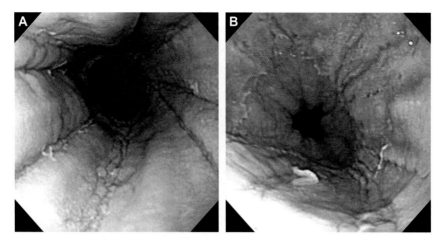

Fig. 11. Overlap findings of allergen- and GERD-induced disease in the same patient. (*A*) Absent vascular pattern and linear furrowing in the proximal esophagus characteristic of allergic eosinophilic esophagitis. (*B*) Multiple erosions at the gastroesophageal junction typical for GERD.

muscle layer (see Fig. 7). The term "felinization" has been applied to this feature, because the appearance is commonly seen in the cat esophagus. In other cases the rings are constant, representing fibrotic stenosis. Strictures of the proximal esophagus are highly suggestive for allergic disease, whereas mid and distal esophageal strictures suggest GERD or overlapping disease (see Fig. 10) [17]. Stenosis involving the entire length of the esophagus, also termed narrow caliber esophagus, is most characteristic of AEE [18]. This long stenosis may be overlooked on barium radiography, because there

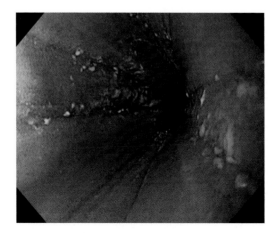

Fig. 12. Narrow-band image of esophagus with absent vascular pattern, linear furrowing, and multiple small plaques of eosinophilic exudate.

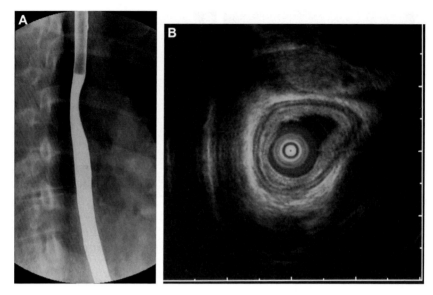

Fig. 13. (A) Barium radiography demonstrating full-length narrowing of the esophagus with smooth contours. (B) High-resolution probe EUS showing narrowed lumen and relative thickening of the mucosa and submucosa. (From Fox VL, Nurko S, Furuta GT. Eosinophilic esophagitis: it's not just kid's stuff. Gastrointest Endosc 2002;56(2):260–70; with permission.)

is no abrupt transition from normal to small caliber (see Fig. 13). Another curious radiologic finding recently reported in association with EE is the Schatzki ring. Nurko and colleagues [30] reported a pediatric radiologic series of Schatzki ring in which 8 of 18 patients (44%) had EE, whereas the remainder had peptic esophagitis. In none of the EE cases compared with 70% of the peptic cases was a true fibrous ring found endoscopically, suggesting a transient narrowing induced by inflammation.

A stenotic lumen may also be overlooked by the endoscopist during initial advancement of the endoscope through the esophagus into the stomach. Resistance to scope advancement may not be appreciated, and longitudinal tearing or splitting of the mucosa is only revealed during withdrawal of the endoscope (see Fig. 14). This increased fragility reported by some investigators is likely a combined consequence of luminal narrowing and reduced tissue compliance caused by subepithelial fibrosis. Aceves and colleagues [31] reported features of structural remodeling, including subepithelial fibrosis in a small case series of children who had EE and esophageal stricture similar to what is seen in airway remodeling in asthma. Thickening of the mucosa and reduced compliance of the wall can also impede tissue sampling. Although normal mucosa easily fills the cupped jaws of biopsy forceps, the toughened mucosa in patients who have EE can be difficult to grasp and requires more forceful application of the forceps against the wall.

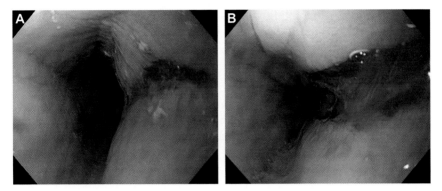

Fig. 14. (*A*) Superficial linear mucosal tear after initial passage of endoscope through the esophagus during diagnostic endoscopy. (*B*) Linear tear reaching deep to the muscle layer after therapeutic balloon dilation in same patient.

Food or foreign body impaction

One of the most common causes of food impaction of the esophagus in children and adults may be chronic EE [15,32]. Food (especially meat) and foreign bodies may become lodged in the esophagus because of strictures or solely from ineffective peristalsis or spasm induced by the underlying inflammation (Fig. 15). Endoscopists should consider the diagnosis of

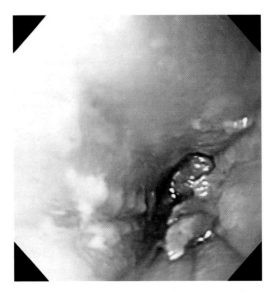

Fig. 15. Endoscopic view of meat impacted in the distal esophagus of a previously asymptomatic adolescent boy. Note the linear furrowing and exudate consistent with eosinophilic esophagitis. (Photo *courtesy of* E. Hait, MD, Boston, MA.)

EE in all patients presenting with food impaction so there are no missed opportunities to establish the correct diagnosis and offer effective therapy.

Summary

The endoscopic findings in EE represent a distinctive yet sometimes subtle pattern of nonerosive inflammatory disease that can involve superficial and deep layers of the esophagus. Early recognition of these findings and their variability can lead to improved care of patients who have esophageal disease.

References

[1] Fox VL, Nurko S, Furuta GT. Eosinophilic esophagitis: it's not just kid's stuff. Gastrointest Endosc 2002;56(2):260–70.

[2] Furuta GT, Liacouras CA, Collins MH, et al. Eosinophilic esophagitis in children and adults: a systematic review and consensus recommendations for diagnosis and treatment. Gastroenterology 2007;133:1342–63.

[3] Straumann A, Bauer M, Fischer B, et al. Idiopathic eosinophilic esophagitis is associated with a T(H)2-type allergic inflammatory response. J Allergy Clin Immunol 2001;108(6): 954–61.

[4] Fogg MI, Ruchelli E, Spergel JM. Pollen and eosinophilic esophagitis. J Allergy Clin Immunol 2003;112(4):796–7.

[5] Spergel JM, Andrews T, Brown-Whitehorn TF, et al. Treatment of eosinophilic esophagitis with specific food elimination diet directed by a combination of skin prick and patch tests. Ann Allergy Asthma Immunol 2005;95(4):336–43.

[6] Ngo P, Furuta GT, Antonioli DA, et al. Eosinophils in the esophagus—peptic or allergic eosinophilic esophagitis? Case series of three patients with esophageal eosinophilia. Am J Gastroenterol 2006;101(7):1666–70.

[7] Kuznetsov K, Lambert R, Rey JF. Narrow-band imaging: potential and limitations. Endoscopy 2006;38(1):76–81.

[8] Goda K, Tajiri H, Ikegami M, et al. Usefulness of magnifying endoscopy with narrow band imaging for the detection of specialized intestinal metaplasia in columnar-lined esophagus and Barrett's adenocarcinoma. Gastrointest Endosc 2007;65(1):36–46.

[9] Lee YC, Lin JT, Chiu HM, et al. Intraobserver and interobserver consistency for grading esophagitis with narrow-band imaging. Gastrointest Endosc 2007;66(2):230–6.

[10] Yanai H, Fujimura H, Suzumi M, et al. Delineation of the gastric muscularis mucosae and assessment of depth of invasion of early gastric cancer using a 20-megahertz endoscopic ultrasound probe. Gastrointest Endosc 1993;39(4):505–12.

[11] Hasegawa N, Niwa Y, Arisawa T, et al. Preoperative staging of superficial esophageal carcinoma: comparison of an ultrasound probe and standard endoscopic ultrasonography. Gastrointest Endosc 1996;44:388–93.

[12] Miller LS, Liu J-B, Collizzo FP, et al. Correlation of high-frequency esophageal ultrasonography and manometry in the study of esophageal motility. Gastroenterology 1995;109: 832–7.

[13] Fox VL, Nurko S, Teitelbaum JE, et al. High-resolution EUS in children with eosinophilic "allergic" esophagitis. Gastrointest Endosc 2003;57(1):30–6.

[14] Liacouras CA, Spergel JM, Ruchelli E, et al. Eosinophilic esophagitis: a 10-year experience in 381 children. Clin Gastroenterol Hepatol 2005;3(12):1198–206.

[15] Sgouros SN, Bergele C, Mantides A. Eosinophilic esophagitis in adults: a systematic review. Eur J Gastroenterol Hepatol 2006;18(2):211–7.

[16] Muller S, Puhl S, Vieth M, et al. Analysis of symptoms and endoscopic findings in 117 patients with histological diagnoses of eosinophilic esophagitis. Endoscopy 2007;39(4):339–44.

[17] Croese J, Fairley SK, Masson JW, et al. Clinical and endoscopic features of eosinophilic esophagitis in adults. Gastrointest Endosc 2003;58(4):516–22.

[18] Vasilopoulos S, Murphy P, Auerbach A, et al. The small-caliber esophagus: an unappreciated cause of dysphagia for solids in patients with eosinophilic esophagitis. Gastrointest Endosc 2002;55(1):99–106.

[19] Lee M, Hodges WG, Huggins TL, et al. Eosinophilic gastroenteritis. South Med J 1996; 89(2):189–94.

[20] Stevoff C, Rao S, Parsons W, et al. EUS and histopathologic correlates in eosinophilic esophagitis. Gastrointest Endosc 2001;54(3):373–7.

[21] Evrard S, Louis H, Kahaleh M, et al. Idiopathic eosinophilic oesophagitis: atypical presentation of a rare disease. Acta Gastroenterol Belg 2004;67(2):232–5.

[22] Furuta K, Adachi K, Kowari K, et al. A Japanese case of eosinophilic esophagitis. J Gastroenterol 2006;41(7):706–10.

[23] Bhutani MS, Moparty B, Chaya CT, et al. Endoscopic ultrasound-guided fine-needle aspiration of enlarged mediastinal lymph nodes in eosinophilic esophagitis. Endoscopy 2007; in press.

[24] Straumann A, Spichtin HP, Bucher KA, et al. Eosinophilic esophagitis: red on microscopy, white on endoscopy. Digestion 2004;70(2):109–16.

[25] Fox VL, Lightdale JR, Mahoney LB, et al. Vascular patterns, narrow band imaging, and esophagitis [abstract]. J Pediatr Gastroenterol Nutr 2007;45:E64.

[26] Straumann A, Beglinger C. Eosinophilic esophagitis: the endoscopist's enigma. Gastrointest Endosc 2006;63(1):13–5.

[27] Remedios M, Campbell C, Jones DM, et al. Eosinophilic esophagitis in adults: clinical, endoscopic, histologic findings, and response to treatment with fluticasone propionate. Gastrointest Endosc 2006;63(1):3–12.

[28] Spechler SJ, Genta RM, Souza RF. Thoughts on the complex relationship between gastroesophageal reflux disease and eosinophilic esophagitis. Am J Gastroenterol 2007;102(6): 1301–6.

[29] Lim JR, Gupta SK, Croffie JM, et al. White specks in the esophageal mucosa: an endoscopic manifestation of non-reflux eosinophilic esophagitis in children. Gastrointest Endosc 2004; 59(7):835–8.

[30] Nurko S, Teitelbaum JE, Husain K, et al. Association of Schatzki ring with eosinophilic esophagitis in children. J Pediatr Gastroenterol Nutr 2004;38(4):436–41.

[31] Aceves SS, Newbury RO, Dohil R, et al. Esophageal remodeling in pediatric eosinophilic esophagitis. J Allergy Clin Immunol 2007;119(1):206–12.

[32] Desai TK, Stecevic V, Chang CH, et al. Association of eosinophilic inflammation with esophageal food impaction in adults. Gastrointest Endosc 2005;61(7):795–801.

ELSEVIER
SAUNDERS

Gastrointest Endoscopy Clin N Am
18 (2008) 59–71

GASTROINTESTINAL
ENDOSCOPY CLINICS
OF NORTH AMERICA

Histopathologic Features of Eosinophilic Esophagitis

Margaret H. Collins, MD[a,b,*]

[a]*Department of Pathology, University of Cincinnati, Cincinnati, Ohio 45221, USA*
[b]*Division of Pathology and Laboratory Medicine, ML1010 B4.180, Cincinnati Center for Eosinophilic Disorders, Cincinnati Children's Hospital Medical Center, 3333 Burnet Avenue, Cincinnati, OH 45229, USA*

Thick epithelium containing large numbers of intraepithelial eosinophils densely aligned near the surface; abnormally long papillae; fibrotic lamina propria containing eosinophils: this is the most characteristic constellation of findings in esophageal mucosal biopsies from patients who have eosinophilic esophagitis (EE). Biopsies showing these findings have been given various descriptors, including allergic esophagitis [1], active esophagitis, and esophagitis with high-grade eosinophilia [2]. The specific pathology diagnosis or descriptor used for such biopsies is less important than understanding that biopsies showing these findings are not pathognomonic of a particular disease, but may be seen in several different diseases. Esophageal histologic findings must be correlated with clinical findings. A biopsy showing these features may occur in patients who have primary or idiopathic EE, hypereosinophilic syndrome, allergy to food or aeroallergens, or a drug reaction [3,4]. Uncommonly, esophageal biopsies resembling the one described are found in patients who have complete resolution of signs and symptoms, endoscopic abnormalities, and pathology following treatment for gastroesophageal reflux disease [5]. More typically, however, the described histology is found in patients who remain symptomatic despite prolonged courses of antireflux therapy.

To more fully appreciate the pathology of EE, the histology of the normal human esophagus is reviewed and illustrated.

---
* Division of Pathology and Laboratory Medicine, ML1010 B4.180, Cincinnati Children's Hospital Medical Center, 3333 Burnet Avenue, Cincinnati, OH 45229.
E-mail address: margaret.collins@cchmc.org

1052-5157/08/$ - see front matter © 2008 Elsevier Inc. All rights reserved.
doi:10.1016/j.giec.2007.09.014   *giendo.theclinics.com*

Normal esophageal histology

Esophageal mucosa is composed of epithelium, lamina propria, and muscularis mucosa (Fig. 1) [6,7]. Normal esophageal epithelium is nonkeratinized stratified squamous epithelium. Lamina propria comprises a connective tissue layer underlying the epithelium. Muscularis mucosa forms a layer beneath the lamina propria. Submucosa is the second layer of the esophageal wall and lies beneath the mucosa, external to the muscularis mucosa. Muscularis propria is external to the submucosa, and the outer surface of the esophagus is bordered by serosa.

Esophageal stratified squamous epithelium consists of several layers (Fig. 2). The basal layer, or zone, normally is composed of up to three layers of oval cells with dark nuclei and little cytoplasm and occupies less than 15% of the total epithelial thickness. More than half of biopsies from asymptomatic adults obtained from the distal 2.5 cm of the esophagus, however, may exhibit basal layer hyperplasia, and approximately one fifth of biopsies obtained from asymptomatic adults more proximally in the esophagus may also exhibit basal layer hyperplasia [8]. These findings suggest that esophageal biopsies from patients who have symptoms of esophageal disease should routinely include sites in addition to the distal esophagus, and, more important, that changes in addition to basal layer hyperplasia should be present to diagnose esophagitis [9]. (See the article by Gonsalves, elsewhere in this issue.)

Cells of the esophageal basal layer proliferate and differentiate into the other layers of the squamous epithelium in the normal process of epithelial cell renewal and in the regeneration that follows injury. The epithelial layer above the basal layer is the prickle cell layer or stratum spinosum, in which intercellular bridges (desmosomes) connect adjacent cells. The functional cell layer of esophageal epithelium is the layer closest to the lumen.

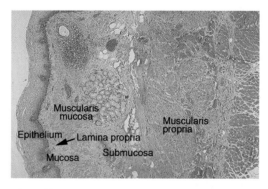

Fig. 1. Transmural view of human esophageal wall. The lumen is at the left and the serosa at the right of the photograph. The squamous epithelium, lamina propria (*with arrow*), muscularis mucosa, submucosa, and muscularis propria are labeled. The mucosa (epithelium plus lamina propria) is also labeled.

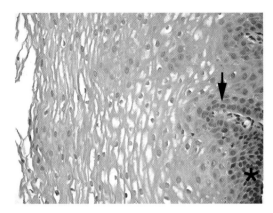

Fig. 2. Normal esophageal epithelium. The normal basal layer (*asterisk*) consists of cells with little cytoplasm and occupies less than 20% of total epithelial thickness. Papillae (*arrow*) extend only a short distance into the epithelium.

The lamina propria is a subepithelial layer of loose connective tissue that contains blood vessels and nerves. Lamina propria forms projections into the epithelium known as papillae that normally are confined to the lower two-thirds of the epithelium (see Fig. 2), but may appear elongated in esophageal biopsies from asymptomatic individuals [8].

The submucosa, like the lamina propria, is composed of loose connective tissue and contains blood vessels and nerves. Muscularis propria is composed of two layers of muscle: the inner circular layer and the outer longitudinal layer, similar to the arrangement in most of the gastrointestinal (GI) tract. The muscularis propria in the upper part of the esophagus is composed of skeletal muscle, in the middle part is composed of skeletal and smooth muscle, and in the distal part is composed of smooth muscle.

Resident leukocytes are normally found in the esophagus, as in the rest of the GI tract. In esophageal epithelium, lymphocytes are usually found above the basal layer, and most are CD3$^+$ and CD8$^+$ T cells [7,10–12]. Langerhans cells are also normally found in esophageal epithelium and stain with S100 and CD1a antibodies. In adult patients undergoing endoscopy for upper tract symptoms, Langerhans cells are more numerous and larger in the distal esophageal epithelium compared with the proximal esophageal epithelium [13]. T and B lymphocytes are normally found in lamina propria and submucosa, and lymphoid aggregates may also be found. Acute inflammatory cells and eosinophils are not normally found in esophageal mucosa [14].

Endoscopic biopsies obtain epithelium, usually but not always full-thickness, and papillae. Most criteria to diagnose EE relate to esophageal epithelial pathology. Lamina propria is seen in a minority of endoscopic biopsies, and even more uncommonly muscularis mucosa and submucosa are seen. Muscularis propria is not included in endoscopic biopsies. Little histologic information is therefore available concerning the muscularis propria in

EE. One case report of a young adult man who had allergies and dysphagia documented esophageal stricture with rupture and dense transmural eosinophilic inflammation [15], including in both epithelium and muscularis propria. This case documents that at least some patients who have EE with significant esophageal epithelial eosinophilic inflammation also have significant esophageal transmural eosinophilic inflammation. Another case report of an 85-year-old man who had esophageal stricture documents dense eosinophilic inflammation in the muscularis propria of the resected esophagus, but little eosinophilic epithelial inflammation [16]. Specific therapy for EE had not been given before resection in that case. Primarily mural eosinophilic inflammation with little epithelial inflammation may represent a subtype of EE that is impossible to diagnose based solely on endoscopic biopsies.

Eosinophilic esophagitis

Biopsy procurement

EE is often patchy, or at least histologically highly variable. Large differences in not only eosinophil number but also other features are often seen among pieces taken from the same site in the esophagus, and even within the same piece. For that reason, multiple biopsies should be obtained. A recent study documented that the sensitivity and specificity of biopsies to diagnose EE in adults increased with increasing numbers of biopsy pieces [17]. Prudent practice is to obtain three pieces from two different sites in the esophagus, including the distal esophagus, plus either mid or proximal esophagus. Mucosa that seems abnormal should be biopsied. If mucosa does not seem abnormal, biopsies should be obtained from apparently normal mucosa in patients clinically suspected of having EE, because biopsies from esophageal mucosa that seems normal at endoscopy may be diagnostic of EE [18]. (See the articles by Gonsalves and Fox, elsewhere in this issue.)

Eosinophilic inflammation

The most characteristic abnormality of biopsies from patients who have EE is large numbers of intraepithelial eosinophils (Fig. 3) (Table 1) [19,20]. There are several methods to count intraepithelial eosinophils in biopsies. The most commonly used method is to count the number that populates the most densely inflamed high-power field (HPF) (400×). This number is referred to as the peak number, and this counting method is suitable for pathologists in daily practice, because the peak number is easily calculated in a short period of time. Some cases, however, require more time and attention, because the number of intraepithelial eosinophils is extremely elevated; several hundred eosinophils are sometimes found in a single HPF. A disadvantage of this method is that it requires viewer selection of the HPF in which eosinophils are counted and that obligatory selection may introduce bias that generates a result that is not the true peak number.

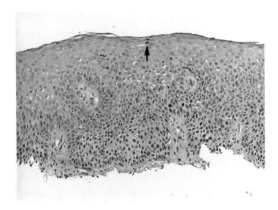

Fig. 3. Eosinophilic esophagitis. The basal layer is thick and prominent, papillae are found close to the lumen, and there are large numbers of intraepithelial eosinophils (*arrow*).

Another method to quantitate eosinophils is to count intraepithelial eosinophils in all HPFs, from which a mean number of eosinophils with standard deviation of the mean can be calculated. Advantages of this method are that an average eosinophil count is obtained, and a peak count (the greatest number recorded among all the counted fields) is also obtained, independent of viewer bias of field selection. Using this method the calculated standard deviations often are large, documenting the variability in inflammation that is striking in some cases. A disadvantage of this method is that it is time-consuming and laborious, particularly in biopsies that are diffusely densely inflamed, and is therefore not practical for daily sign-out.

A third method is to count intraepithelial eosinophils in several adjacent HPFs in the area that seems most densely inflamed. This method is less laborious and time-consuming than counting all HPFs, but it does not eliminate field selection bias.

In large series ($\geq$ 10 patients), the threshold number of intraepithelial eosinophils used to define EE has been a peak count of $\geq$ 15/HPF [21–26], $\geq$ 20/HPF [2,18,27–33], $\geq$ 24/HPF peak count [34–37] or $\geq$ 30/HPF [38], and a peak count of either 25 eosinophils in one HPF or 15 eosinophils in two HPFs [39]. In some series, the diagnosis of EE was based on counting more than one, or all, HPFs in a biopsy [34,36,40–43].

Table 1
Histologic features of eosinophilic esophagitis

Feature	Normal	Eosinophilic esophagitis
Basal layer	10%–15% total thickness	>20% total thickness
Papillae	Lower third of epithelium	Upper third of epithelium
Inflammatory cells	Rare eosinophils	Numerous eosinophils
Lamina propria	Loose connective tissue	Dense collagen

Although there is not a universally agreed on threshold number or method to generate that number, most studies reporting at least several patients have used a peak of 15/HPF as the threshold number of eosinophils to diagnose EE. Biopsies from patients who have gastroesophageal reflux disease, however, may contain 15 or more eosinophils/HPF [2,5], and therefore 15/HPF may be too small to diagnose EE and could result in patients who have GERD being diagnosed with EE. Using a higher peak threshold number ensures a purer population and is more appropriate for research and therapeutic protocols. More important than setting any threshold number is realizing that there is not a magic number, at least not currently, that is pathognomonic of a particular cause of EE. Instead it is important to emphasize that a differential diagnosis exists and correlation with clinical information is required for proper diagnosis [44].

The distribution of intraepithelial eosinophils in patients who have EE is also characteristic. Eosinophils may be present in aggregates or microabscesses [1,23,24,29,30,39,41,43] generally in the biopsies that are mostly intensely inflamed with eosinophils (Fig. 4) [29]. Three studies determined that eosinophilic microabscesses, defined as aggregates of four or more eosinophils, were found exclusively in patients affected by EE and not in those who had GERD [1,39,43]. Eosinophils also align linearly in the upper third of the epithelium, parallel to the epithelial surface, so-called "surface layering" [1,2,23,24,29,39,41,43,45–47], or on the surface (Fig. 5) [28]. In adults who have EE and who were followed for several years, the number of intraepithelial eosinophils declined but did not become normal [48].

Extracellular eosinophil granules are often found in EE [2,23,29,33,39], most commonly in intensely inflamed biopsies [29], but also in those not intensely inflamed. Extracellular granules may result from mechanical trauma to the tissue [14,49] and should not be included in counts, unless the granules

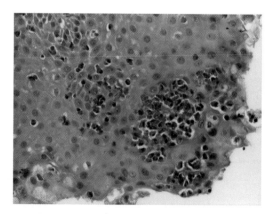

Fig. 4. Eosinophil microabscesses. Large aggregates of eosinophils are found near the surface of esophageal squamous epithelium.

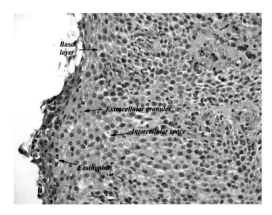

Fig. 5. Basal layer hyperplasia, surface layering, extracellular granules, edema. The basal layer extends almost to the surface in eosinophilic esophagitis (*label*). Eosinophils (*label*) are found in rows near the epithelial surface. Numerous extracellular eosinophil granules (*label*) are seen scattered among eosinophils and epithelial cells. Intercellular spaces are widened, consistent with epithelial edema (*label*).

form a discrete structure that might represent an asymmetric cut through an eosinophil (see Fig. 5). Deposition of major basic protein (MBP) is another measure of eosinophil degranulation, and increased extracellular MBP deposition has been found in the esophageal mucosa of children [33] who have EE and adults who have EE compared to those who have GERD [12,39,43].

Epithelial alterations

Evaluating epithelial changes is often difficult because of poor orientation of biopsy pieces. Tissue fragments obtained endoscopically are so small that luminal and cut surfaces cannot be discerned after the pieces have been placed in fixative. Pieces that are properly oriented by the endoscopist before fixation may separate from the surface on which they are placed and proper orientation cannot be discerned even on those pieces. Nevertheless, some pieces or parts of pieces are usually able to be evaluated for features affected by orientation.

Esophageal squamous epithelium generally shows the most impressive changes in areas of the greatest eosinophilic inflammation. In a large study of esophageal biopsies from infants who had GERD, only biopsies that had abnormal epithelium determined morphometrically had eosinophils [50]. The basal layer may become so hyperplastic in EE [1,2,19,32,39,41,43,45, 46,48] that it occupies virtually all of the total epithelial thickness, which often is greater than normal (Fig. 5). MIB1 antibody decorates the cell cycle antigen Ki-67 that is absent from cells in G0 and documents epithelial cell proliferation in biopsies showing EE [33,34].

Intercellular edema [24,39] may be so marked that intercellular bridges in cells in the prickle cell layer that are usually invisible by light microscopy in normal esophageal epithelium become apparent (Fig. 5) [51]. Epithelial integrity may be compromised in epithelium showing dilated intercellular spaces [52]. Passive permeability manifested as increased mannitol transport is increased in rabbit esophageal epithelium that exhibits dilated intercellular spaces, even without cell necrosis or inflammation [53].

Proper evaluation of papillary length also depends on orientation and is not possible or reliable in many biopsies. Some investigators require three adjacent well-oriented papillae to properly evaluate esophageal biopsies for mucosal changes, including elongated papillae [1,41,43]. In well-oriented sections, papillae in EE often are seen higher in the epithelium than normal, especially in pieces that show marked basal layer hyperplasia (see Fig. 3) [1,2,19,39,45,47,48].

Lamina propria

In most biopsies, nonpapillary, ie, subepithelial, lamina propria is not included. Lamina propria is subject to squeeze artifact during biopsy procurement, especially if only a small amount is present. Nevertheless, in cases that include sufficient lamina propria for meaningful evaluation, the loose connective tissue that characterizes normal lamina propria may be obviously replaced by dense collagen (Fig. 6) [33,39,48]. This change is a manifestation of significant esophageal remodeling and may contribute to esophageal dysfunction. Increased immunohistochemical expression of TGF-B1 and its signaling molecule phosphorylated SMAD2/3 in biopsies from patients who have EE implicates these cytokines in the genesis of lamina propria fibrosis [33]. The occurrence of esophageal remodeling in pediatric patients who have EE indicates that a prolonged course of the disease is not required

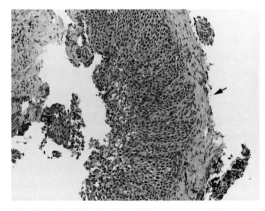

Fig. 6. Lamina propria fibrosis. The subepithelial lamina propria (*arrow*) contains thick collagen fibers.

for induction of remodeling in the form of fibrosis. Eosinophils and other inflammatory cells may be numerous in the lamina propria in biopsies showing EE [2,24,39] and in an animal model of EE [54]. It is important to remember that the threshold number to diagnose EE histologically is based on the number of intraepithelial eosinophils only—the number of eosinophils in connective tissue in papillae or in subepithelial lamina propria is not included in the count. Intravascular eosinophils are also not counted, because they may merely reflect the blood eosinophil count. Eosinophils that are on the surface of the epithelium, especially if admixed with shed epithelial cells, may be included in the counts. Muscularis mucosa and submucosa are uncommonly included in esophageal biopsies, but in biopsies in which they are included, if eosinophilic inflammation is present in the lamina propria it is often seen in those structures also. Eosinophils in muscularis mucosa or submucosa are not included in the intraepithelial eosinophil count.

Other inflammatory cells (also see the article by Chehade)

Inflammatory cells in addition to eosinophils may be increased in EE. T lymphocytes [1,12,34,35,43,46,55], mast cells [12,25,35,55,56], and dendritic cells [46] have been shown to be increased. Occasionally acute inflammatory cells are seen, but they are generally not numerous [1,2,39,57].

Biopsies from other sites

Currently the definition of EE does not include specific recommendations concerning quantifying eosinophils in biopsies from non-esophageal sites or the significance of eosinophilia in those sites [44]. Many studies include the fact that in the patients reported with EE, biopsies from their stomach and duodenum were normal [1,2,18–20,22,24–26,28–31,38–43,45–48,55]. Biopsies should be obtained from stomach and duodenum to identify pathology at those sites that may require treatment, such as gastritis caused by *Helicobacter pylori*, celiac disease, evidence of inflammatory bowel disease, and the like. In larger EE studies, some investigators eliminated patients who had eosinophilia in non-esophageal biopsies from their analysis of EE [22,38,40,43]. One study of cytokine expression in EE biopsies showed differences between biopsies from patients who had EE who did not have extraesophageal eosinophilia compared with those who did [26], supporting the concept that there may be molecular differences between isolated EE and EE associated with eosinophilic inflammation in other sites. Biopsies from extraesophageal sites should be obtained at follow-up endoscopies of patients who have EE, because eosinophilic inflammation is found frequently in those sites after the initial diagnosis of EE [37].

Response to therapy

Although the degree of inflammation and epithelial alterations may be impressive in EE biopsies, these changes are reversible, as documented in biopsies obtained following therapy targeted specifically at EE [12,18,19,22,28,34,36,40,42,46,58,59] (Fig. 7). Relapse is common, however, if specific therapy is eliminated [18,22,30,37]. (See the articles by Spergel and Shuker, Liacouras, and Aceves and colleagues, elsewhere in this issue.)

Basic research in eosinophilic esophagitis

Intranasal but not oral or intragastric allergen causes EE in mice (eosinophilic infiltrates with extracellular granules, and epithelial hyperplasia), which is attenuated in the absence of eotaxin and ablated in the absence of IL-5 [54]. Mice that overexpress IL-5 develop EE, which is attenuated in the absence of eotaxin-1 [60]. Intratracheal IL-13 induces EE in mice, and IL-5, eotaxin-1, and STAT6 are required for the EE to develop [61]. This body of work strongly suggests that Th2-associated cytokines are important in the pathogenesis of EE and provides experimental groundwork for novel clinical trials to treat EE in humans [58,59]. (See the articles by Blanchard and Rothenberg, and Chehade, elsewhere in this issue.)

Genome-wide microarray expression analysis of esophageal biopsies from patients who have EE showed that eotaxin-3 is the gene most highly induced compared with normal biopsies [35]. Epithelial cells from patients who have EE express eotaxin-3 mRNA, but epithelial cells in biopsies from patients who do not have EE do not express eotaxin-3 [35]. Furthermore, a single nucleotide polymorphism at the 3' untranslated region of the eotaxin-3 gene associates with EE [35]. These data provide the basis for further studies in EE.

The future

Although much is known about EE, much remains to be discovered. Continuing evolution of our understanding of this disease requires

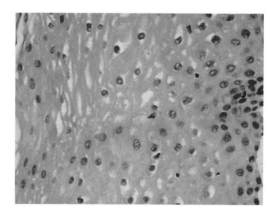

Fig. 7. Response to therapy. With successful treatment, all inflammation disappears and epithelial alterations revert to normal.

collaboration between pathologists and clinicians caring for patients who have EE. Recently a group of such clinicians and pathologists proposed diagnostic and treatment guidelines for EE based on a literature review and expert opinion [44]. Continued such efforts will advance clinical and basic science knowledge of this disease, increasing the ability to effectively treat, and hopefully prevent, EE.

References

[1] Walsh SV, Antonioli DA, Goldman H, et al. Allergic esophagitis in children. A clinicopathological entity. Am J Surg Pathol 1999;23:390–6.
[2] Attwood SEA, Smyrk TC, Demeester TR, et al. Esophageal eosinophilia with dysphagia. A distinct clinicopathologic syndrome. Dig Dis Sci 1993;1:109–16.
[3] Rothenberg ME. Eosinophilic gastrointestinal disorders (EGID). J Allergy Clin Immunol 2004;113:11–28.
[4] Rothenberg ME, Mishra A, Collins MH, et al. Pathogenesis and clinical features of eosinophilic esophagitis. J Allergy Clin Immunol 2001;108:891–4.
[5] Ngo P, Furuta GT, Antonioli DA, et al. Eosinophils in the esophagus—peptic or allergic eosinophilic esophagitis? Case series of three patients with esophageal eosinophilia. Am J Gastroenterol 2006;101:1666–70.
[6] DeNardi FG, Riddell RH. Esophagus. In: Sternberg SS, editor. Histology for pathologists. 2nd edition. Philadelphia: Lippincott-Raven; 1997. p. 461–80.
[7] Fenoglio-Preiser CM, Noffsinger AE, Stemmermann GN, et al, editors. Gastrointestinal pathology. An atlas and text. 2nd edition. Philadelphia: Lippincott-Raven; 1999. p. 1–29.
[8] Weinstein WM, Bogoch ER, Bowes KL. The normal human esophageal mucosa: a histological reappraisal. Gastroenterology 1975;68:40–4.
[9] Cooper HS, Dayal Y, Gourley WK, et al. Proceedings of the 1988 subspecialty conference on gastrointestinal pathology at the USCAP. Diagnostic nonproblems in gastrointestinal biopsy pathology. Mod Pathol 1989;2(2):244–59.
[10] Mangano MM, Antonioli DA, Schnitt SJ, et al. Nature and significance of cells with irregular nuclear contours in esophageal mucosal biopsies. Mod Pathol 1992;5(2):191–6.
[11] Wang HH, Mangano MM, Antonioli DA. Evaluation of T-lymphocytes in esophageal mucosal biopsies. Mod Pathol 1994;7(1):55–8.
[12] Lucendo AJ, Navarro M, Comas C, et al. Immunophenotypic characterization and quantification of the epithelial inflammatory infiltrate in eosinophilic esophagitis through stereology. Am J Surg Pathol 2007;31(4):598–606.
[13] Zavala WD, De Simone DS, Sacerdote FL, et al. Variation in Langerhans cell number and morphology between the upper and lower regions of the human esophageal epithelium. Anat Rec 2002;268:360–4.
[14] DeBrosse CW, Case JW, Putnam PE, et al. Quantity and distribution of eosinophils in the gastrointestinal tract of children. Pediatr Dev Pathol 2006;9:210–8.
[15] Riou PJ, Nicholson AG, Pastorino U. Esophageal rupture in a patient with idiopathic eosinophilic esophagitis. Ann Thorac Surg 1996;62:1854–6.
[16] Stevoff C, Rao S, Parson W, et al. EUS and histopathologic correlates in eosinophilic esophagitis. Gastrointest Endosc 2001;54:373–7.
[17] Gonsalves N, Policarpio-Nicolas M, Zhang Q, et al. Histologic variability and endoscopic correlates in adults with eosinophilic esophagitis. Gastrointest Endosc 2006;64:313–9.
[18] Liacouris CA, Spergel JM, Ruchelli E, et al. Eosinophilic esophagitis: a 10-year experience in 381 children. Clin Gastroenterol Hepatol 2005;3:1198–206.
[19] Kelly KJ, Lazenby AJ, Rowe PC, et al. Eosinophilic esophagitis attributed to gastroesophageal reflux? Improvement with an amino acid-based formula. Gastroenterology 1995;109: 1503–12.

[20] Ruchelli E, Wenner W, Voytek T, et al. Severity of esophageal eosinophilia predicts response to conventional gastroesophageal reflux therapy. Pediatr Dev Pathol 1999;2:15–8.

[21] Lim JR, Gupta SK, Croffie JM, et al. White specks in the esophageal mucosa: an endoscopic manifestation of non-reflux eosinophilic esophagitis in children. Gastrointest Endosc 2004; 59:835–8.

[22] Spergel JM, Andrews T, Brown-Whitehorn TF, et al. Treatment of eosinophilic esophagitis with specific food elimination diet directed by a combination of skin prick and patch tests. Ann Allergy Asthma Immunol 2005;95:336–43.

[23] Fox VL, Nurko S, Teitelbaum JE, et al. High-resolution EUS in children with eosinophilic "allergic" esophagitis. Gastrointest Endosc 2003;57:30–6.

[24] Potter JW, Saeian K, Staff D, et al. Eosinophilic esophagitis in adults: an emerging problem with unique esophageal features. Gastrointest Endosc 2004;59:355–61.

[25] Gupta SK, Fitzgeral JF, Kondratyuk T, et al. Cytokine expression in normal and inflamed esophageal mucosa: a study into the pathogenesis of allergic eosinophilic esophagitis. J Pediatr Gastroenterol Nutr 2006;42:22–6.

[26] Gupta SK, Peters-Golden M, Fitzgerald JF, et al. Cysteinyl leukotriene levels in esophageal mucosal biopsies of children with eosinophilic inflammation. Are they all the same? Am J Gastroenterol 2006;101:1125–8.

[27] Steiner SJ, Gupta SK, Croffie JM, et al. Correlation between number of eosinophils and reflux index on same day esophageal biopsy and 24-hour esophageal pH monitoring. Am J Gastroenterol 2004;99:801–5.

[28] Markowitz JE, Spergel JM, Ruchelli E, et al. Elemental diet is an effective treatment for eosinophilic esophagitis in children and adolescents. Am J Gastroenterol 2003;98: 777–82.

[29] Cheung KM, Oliver MR, Cameron DJS, et al. Esophageal eosinophilia in children with dysphagia. J Pediatr Gastroenterol Nutr 2003;37:498–503.

[30] Arora AS, Perrault J, Smyrk TC. Topical corticosteroid treatment of dysphagia due to eosinophilic esophagitis in adults. Mayo Clin Proc 2003;78:830–5.

[31] Zimmerman SL, Levine MS, Rubesin SE, et al. Idiopathic eosinophilic esophagitis in adults: the ringed esophagus. Radiology 2005;236:159–65.

[32] Steiner SJ, Kernek KM, Fitzgerald JF. Severity of basal cell hyperplasia differs in reflux versus eosinophilic esophagitis. J Pediatr Gastroenterol Nutr 2006;42:506–9.

[33] Aceves SS, Newbury RO, Dohil R, et al. Esophageal remodeling in pediatric eosinophilic esophagitis. J Allergy Clin Immunol 2007;119:206–12.

[34] Noel RJ, Putnam PE, Collins MH, et al. Clinical and immunopathologic effects of swallowed fluticasone for eosinophilic esophagitis. Clin Gastroenterol Hepatol 2004;2:568–75.

[35] Blanchard C, Wang N, Stringer KF, et al. Eotaxin-3 and a uniquely conserved gene-expression profile in eosinophilic esophagitis. J Clin Invest 2006;116:536–47.

[36] Konikoff MR, Noel RJ, Blanchard C, et al. A randomized, double-blind, placebo-controlled trial of fluticasone propionate for pediatric eosinophilic esophagitis. Gastroenterology 2006; 131:1381–91.

[37] Assa'ad AH, Putnam PE, Collins MH, et al. Pediatric patients with eosinophilic esophagitis: an 8-year follow-up. J Allergy Clin Immunol 2007;119:731–8.

[38] Croese J, Fairley SK, Masson JW, et al. Clinical and endoscopic features of eosinophilic esophagitis in adults. Gastrointest Endosc 2003;58:516–22.

[39] Parfitt JR, Gregor JC, Suskin NG, et al. Eosinophilic esophagitis in adults: distinguishing features from gastroesophageal reflux disease: a study of 41 patients. Mod Pathol 2006;19: 90–6.

[40] Liacouris CA, Wenner WJ, Brown K, et al. Eosinophilic esophagitis in children: successful treatment with oral corticosteroids. J Pediatr Gastroenterol Nutr 1998;26:380–5.

[41] Nurko S, Tetelbaum JE, Husain K, et al. Association of Schatzki ring with eosinophilic esophagitis in children. J Pediatr Gastroenterol Nutr 2004;38:436–41.

[42] Remedios M, Campbell C, Jones DM, et al. Eosinophilic esophagitis in adults: clinical, endoscopic, histologic findings, and response to treatment with fluticasone propionate. Gastointest Endosc 2006;63:3–12.

[43] Desai TK, Stecevic V, Chang C-H, et al. Association of eosinophilic inflammation with esophageal food impaction in adults. Gastrointest Endosc 2005;61:795–801.

[44] Furuta GT, Liacouras CA, et al. First International Gastrointestinal Eosinophil Research Symposium (FIGERS) Subcommittees. Related Articles, Links Eosinophilic esophagitis in children and adults: a systematic review and consensus recommendations for diagnosis and treatment. Gastroenterology 2007;133(4):1342–63.

[45] Orenstein SR, Shalaby TM, DiLorenzo C, et al. The spectrum of pediatric eosinophilic esophagitis beyond infancy: a clinical series of 30 children. Am J Gastroenterol 2000;95:1422–30.

[46] Teitelbaum JE, Fox VL, Twarog FJ, et al. Eosinophilic esophagitis in children: immunopathological analysis and response to fluticasone propionate. Gastroenterology 2002;122:1216–25.

[47] Sant'Anna AMGA, Fournet JC, Yazbeck S, et al. Eosinophilic esophagitis in children: symptoms, histology, and pH probe results. J Pediatr Gastroenterol Nutr 2004;39:373–7.

[48] Straumann A, Spichtin HP, Grize L, et al. Natural history of primary eosinophilic esophagitis: a follow-up of 30 adult patients for up to 11.5 years. Gastroenterology 2003;125:1660–9.

[49] Kato M, Kephart GM, Talley NJ, et al. Eosinophil infiltration and degranulation in normal human tissue. Anat Rec 1998;252:418–25.

[50] Sabri MT, Hussain SZ, Shalaby TM, et al. Morphometric histology for infant gastroesophageal reflux disease: evaluation of reliability in 497 esophageal biopsies. J Pediatr Gastroenterol Nutr 2007;44:27–34.

[51] Ravelli AM, Villanacci V, Ruzzenenti N, et al. Dilated intercellular spaces: a major morphological feature of esophagitis. J Pediatr Gastroenterol Nutr 2006;42:510–5.

[52] Tobey NA. How does the esophageal epithelium maintain its integrity? Digestion 1995;56(suppl 1):45–50, 1995.

[53] Orlando RC, Powell DW, Carney CN. Pathophysiology of acute acid injury in rabbit esophageal epithelium. J Clin Invest 1981;68:286–93.

[54] Mishra A, Hogan SP, Brandt EB, et al. An etiological role for aeroallergens and eosinophils in experimental esophagitis. J Clin Invest 2001;107:83–90.

[55] Straumann A, Bauer M, Fischer B, et al. Idiopathic eosinophilic esophagitis is associated with a TH2-type allergic inflammatory response. J Allergy Clin Immunol 2001;108:954–61.

[56] Kirsch R, Bokhary R, Marcon MA, et al. Activated mucosal mast cells differentiated eosinophilic (allergic) esophagitis from gastroesophageal reflux disease. J Pediatr Gastroenterol Nutr 2007;44:20–6.

[57] Gupta SK, Fitzgerald JF, Chong SKF, et al. Vertical lines in distal esophageal mucosa (VLEM): a true endoscopic manifestation of esophagitis in children? Gastrointest Endosc 1997;45:485–9.

[58] Garrett JK, Jameson SC, Thomson B, et al. Anti-interleukin-5 (mepolizumab) therapy for hypereosinophilic syndromes. J Allergy Clin Immunol 2004;113:115–9.

[59] Stein ML, Collins MH, Villaneuva JM, et al. Anti-IL-5 (mepolizumab) therapy for eosinophilic esophagitis. J Allergy Clin Immunol 2006;118:1312–9.

[60] Mishra A, Hogan SP, Brandt EB, et al. IL-5 promotes eosinophil trafficking to the esophagus. J Immunol 2002;168:2464–9.

[61] Mishra A, Rothenberg ME. Intratracheal IL-13 induces eosinophilic esophagitis by an IL-5, eotaxin-1, and STAT6-dependent mechanism. Gastroenterology 2003;125:1419–27.

GASTROINTESTINAL
ENDOSCOPY CLINICS
OF NORTH AMERICA

ELSEVIER
SAUNDERS

Gastrointest Endoscopy Clin N Am
18 (2008) 73–89

Esophageal Dysmotility in Patients Who Have Eosinophilic Esophagitis

Samuel Nurko, MD, MPH*, Rachel Rosen, MD, MPH

Center for Motility and Functional Gastrointestinal Disorders, Children's Hospital Boston, Hunnewell – Ground, 300 Longwood Avenue, Boston, MA 02115, USA

One of the primary presenting symptoms in patients who have eosinophilic esophagitis (EE) is dysphagia. Even though it is a very common symptom, its etiology is unclear. In some cases it is related to anatomic problems such as strictures. In most patients, however, there is no underlying anatomic problem, raising the possibility that there may be an underlying esophageal motility disturbance. There is very limited information regarding esophageal motility patterns in patients who have EE, but in recent years a small number of basic and clinical studies have begun to explore the cause for this dysphagia.

This article reviews the existing data focusing on motility alterations in patients who have EE and its pathophysiologic meaning.

Dysphagia

Intermittent dysphagia and food impactions are the most common presenting symptoms associated with EE in older children and adults. In a report of 103 children, 26% of patients (mean age, 13 years) presented with dysphagia and 6.8% (mean age, 16 years) presented with food impaction [1]. Other pediatric series have found that food impaction was the initial presenting symptom in up to 20% of the patients [2]. In adults, the main presenting symptom is dysphagia, which has been reported in 29% to 100% of patients [3].

Dysphagia in patients who have EE is usually long standing, may be intermittent, and is resistant to therapy with acid blockade. It may be

This work was supported in part by the Pappas Foundation and by NIH grant 1K23DK073713-01A1.

* Corresponding author.

E-mail address: samuel.nurko@childrens.harvard.edu (S. Nurko).

secondary to focal and diffuse esophageal narrowing consistent with esophageal strictures, rings, or a small-caliber esophagus [4–6], or the presence of a Schatzki ring (SR). If anatomic problems are excluded, dysphagia may be caused by esophageal dysmotility, which is the main focus of this article.

Etiopathogenesis of esophageal dysmotility

The etiopathogenesis of esophageal dysmotility is not well understood. It may be related to the eosinophilic infiltration of the esophageal mucosa and its interactions with the microenvironment. Studies in which full-thickness biopsies were performed in patients who had EE found eosinophilic infiltration in all esophageal layers [7–11].

The exact mechanism by which eosinophilic infiltration may produce esophageal dismotility is not certain, but several speculations exist. First, co-culture of fibroblasts with eosinophils results in increased contraction of the fibroblasts, which may result in abnormal motility [12]. Second, eosinophil degranulation has been associated with axonal necrosis, which may have an impact on esophageal motility [11,13,14]. Third, eosinophil-derived major basic protein binds muscarinic acetylcholine receptors that can lead to smooth muscle contraction and subsequent dysmotility [15,16]. Fourth, gastric eosinophilia is associated with dysmotility, although the direct cause is uncertain [17]; some data suggest that the inflammatory cytokines interleukin 1 and interleukin 6 inhibit acetylcholinesterase release and result in esophageal dysmotility in animal models of esophagitis, but their role in EE in humans is unknown [18].

Although endoscopic ultrasound data show increased esophageal wall thickness as well as expansion of the mucosa, submucosa, and muscularis propria in patients who have EE [19], recent data suggest that the expression of one of the most potent eosinophil chemoattractants, eotaxin-3, is increased only in the epithelial cells of the esophagus. This finding suggests that esophageal-mediated inflammation may begin in the epithelium and that the resultant damage to the submucosa may be a secondary effect [20]. Activated eosinophils also may have a potential role in fibroblast proliferation and/or collagen deposition, producing secondary fibrosis, especially because eosinophils have been shown to have profibrogenic properties [21]. This possibility is discussed in the article by Chehade, elsewhere in this issue.

Apart from the role of the eosinophil as the offender in esophageal motility alterations, mast cells may exert a negative effect on esophageal motility. Mast cells are located in the esophagus and are present in higher numbers in patients who have EE; the expression of mast cell genes also is increased in patients who have EE [20] Mast cells exert an effect on fibrosis by releasing proinflammatory mediators such as tumor necrosis factor-alpha, tumor necrosis factor-beta, and tryptase, and they can independently produce type IV collagen [22,23]. Additionally, the activation of acetylcholine by histamine released from mast cells in the esophageal wall may cause contraction of the muscle fibers in the muscularis mucosa, resulting in uncoordinated contractions or hypocontraction [24]. (See the articles by Chehade, and Blanchard and Rothenberg, elsewhere in this issue.)

It is not clear if the motility abnormalities are specific to EE or are secondary to nonspecific eosinophilic infiltration [9,11,25]. Much of the data available on the role of eosinophils in the dysmotility are derived from models of the esophagus that are nonallergic in origin or are derived from studies of eosinophils in different organ systems. Additional studies are needed in patients who have EE and in models with an allergic foundation.

Esophageal motility abnormalities

Stationary esophageal manometry

Esophageal motility has not been well characterized in patients who have EE. The results of stationary manometry are varied and include findings ranging from normal peristalsis to ineffective peristalsis (particularly after meals), including simultaneous and high-amplitude esophageal body contractions, achalasia, diffuse esophageal spasms, tertiary contractions, aperistalsis, nonspecific motor disorders, nutcracker esophagus, and high-amplitude contractions, particularly in the lower esophagus [26].

In the initial report by Attwood and colleagues [26], 10 of 12 patients had abnormal esophageal peristalsis by stationary manometry; two had diffuse esophageal spasm, 2 had nutcracker esophagus, 3 had a mean amplitude of contractions that was less than the 2.5 percentile of normal, and 4 had contractions of short duration. All 12 patients had normal lower esophageal sphincter pressure and function [26]. In a report from 1978, Landres and colleagues [8] described a patient who had vigorous achalasia and who had underlying severe eosinophilic infiltration of the esophageal mucosa. In that case the symptoms probably were related to the achalasia, but the finding suggested that EE may predispose a patient to a motor esophageal disorder. Dobbins and colleagues [27] described one patient who had EE who had esophageal spasm.

Since the initial reports, at least 19 adult and 3 pediatric studies have reported the results of esophageal manometry. Esophageal manometry has been reported in 144 patients (115 adults and 29 children). The studies are summarized in Table 1.

Most of the abnormalities have been described in adults, although, as can be seen in Table 1, one third of children also may have peristaltic abnormalities during stationary manometry. Primary motility disorders were rare but were found in 12 adult patients who had EE: 2 of these patients had achalasia, 7 had diffuse esophageal spasm, and 3 had nutcracker esophagus. The remaining abnormalities were largely nonspecific and mainly affected the peristalsis. Of the 144 patients, 129 had a normal lower esophageal sphincter

Table 1
Studies that performed stationary esophageal manometry in adults and children who had eosinophilic esophagitis

Author/year [Ref]	N	Lower esophageal sphincter				Esophageal peristalsis				Other diagnoses		
		Normal	Hypo-tensive	Hyper-tensive	Abnormal relaxation	Normal	High-amplitude	Abnormal peristalsis NSMD	Type of abnormal peristalsis	Achalasia	DES	Nutcracker
Adults												
Dobbins, et al 1977 [27]	1	1	—	—	—	—	1	—		—	1	—
Landres, et al 1978 [8]	1	—	—	1	1	—	1	—	Simultaneous contractions	1	—	—
Feczko, et al 1985 [43]	—	1	—	—	—	—	—	1	Simultaneous contractions	—	—	—
Attwood, et al 1993 [26]	12	12	—	—	—	1	—	7	3 low amplitude; 4 short duration	—	2	2
Vitellas, et al 1993 [44]	13	12	—	1	—	12	1	—		—	1	—
Borda, et al 1996 [45]	1	1	—	—	—	—	—	1	Absent peristalsis	—	—	—
Hempel, et al 1996 [38]	1	—	1	—	—	—	—	—		—	1	—
Arora, et al 2003 [46]	6	6	—	—	—	4	1	1		—	—	1
Croese, et al 2003 [47]	13	13	—	—	—	8	—	5		—	—	—
Stevoff, et al 2001 [11]	1	—	1	—	—	—	—	1	Aperistalsis upper and middle esophagus, simultaneous lower esophagus	—	—	—

Study											
Vasilopoulos, et al 2002 [48]	4	4	—	—	—	4	—	—	—	—	—	—
Kaplan, et al 2003 [49]	5	5	—	—	—	4	—	—	—	—	—	—
Straumann, et al 2003 [50]	3	3	—	—	—	3	—	—	—	—	—	—
Evrard, et al 2004 [9]	—	—	—	1	1	—	—	—	—	1	1	—
Cantu, et al 2005 [51]	2	2	—	—	—	1	—	1	Absence of peristalsis middle esophagus	—	—	—
Remedios, et al 2006 [52]	23	15	8	—	—	19	3	1	Aperistalsis	—	—	—
Furuta, et al 2006 [53]	1	—	—	—	—	—	1	1	Ineffective peristalsis, simultaneous contractions	—	—	—
Gonsalves, et al 2006 [54]	15	15	—	—	—	5	—	9	—	1	1	—
Lucendo, et al 2007 [55]	12	10	2	—	—	2	3	7	6 severe interrupted peristalsis, low amplitude contractions; 1 simultaneous	—	—	—
Total (Adults)	115	100	12	3	2	63	11	35	—	2	7	3

(continued on next page)

Table 1 (continued)

Author/year [Ref]	N	Lower esophageal sphincter				Esophageal peristalsis				Other diagnoses		
		Normal	Hypo-tensive	Hyper-tensive	Abnormal relaxation	Normal	High-amplitude	Abnormal peristalsis NSMD	Type of abnormal peristalsis	Achalasia	DES	Nutcracker
Children												
Orenstein, et al 2000 [56]	1	1	—	—	—	1	—	—	—	—	—	—
Cheung, et al 2003 [57]	11	11	—	—	—	11	—	—	—	—	—	—
Nurko, et al 2006 [36]	17	17	—	—	—	10	—	7	Ineffective peristalsis, low amplitude	—	—	—
Total children	29	29	—	—	—	22	—	7	—	—	—	—
Total adults and children	144	129	12	3	2	85	11	42	—	2	7	3

Abbreviations: DES, diffuse esophageal spasms; NEMD, nonspecific motility disorders.

tone. The lower esophageal sphincter was hypotensive with normal relaxation in 12 patients and was hypertensive with normal relaxation in 3 patients. There was incomplete relaxation in 2 patients who had a diagnosis of achalasia. Nonspecific peristaltic abnormalities (tertiary contractions, low amplitude, ineffective peristalsis) were reported in 42 of 144 patients (35 adults and 7 children), and high-amplitude contractions were reported in 11 patients (all adults). Hence, abnormal esophageal manometry was found in 59 patients who underwent this procedure (41%). No prospective large studies have been performed to determine if the manometric abnormalities result in abnormal esophageal transit or if the severity of histologic disease correlates with manometric abnormalities or the severity of dysphagia.

Some investigators suggest there may be different phases in the development of esophageal motor abnormalities. Initially the motility is normal, and then motor alterations develop with hyperperistaltic or spastic abnormalities that eventually evolve into abnormal peristalsis with low-amplitude simultaneous contractions [28]. This evolution has been observed in other disorders affecting esophageal function, such as gastroesophageal reflux disease (GERD) or achalasia [28].

Studies with high-resolution manometry

High-resolution manometry offers some advantages over standard manometry; the catheters have more recording sites and less space between them, allowing the clinician to define the intraluminal pressures completely and to reduce movement-related artifacts [29,30]. The technology allows seamless, dynamic representation of peristalsis at every axial position within and across the esophagus, although the role of this additional data in clinical management is unclear [29,30]. Recent studies showed that high-resolution manometry predicted the presence of abnormal bolus transport more accurately than conventional manometry and identified clinically important motor dysfunction that was not detected by standard manometry and radiography [31]. In a recent study using high-resolution manometry in 24 patients who had EE, Chen and colleagues [32] report that the most common motility abnormality was elevation in peristaltic velocity; subsets of patients had failed esophageal peristalsis and impaired relaxation of the lower esophageal sphincter junction, and one patient had a significantly elevated esophageal contractile pressure (Table 2).

Studies with combined esophageal impedance and manometry

Technological advances have allowed the pairing of impedance sensors with pressure sensors in a single catheter. The addition of impedance provides insight into the transit of liquid, viscous, and solid food in the

Table 2
Summary of prolonged and high-resolution manometry studies

Author/year [Ref.]	N	Age (Years)	Findings
24-hour prolonged pH/manometry			
Luis, et al 2006 [58]	13	Median: 12 (range, 7.6–14.4)	Normal lower esophageal sphincter 10% had high-amplitude contractions in the distal esophagus. All patients had an increased mean duration (> 7 s) of the esophageal contractions as compared with controls.
Nurko, et al 2006 [36]	17	Mean: 9.7 ± 1.1	High number of high-amplitude contractions. Significant decrease in complete peristaltic waves, as well as a significant increase in ineffective peristalsis, both during fasting and during meals as compared with controls. Symptoms highly correlated with ineffective peristalsis.
High-resolution manometry			
Chen, et al 2007 [32]	24	Mean: 42 (range, 14–80)	Elevation in esophageal peristaltic velocity. Subsets of patients had failed esophageal peristalsis and impaired esophago-gastric junction relaxation. One patient had a significantly elevated esophageal contractile pressure.

esophagus and its relationship with esophageal peristalsis. The sensors provide information about the transit time of substances down the esophagus and can identify areas of the esophagus that retain ingested contents, suggesting impaired motility. Studies in adults showed that manometric evidence demonstrating ineffective peristalsis might underestimate the true bolus clearance; thus the combination of impedance with manometry may be a more sensitive technique for assessing esophageal function and evaluating patients who have dysphagia [33–35]. The combined used of manometry and impedance has shown that approximately 97% of normal peristaltic swallows have normal bolus transit, but almost half of manometrically ineffective swallows also have normal bolus transit, suggesting that motility abnormalities may not be representative of true esophageal function [35]. Preliminary information in children has shown that effective bolus clearance by impedance was present in 75% of swallows that had ineffective peristalsis [34].

Although no large studies have been completed in patients who have EE, preliminary data from Children's Hospital, Boston suggests that this new technology may help clarify the degree of esophageal dysfunction in patients who have EE. Figs. 1–3 show a normal swallow with good clearance of the esophagus as detected by impedance (see Fig 1), a swallow with evidence of esophageal spasm with normal esophageal clearance (see Fig 2), and a swallow with abnormal peristalsis and poor esophageal clearance (see Fig 3).

Studies with prolonged esophageal manometry

The majority of patients who have EE and dysphagia have normal esophageal stationary manometry. Although this result may reflect a limitation of the technology, other possibilities explaining the normal results include the study's short duration, its performance during fasting rather than meal periods, and the lack of symptoms that typically occur during the short study duration. Prolonged esophageal manometry, conducted over 24 hours, allows the clinician to measure motility during meal periods and provides more opportunities to capture symptoms with the catheter in place (see Table 2).

The authors performed 24 ambulatory pH/manometry measurements on 17 children who had EE and compared these findings with findings in control patients and children who had GERD (see Table 2). All controls and children who had GERD had a normal stationary manometry, but 41%

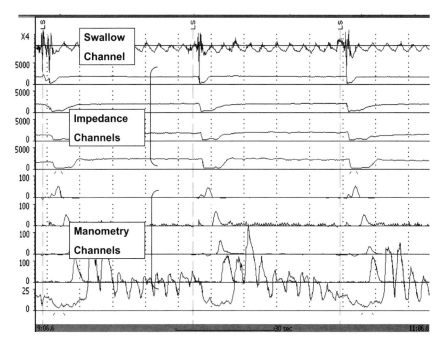

Fig. 1. Normal esophageal peristalsis with good esophageal clearance as evidenced by a drop in impedance followed by a subsequent return to baseline in all of the impedance channels.

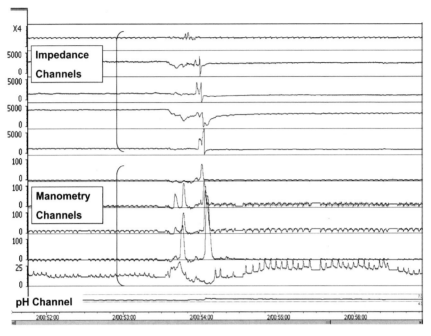

Fig. 2. A high-amplitude contraction in the distal esophagus with normal esophageal clearance as evidenced by drop in impedance followed by a subsequent return to baseline in all of the impedance channels.

of those who had EE had nonspecific peristaltic abnormalities. Patients who had EE had a significantly higher percent of ineffective peristalsis (Fig. 4), high-amplitude contractions (> 180 mm Hg) (Fig. 5), and isolated contractions in a 24-hour period than did control patients [36]. Abnormal esophageal peristaltic events correlated with dysphagia during the study. In the authors' case series, there were no motility abnormalities in patients who had documented peptic esophagitis, suggesting that inflammation alone was not responsible for the motor abnormalities [37].

Effect of treatment on esophageal motility abnormalities

It is not clear if nonspecific motor abnormalities are responsible for the dysphagia, and it has been suggested the abnormalities found during stationary manometry may be nonspecific. Three case reports and one prospective study tried to establish if the motor abnormalities would disappear after successful treatment (Table 3). In one case report of a patient who had achalasia and EE, normal peristalsis returned after myotomy. Two other patients experienced resolution of nonspecific motor abnormalities after treatment with either systemic or swallowed steroids [28,38]. In the only prospective

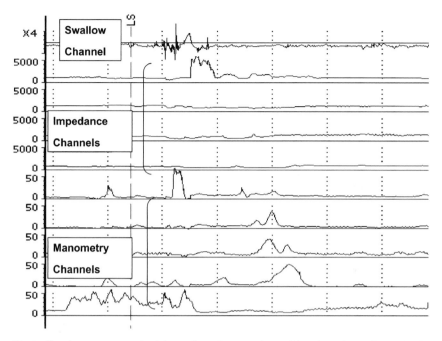

Fig. 3. Simultaneous, nonperistaltic esophageal contractions with no impedance changes in the esophagus indicating poor esophageal clearance.

study, Lucendo [28] reported the manometric abnormalities in 12 patients. Nine of those patients had abnormal esophageal peristalsis before treatment: Six had a nonspecific esophageal motor disorder characterized by up to 80% of nontransmitted or very-low-amplitude waves in the distal esophagus, and 3 had high-amplitude contractions in the distal esophagus. Of those nine patients, esophageal manometry was repeated in seven patients after successful treatment with fluticasone; in all seven patients, the esophageal motor problems and the dysphagia had improved. The investigators found a significant increase in the number of normal peristaltic waves ($P = .018$) as well as a significant decrease in nontransmitted and high-amplitude waves. Although the data are limited to a small number of individual cases, treatment of the EE does seem to improve manometric abnormalities and the associated symptom of dysphagia.

Other possible explanations for the dysphagia

It often is difficult to determine if subtle motor abnormalities are responsible for symptoms; adult studies have shown that nonspecific motor disorders do not consistently result in functional abnormalities [35]. As mentioned previously, patients who have EE have a high incidence of

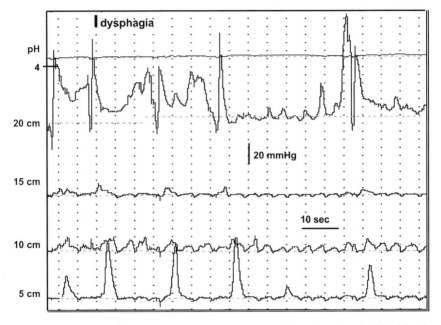

Fig. 4. Tracing from a 24-hour manometry showing absent mid-esophageal peristalsis with a simultaneous symptom of dysphagia.

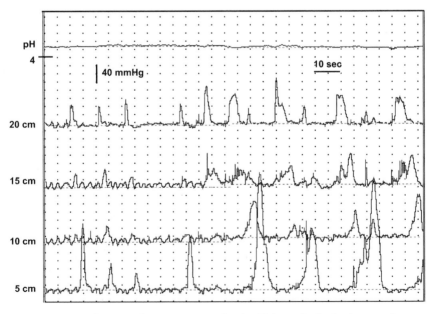

Fig. 5. Tracing from a 24-hour manometry showing high-amplitude distal contractions.

Table 3
Studies in which esophageal manometry was performed before and after treatment for
eosinophilic esophagitis

Author/year [Ref]	N	Peristalsis before treatment	Treatment	Peristalsis after treatment
Landres, et al 1978 [8]	1	Vigorous achalasia	Myotomy	Normal peristalsis Normal LES pressure
Hempel & Elliott 1996 [38]	1	Low LES DES	Systemic steroids	Low LES Normal peristalsis
Lucendo 2006 [28]	1	Absent distal 2/3 Low-amplitude simultaneous waves	Fluticasone	80% normal
Lucendo, et al 2007 [55]	12	6 severe abnormal peristalsis 1 mildly abnormal peristalsis 3 high amplitude contractions	Fluticasone	7 patients with abnormal baseline manometry had a repeat test. In all there was significant improvement in number of peristaltic waves.

Abbreviations: DES, diffuse esophageal spasms; LES, Lower esophageal sphincter.

esophageal narrowing and strictures that may represent diffuse thickening of the muscularis propria or a functional constriction related to the marked infiltration of the myenteric plexus [11]. It also has been postulated that the eosinophilic infiltrate leads to edema and inflammation, perhaps evolving over time to fibrosis. Straumann and colleagues [39] demonstrated architectural alteration and increased fibrous tissue in some patients who had long-standing EE; the result is the narrow-bore esophagus. Endoscopic ultrasound studies have demonstrated the full-thickness nature of the condition. Chehade and colleagues [40] also demonstrated fibrosis in a significant proportion of children who had EE, and they reported that fibrosis was associated with the presence of dysphagia.

The dysphagia also could be related to mucosal plication. The authors recently described a series of 18 patients who had SR diagnosed by upper gastrointestinal series. Eight of the patients who had SR (44%) fulfilled criteria for EE, including lack of response to acid blockade, normal pH-probe monitoring of the distal esophagus, esophageal exudates and furrows, and severe eosinophilic inflammation of the esophageal mucosa [41]. These eight children who had EE, however, did not have any endoscopic evidence of a SR, despite an abnormal upper gastrointestinal series. One hypothesis is that the ring appears and disappears as the longitudinal muscle of the esophagus contracts and relaxes below a redundant, overlying mucosa [42]. Another hypothesis is that including mucosal edema and/or thickening of redundant, inflamed esophageal mucosa may result in the appearance of a SR.

The authors' previous work supports this speculation, because endoscopic ultrasonographic evidence suggests that eosinophilic inflammation associated with EE extends beyond the squamous epithelium and into the esophageal submucosa, and that muscularis propria can be consistent with deep tissue edema and lack of tissue compliance [19]. In a study that used high-resolution ultrasound to compare esophageal tissue in 11 children who had EE and 8 normal controls, the authors determined that children who had EE developed significant esophageal wall expansion, with thickening of the total wall, mucosa, submucosa, and muscularis propria [19].

Adult data also suggest that the inflammation extends deep into the esophageal layers. Several case reports show evidence of eosinophils penetrating into all of the esophageal layers and even into the paraesophageal connective tissue [9–11].

Summary

The ethiopathogenesis of the dysphagia in patients who have EE is probably multifactorial. Primary motility disorders such as achalasia or diffuse esophageal spasms, as well as nonspecific motility disorders including abnormal peristalsis and high-amplitude contractions, have been described. These abnormalities probably result from the interactions between eosinophils and mast cells with the esophageal microenvironment. Even though some of the observed motility abnormalities improve after medical therapy, it is not clear if they are responsible for symptom improvement. Future studies are needed to determine the interrelationship between eosinophilic infiltration, abnormal motility testing, and symptoms of dysphagia.

References

[1] Noel RJ, Putnam PE, Collins MH, et al. Clinical and immunopathologic effects of swallowed fluticasone for eosinophilic esophagitis. Clin Gastroenterol Hepatol 2004;2(7): 568–75.

[2] Khan S, Orenstein SR, Di Lorenzo C, et al. Eosinophilic esophagitis. Strictures, impactions, dysphagia. Dig Dis Sci 2003;48:22–9.

[3] Sgouros SN, Bergele C, Mantides A. Eosinophilic esophagitis in adults: a systematic review. Eur J Gastroenterol Hepatol 2006;18(2):211–7.

[4] Walsh SV, Antonioli DA, Goldman H, et al. Allergic esophagitis in children: a clinicopathological entity. Am J Surg Pathol 1999;23(4):390–6.

[5] Teitelbaum JE, Fox VL, Twarog FJ, et al. Eosinophilic esophagitis in children: immunopathological analysis and response to fluticasone propionate. Gastroenterology 2002; 122(5):1216–25.

[6] Fox VL, Nurko S, Furuta GT. Eosinophilic esophagitis: it's not just kid's stuff. Gastrointest Endosc 2002;56:260–70.

[7] Nicholson AG, Li D, Pastorino U, et al. Full thickness eosinophilia in oesophageal leiomyomatosis and idiopathic eosinophilic oesophagitis. A common allergic inflammatory profile? J Pathol 1997;183(2):233-6.

[8] Landres RT, Kuster GR, Strum W. Eosinophilic esophagitis in a patient with vigorous achalasia. Gastroenterol 1978;74:1298-301.

[9] Evrard S, Louis H, Kahaleh M, et al. Idiopathic eosinophilic oesophagitis: atypical presentation of a rare disease. Acta Gastroenterol Belg 2004;67(2):232-5.

[10] Riou PJ, Nicholson AG, Pastorino U. Esophageal rupture in a patient with idiopathic eosinophilic esophagitis. Ann Thorac Surg 1996;62(6):1854-6.

[11] Stevoff C, Rao S, Parsons W, et al. EUS and histopathologic correlates in eosinophilic esophagitis. Gastrointest Endosc 2001;54:373-7.

[12] Zagai U, Skold CM, Trulson A, et al. The effect of eosinophils on collagen gel contraction and implications for tissue remodeling. Clin Exp Immunol 2004;135(3):427-33.

[13] Dvorak AM, Onderdonk AB, McLeod RS, et al. Ultrastructural identification of exocytosis of granules from human gut eosinophils in vivo. Int Arch Allergy Immunol 1993;102(1):33-45.

[14] Tottrup A, Fredens K, Funch-Jensen P, et al. Eosinophil infiltration in primary esophageal achalasia. A possible pathogenic role. Dig Dis Sci 1989;34(12):1894-9.

[15] Hogan SP, Mishra A, Brandt EB, et al. A pathological function for eotaxin and eosinophils in eosinophilic gastrointestinal inflammation. Nat Immunol 2001;2(4):353-60.

[16] Gundel RH, Letts LG, Gleich GJ. Human eosinophil major basic protein induces airway constriction and airway hyperresponsiveness in primates. J Clin Invest 1991;87(4):1470-3.

[17] Martin ST, Collins CG, Fitzgibbon J, et al. Gastric motor dysfunction: is eosinophilic mural gastritis a causative factor? Eur J Gastroenterol Hepatol 2005;17(9):983-6.

[18] Cao W, Cheng L, Behar J, et al. Proinflammatory cytokines alter/reduce esophageal circular muscle contraction in experimental cat esophagitis. Am J Physiol Gastrointest Liver Physiol 2004;287(6):G1131-9.

[19] Fox VL, Nurko S, Teitelbaum JE, et al. High-resolution EUS in children with eosinophilic "allergic" esophagitis. Gastrointest Endosc 2003;57(1):30-6.

[20] Blanchard C, Wang N, Stringer KF, et al. Eotaxin-3 and a uniquely conserved gene-expression profile in eosinophilic esophagitis. J Clin Invest 2006;116(2):536-47.

[21] Levi-Schaffer F, Garbuzenko E, Rubin A, et al. Human eosinophils regulate human lung- and skin-derived fibroblast properties in vitro: a role for transforming growth factor beta (TGF-beta). Proc Natl Acad Sci USA 1999;96(17):9660-5.

[22] Ruger B, Dunbar PR, Hasan Q, et al. Human mast cells produce type VIII collagen in vivo. Int J Exp Pathol 1994;75(6):397-404.

[23] Xu X, Rivkind A, Pikarsky A, et al. Mast cells and eosinophils have a potential profibrogenic role in Crohn disease. Scand J Gastroenterol 2004;39(5):440-7.

[24] Mann NS, Leung JW. Pathogenesis of esophageal rings in eosinophilic esophagitis. Med Hypotheses 2005;64(3):520-3.

[25] D'Alteroche L, Bourlier P, Picon L, et al. [Myotomy for esophageal muscular hypertrophy with eosinophil infiltration of the esophagus associated with toxocariasis revealed by esophageal motor disorder]. Gastroenterol Clin Biol 1998;22(5):541-5 [in French].

[26] Attwood SE, Smyrk TC, DeMeester TR, et al. Esophageal eosinophilia with dysphagia. A distinct clinicopathologic syndrome. Dig Dis Sci 1993;38:109-16.

[27] Dobbins JW, Sheahan D, Behar J. Eosinophilic gastroenteritis with esophageal involvement. Gastroenterol 1977;72:1312-6.

[28] Lucendo AJ. Motor disturbances participate in the pathogenesis of eosinophilic oesophagitis, beyond the fibrous remodeling of the oesophagus. Aliment Pharmacol Ther 2006;24(8):1264-7.

[29] Ghosh SK, Pandolfino JE, Zhang Q, et al. Quantifying esophageal peristalsis with high-resolution manometry: a study of 75 asymptomatic volunteers. Am J Physiol Gastrointest Liver Physiol 2006;290(5):G988-97.

[30] Pandolfino JE, Ghosh SK, Zhang Q, et al. Quantifying EGJ morphology and relaxation with high-resolution manometry: a study of 75 asymptomatic volunteers. Am J Physiol Gastrointest Liver Physiol 2006;290(5):G1033–40.

[31] Fox M, Hebbard G, Janiak P, et al. High-resolution manometry predicts the success of oesophageal bolus transport and identifies clinically important abnormalities not detected by conventional manometry. Neurogastroenterol Motil 2004;16(5):533–42.

[32] Chen J, Ghosh S, Pandolfino J, et al. Esophageal dysmotility in eosinophilic esophagitis: analysis using high resolution esophageal manometry. Gastroenterology 2007;132(Suppl): A-6.

[33] Nguyen NQ, Tippett M, Smout AJ, et al. Relationship between pressure wave amplitude and esophageal bolus clearance assessed by combined manometry and multichannel intraluminal impedance measurement. Am J Gastroenterol 2006;101(11):2476–84.

[34] Rosen R, Nurko S. Do abnormalities in peristalsis result in abnormal esophageal clearance? Use of esophageal function testing (EFT) a novel technology to evaluate dysphagia in children. Gastroenterology 2006;130(Suppl 2):A-192–3.

[35] Tutuian R, Castell DO. Combined multichannel intraluminal impedance and manometry clarifies esophageal function abnormalities: study in 350 patients. Am J Gastroenterol 2004;99(6):1011–9.

[36] Nurko SS, Fox VL, Furuta GT. Esophageal motor abnormalities in patients with eosinophilic esophagitis. A study using prolonged esophageal pH/manometry. Neurogastroenterol Motil 2006;18:751.

[37] Chitkara D, Fortunato C, Nurko S. Esophageal motor activity in children with gastroesophageal reflux disease and esophagitis. J Pediatr Gastroenterol Nutr 2005;40:70–5.

[38] Hempel SL, Elliott DE. Chest pain in an aspirin-sensitive asthmatic patient. Eosinophilic esophagitis causing esophageal dysmotility. Chest 1996;110:1117–20.

[39] Straumann A, Spichtin H, Bucher KA, et al. Natural history of primary eosinophilic esophagitis: a follow-up of 30 adult patients for up to 11.5. Gastroenterol 2003;125:1660–9.

[40] Chehade M, Sampson H, Morotti R, et al. Esophageal subepithelial fibrosis in children with eosinophilic esophagitis. J Pediatr Gastrointest Nutr 2007;45:319–28.

[41] Nurko S, Teitelbaum JE, Husain K, et al. Association of Schatzki ring with eosinophilic esophagitis in children. J Pediatr Gastroenterol Nutr 2004;38:436–41.

[42] Chandrahasan AC, Lester PD, Johnson S, et al. Esophagogastric ring: why and when we see it, and What it implies: a radiologic-pathologic correlation. South Med J 1992;85(10):946–52.

[43] Feczko P, Halpert R, Zonca M. Radiographic abnormalities in eosinophilic esophagitis. Gastrointest Radiol 1985;10:321–4.

[44] Vitellas KM, Bennett WF, Bova JG, et al. Idiopathic eosinophilic esophagitis. Radiology 1993;186(3):789–93.

[45] Borda F, Jimenez FJ, Martinez-Penuela JM, et al. Eosinophilic esophagitis: an underdiagnosed entity? Rev Esp Enferm Dig 1996;88:701–4.

[46] Arora AS, Perrault J, Smyrk TC. Topical corticosteroid treatment of dysphagia due to eosinophilic esophagitis in adults. Mayo Clin Proc 2003;78(7):830–5.

[47] Croese J, Fairley SK, Masson JW, et al. Clinical and endoscopic features of eosinophilic esophagitis in adults. Gastrointest Endosc 2003;58:516–22.

[48] Vasilopoulos S, Murphy P, Auerbach A, et al. The small-caliber esophagus: an unappreciated cause of dysphagia for solids in patients with eosinophilic esophagitis. Gastrointest Endosc 2002;55(1):99–106.

[49] Kaplan M, Mutlu EA, Jakate S, et al. Endoscopy in eosinophilic esophagitis: "feline" esophagus and perforation risk. Clin Gastroenterol Hepatol 2003;1(6):433–7.

[50] Straumann A, Spichtin HP, Grize L, et al. Natural history of primary eosinophilic esophagitis: a follow-up of 30 adult patients for up to 11.5 years. Gastroenterology 2003;125(6): 1660–9.

[51] Cantu P, Velio P, Prada A, et al. Ringed oesophagus and idiopathic eosinophilic oesophagitis in adults: an association in two cases. Dig Liver Dis 2005;37(2):129–34.

[52] Remedios M, Campbell C, Jones DM, et al. Eosinophilic esophagitis in adults: clinical, endoscopic, histologic findings, and response to treatment with fluticasone propionate. Gastrointest Endosc 2006;63(1):3–12.

[53] Furuta K, Adachi K, Kowari K, et al. A Japanese case of eosinophilic esophagitis. J Gastroenterol 2006;41(7):706–10.

[54] Gonsalves N, Policarpio-Nicolas M, Zhang Q, et al. Histopathologic variability and endoscopic correlates in adults with eosinophilic esophagitis. Gastrointest Endosc 2006;64(3): 313–9.

[55] Lucendo AJ, Castillo P, Martin-Chavarri S, et al. Manometric findings in adult eosinophilic oesophagitis: a study of 12 cases. Eur J Gastroenterol Hepatol 2007;19(5):417–24.

[56] Orenstein SR, Shalaby TM, Di Lorenzo C, et al. The spectrum of pediatric eosinophilic esophagitis beyond infancy: a clinical series of 30 children. Am J Gastroenterol 2000; 95(6):1422–30.

[57] Cheung KM, Oliver MR, Cameron DJ, et al. Esophageal eosinophilia in children with dysphagia. J Pediatr Gastroenterol Nutr 2003;37(4):498–503.

[58] Luis AL, Rinon C, Encinas JL, et al. Non stenotic food impaction due to eosinophilic esophagitis: a potential surgical emergency. Eur J Pediatr Surg 2006;16(6):399–402.

GASTROINTESTINAL
ENDOSCOPY CLINICS
OF NORTH AMERICA

Gastrointest Endoscopy Clin N Am
18 (2008) 91–98

ELSEVIER
SAUNDERS

Otorhinolaryngologic Manifestations of Eosinophilic Esophagitis

Dana M. Thompson, MD[a],*,
Laura J. Orvidas, MD[b,c]

[a]Division of Pediatric Otolaryngology, Cincinnati Children's Hospital Medical Center,
University of Cincinnati, 3333 Burnet Avenue, Cincinnati, OH 45229, USA
[b]Mayo Clinic, Mayo Eugenio Litta Children's Hospital, Rochester, MN, USA
[c]Mayo Clinic College of Medicine, 200 First Street SW, Rochester, MN 55905, USA

Eosinophilic Esophagitis (EE) is a chronic inflammatory disorder of the esophagus that rapidly is emerging as a distinct clinical disease entity of importance [1]. Although the presenting symptoms usually are gastrointestinal in nature, recent reports highlight the spectrum of associated symptoms outside of the esophagus [2,3]. Extraesophageal symptoms include upper airway and respiratory symptoms of rhinitis, sinusitis, pneumonia, wheezing, globus, hoarseness, dysphonia, and cough. Additionally, EE is attributed as an etiologic factor in upper airway diseases managed by otolaryngologists. These laryngeal diseases include subglottic stenosis (SGS) [4–7], vocal fold nodules [7,8], recurrent croup [7,9], and chronic laryngeal edema refractory to traditional gastroesophageal reflux therapy [4,5]. The purpose of this report is to review the associated symptoms and diseases seen in an otolaryngology practice that are related to EE and to review the potential associated pathophysiologic mechanisms.

Rhinosinusitis

Allergic rhinitis is an IgE-dependent disease. An allergen enters the nasal cavity, triggering an IgE-dependent reaction and the release of histamine, leading to mucus secretion, itching, sneezing, and nasal drainage. The allergen trigger activates a complex sequence of events that involves multiple

* Corresponding author. Cincinnati Children's Hospital Medical Center, 3333 Burnet Avenue, Cincinnati, OH 45229.
   E-mail address: dana.thompson@cchmc.org (D.M. Thompson).

components of the immune response. Sinusitis often is preceded by rhinitis and rarely occurs without concurrent rhinitis; thus, the term, "rhinosinusitis," is most appropriate to describe the disease. Symptoms include nasal obstruction, nasal congestion, nasal discharge, nasal purulence, postnasal drip, facial pressure and pain, alteration in the sense of smell, cough not caused by asthma, fever, halitosis, pharyngitis, and headache.

Nasal symptoms and rhinosinusitus are reported in 19% to 25% of children who have EE [2,3] Whether or not these children have an allergen as the antigenic trigger is unknown. Up to 62% of the children, however, have a personal or family history of allergy [2,3]. There are several common features that may link rhinosinusitis and EE. Common symptoms are chronic cough, hoarseness, and dysphagia. Common concurrent diseases are allergic rhinitis, allergic conjunctivitis, asthma, and atopic diseases, such as eczema and food allergy.

Eosinophilic inflammation is the major histologic hallmark of allergic and nonallergic rhinosinusitis and EE. Tissue response to eosinophil activation likely is the common pathophysiologic link between the two diseases. The response of nasal sinus mucosa to eosinophil activation in patients who have chronic rhinosinusitis [10,11] is similar to the pathophysiolgic response of mucosal inflammation seen in asthma [12] and EE [13,14]. In all three diseases, the eosinophil, major basic protein (MBP), likely exerts cytotoxic effects on sinus tissue, including smooth muscle hypertrophy, basement membrane thickening, and erosion of the epithelium (Fig. 1). The cause and effect relationship of EE and rhinosinusitis has not been studied. It is unlikely that EE causes rhinosinusitis. The more likely mechanism is eosinophil activation by allergen triggers that enter the upper aerodigestive tract through the nose and mouth as aeroallergens. Chronic exposure to the aeroallergens in the nose leads to rhinosinusitus. It is likely that most allergens that enter through the oronasal cavity are swallowed. In predisposed individuals, once an allergen enters the esophagus, the same eosinophil cytotoxic tissue damage may cause esophageal mucosal damage and EE.

Laryngeal diseases and eosinophilic esophagitis

Laryngeal symptoms of EE include hoarseness, cough, croup, globus sensation, and sleep-disordered breathing. The larynx is a prime target as it is located at the interface of the oronasal cavity and the esophagus. The younger a child, the closer the relationship of the larynx to the nasal cavity and esophagus. Any antigenic stimulation of eosinophils in the nose or esophagus has high potential to affect the larynx. Most patients who have diffuse laryngeal edema are assumed to have extra-esophageal acid reflux disease as the cause [15,16]. Recent reports describe patients, however, who had persistent laryngeal disease refractory to maximal acid

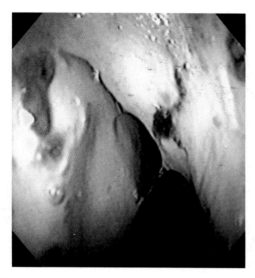

Fig. 1. Anterior rhinoscopy view of the nasal mucosa in a child who had EE and allergic rhinitis with rhinosinusitis. Findings of eosinophilic cytotoxic damage include mucosal erosion, ulceration, and bleeding.

reflux therapy who eventually were diagnosed with EE. Aggressive treatment of EE resulted in reversal or improvement in the laryngeal symptoms [4,5,7,9]. The patient characteristics and comorbidities in patients who have EE-associated laryngeal disease are similar to those who have gastrointestinal symptoms. They commonly present with persistent symptoms that are attributed to GERD. There is a male predominance. Many have a history of allergic rhinitis, atopy, and asthma. Some have elevated peripheral eosinophil counts or total IgE levels. Similar to patients who have typical gastrointestinal symptoms of EE, those who have laryngeal symptoms may go unrecognized; thus, a high index of suspicion is required.

The pathophysiology of EE-associated laryngeal disease is poorly understood. It is plausible that the larynx is affected by allergen stimulation of the eosinophils present in the sinonasal cavity leading to post nasal drainage and soiling of the larynx. This could explain symptoms of chronic cough, throat clearing, and globus sensation. Just as reflux of acid into the laryngopharyngeal region causes laryngeal disease, it is plausible that reflux of the cytokines or granule proteins released from eosinophils present in the esophagus into the larynx leads to chronic laryngeal edema. This could explain the visual findings of diffuse laryngeal edema and supra-arytenoid tissue prolapse into the glottis seen in some patients who have EE (Fig. 2). The diffuse laryngeal edema can lead to hoarseness and sleep-disordered breathing in addition to the laryngeal symptoms discussed previously.

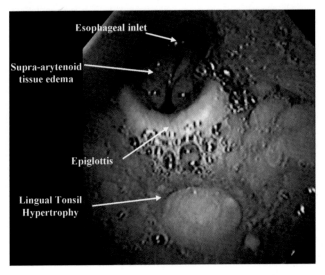

Fig. 2. Flexible laryngoscopy of the larynx in a child who had EE and symptoms of globus, dysphagia, hoarseness, and sleep-disordered breathing. Findings include diffuse laryngeal edema, prolapse of the supra-arytenoid tissue into the glottic inlet obstructing the view of the vocal folds, edema of the posterior glottic tissue near the entry to the esophagus, and lingual tonsil hypertrophy.

Subglottic stenosis

Chronic inflammatory changes in the subglottic region lead to stenosis and airway obstruction. The etiology is complex and multifactorial. Direct trauma from prolonged endotracheal intubation, combined with infection and gastroesophageal reflux disease, is the most common proceeding sequence of events. Patients who have SGS present with symptoms of stridor, cough, croup, and airway obstruction. Severe stenoses require surgical intervention for correction. The first report of EE and SGS was in a child who had failed multiple laryngotracheal reconstructive procedures despite meticulous surgical care and control for GERD [5]. Subsequent reports verify this association [4,6]. In many institutions, a full diagnostic evaluation for EE and treatment, if EE is present, has become the standard of care for airway surgeons before attempts at laryngotracheal reconstruction. Some patients who have recurrent croup-like illnesses may have less severe forms of SGS. EE is reported in children in association with SGS and recurrent croup (discussed later).

Recurrent croup

Recurrent or spasmodic croup is an entity that is understood poorly. The typical presentation is a sudden onset of inspiratory stridor, accompanied by a barky cough and dyspnea that usually occurs at night. Compared with isolated acute croup (laryngotracheobronchitis), fever usually is absent and a preceding viral prodrome may or may not be present. The same upper respiratory tract infection or virus causing mild symptoms in one child and resulting in croup in another questions the role of other endogenous or exogenous factors in the recurrence of the disease process and etiology. Many of the triggers of recurrent croup are associated with and implicated in the etiology of EE, namely sensitization to environmental allergens and asthma [2–4,7,13,14,17–19]. This connection begs the question of the mechanistic association of EE to recurrent croup. The pathophysiologic commonality again is the eosinophil. Once the antigen enters the aerodigestive tract, the eosinophil can releases cytotoxic mediators that cause tissue injury and inflammation [14]. Specific to the symptoms of croup are the effects of the release of the cytotoxic granule proteins, eosinophilic cationic protein (ECP) and MBP, and the neuromediator, substance P. Release of ECP leads to tissue injury and inflammation. Serum ECP levels are accepted as a reflection of eosinophilic activation and allergic inflammation in asthma and other allergic diseases [20,21]. Serum ECP levels also may increase in some viral infections [20,22]. A recent study shows that serum ECP levels are elevated in patients who have acute and recurrent croup [20]. This same study showed higher ECP levels in patients who had recurrent croup compared with those who had isolated croup, suggesting exposure to eosinophils. It is plausible that prolonged exposure of eosinophils is the direct result of EE. Similar to ECP, MBP exerts a significant cytotoxic injury to mucosa. MBP-associated changes also are documented in patients who have EE [4,23,24]. It is plausible that the deleterious effects of these two cytotoxic granule proteins have a pathophysiologic role in the laryngeal inflammation and the obstructive airway symptoms in patients who have EE and recurrent croup.

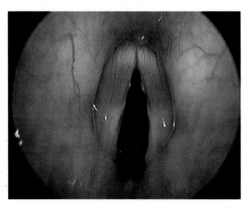

Fig. 3. Endoscopic view of the larynx and vocal folds demonstrating vocal fold nodules in a child who had recurrent croup and EE.

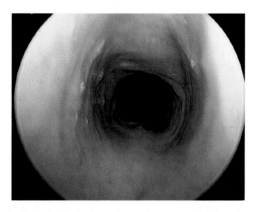

Fig. 4. Grade I SGS and tracheal cobblestoning and inflammation in a child who had recurrent spasmodic croup and EE.

The neuromediator, substance P, is released in response to eosinophil activation [14]. Substance P is a known potent activator of laryngeal vagal responses of apnea and laryngospasm [25–27], another plausible mechanism of recurrent barky cough in patients who have EE. The act of recurrent coughing may lead to vocal fold nodule formation, a finding reported in children who have EE [7–9].

Airway endoscopy findings in patients who have recurrent croup and EE include diffuse laryngeal edema, vocal fold nodules (Fig. 3), and laryngeal ventricular obliteration. Some of these patients are found to have grade I and grade II SGS (Fig. 4). Children who have recurrent croup refractory to other modes of therapy should be evaluated for EE. Their symptoms abate once successfully identified and treated [9].

Summary

Similar to gastrointestinal symptoms of EE, symptoms of otorhinolaryngologic disease associated with EE often are refractory to traditional treatment of gastroesophageal reflux disease. Patient demographics and characteristics often are similar. Clinicians must maintain a high index of suspicion to accurately diagnose and manage airway findings related to EE. Team collaboration between otolaryngologists, allergists, and gastroenterologists will assure the best treatment in this select group of predisposed patients.

References

[1] Furuta GT, Liacouras CA, Collins MH, et al. Eosinophilic esophagitis in children and adults: a systematic review and consensus recommendations for diagnosis and treatment. Gastroenterology 2007;133:1342–63.
[2] Dauer EH, Freese DK, El-Youssef M, et al. Clinical characteristics of eosinophilic esophagitis in children. Ann Otol Rhinol Laryngol 2005;114:827–33.

[3] Orenstein SR, Shalaby TM, Di Lorenzo C, et al. The spectrum of pediatric eosinophilic esophagitis beyond infancy: a clinical series of 30 children. Am J Gastroenterol 2000;95: 1422–30.

[4] Dauer EH, Ponikau JU, Smyrk TC, et al. Airway manifestations of pediatric eosinophilic esophagitis: a clinical and histopathologic report of an emerging association. Ann Otol Rhinol Laryngol 2006;115:507–17.

[5] Hartnick C, Liu J, Cotton R, et al. Subglottic stenosis complicated by allergic esophagitis: case report. Ann Otol Rhinol Laryngol 2002;111:57–60.

[6] Johnson LB, Rutter MJ, Putnam PE, et al. Airway stenosis and eosinophilic esophagitis. Presented at the 83rd Annual Meeting of the American Broncho-Esophagological Association. Nashville, Tennessee; May 3–4, 2003. p. 137.

[7] Thompson DM, Arora AS, Romero Y, et al. Eosinophilic esophagitis: its role in aerodigestive tract disorders. Otolaryngol Clin North Am 2006;39:205–21.

[8] Mandell DL, Yellon RF. Synchronous airway lesions and esophagitis in young patients undergoing adenoidectomy. Arch Otolaryngol Head Neck Surg 2007;133:375–8.

[9] Thompson DM, Orvidas LJ. Eosinophilic esophagitis: a cause of recurrent spasomidic croup symptoms. Arch Otolaryngol Head Neck Surg 2007; in review.

[10] Ponikau JU, Sherris DA, Kephart GM, et al. Striking deposition of toxic eosinophil major basic protein in mucus: implications for chronic rhinosinusitis. J Allergy Clin Immunol 2005; 116:362–9.

[11] Ponikau JU, Sherris DA, Kephart GM, et al. Features of airway remodeling and eosinophilic inflammation in chronic rhinosinusitis: is the histopathology similar to asthma? J Allergy Clin Immunol 2003;112:877–82.

[12] Gleich GJ. The eosinophil and bronchial asthma: current understanding. J Allergy Clin Immunol 1990;85:422–36.

[13] Rothenberg ME. Eosinophilic gastrointestinal disorders (EGID). J Allergy Clin Immunol 2004;113:11–28.

[14] Rothenberg ME, Mishra A, Collins MH, et al. Pathogenesis and clinical features of eosinophilic esophagitis. J Allergy Clin Immunol 2001;108:891–4.

[15] Koufman JA. Laryngopharyngeal reflux is different from classic gastroesophageal reflux disease. Ear Nose Throat J 2002;81:7–9.

[16] Koufman JA, Aviv JE, Casiano RR, et al. Laryngopharyngeal reflux: position statement of the committee on speech, voice, and swallowing disorders of the American Academy of Otolaryngology-Head and Neck Surgery. Otolaryngol Head Neck Surg 2002;127: 32–5.

[17] Arora AS, Yamazaki K. Eosinophilic esophagitis: asthma of the esophagus? Clin Gastroenterol Hepatol 2004;2:523–30.

[18] Mishra A, Hogan SP, Brandt EB, et al. An etiological role for aeroallergens and eosinophils in experimental esophagitis. J Clin Invest 2001;107:83–90.

[19] Spergel JM, Beausoleil JL, Mascarenhas M, et al. The use of skin prick tests and patch tests to identify causative foods in eosinophilic esophagitis. J Allergy Clin Immunol 2002;109: 363–8.

[20] Cetinkaya F, Cakir M. Serum ECP and total IgE levels in children with acute laryngotracheobronchitis. Int J Pediatr Otorhinolaryngol 2005;69:493–6.

[21] Koller DY, Herouy Y, Gotz M, et al. Clinical value of monitoring eosinophil activity in asthma. Arch Dis Child 1995;73:413–7.

[22] Reijonen TM, Korppi M, Kuikka L, et al. Serum eosinophil cationic protein as a predictor of wheezing after bronchiolitis. Pediatr Pulmonol 1997;23:397–403.

[23] Desai TK, Stecevic V, Chang C-H, et al. Association of eosinophilic inflammation with esophageal food impaction in adults. Gastrointest Endosc 2005;61:795–801.

[24] Furuta GT, Walsh S, Antonioli DA, et al. Eosinophil derived major basic protein deposition occurs in idiopathic eosinophilic esophagitis. Gastroenterology 1998;114:A126.

[25] Bauman NM, Wang D, Sandler AD, et al. Response of the cricothyroid and thyroarytenoid muscles to stereotactic injection of substance P into the region of the nucleus tractus solitarius in developing dogs. Ann Otol Rhinol Laryngol 2000;109:1150–6.

[26] Prabhakar NR, Runold M, Yamamoto Y, et al. Effect of substance P antagonist on the hypoxia-induced carotid chemoreceptor activity. Acta Physiol Scand 1984;121:301–3.

[27] Sun QJ, Berkowitz RG, Goodchild AK, et al. Substance P inputs to laryngeal motoneurons in the rat. Respir Physiol Neurobiol 2003;137:11–8.

ELSEVIER
SAUNDERS

Gastrointest Endoscopy Clin N Am
18 (2008) 99–118

GASTROINTESTINAL
ENDOSCOPY CLINICS
OF NORTH AMERICA

The Natural History and Complications of Eosinophilic Esophagitis

Alex Straumann, MD

*Department of Gastroenterology, Kantonsspital Olten, Roemerstrasse 7,
4600 Olten, Switzerland*

Eosinophilic esophagitis (EE) is a relatively newly recognized disorder, with the first comprehensive descriptions of this inflammatory esophageal disease published less than 15 years ago [1–3]. Within this relatively short time frame, EE has become a well-recognized and clearly defined clinico-pathologic entity. Symptoms revolve around the esophagus, where eosino-philic accumulation occurs. Long-term administration of proton-pump inhibitors alleviates neither symptoms nor eosinophilia [4]. Initially thought to be a rare curiosity, EE has emerged as one of the most common causes of dysphagia and esophageal food impaction in adults [5]. In children, the lat-est incidence rates may even exceed those of pediatric inflammatory bowel disease [6]. Despite enormous research activity, the natural history, the long-term prognosis, and the complications of EE still remain poorly under-stood [7].

General considerations about the natural history of a disease

Characterization of the natural history of a disease

The two terms "natural history" and "natural course" of a disease are used widely in medical literature, but a precise definition is hard to find. A simple paraphrase, "the course of a disease left untreated," is usually ac-cepted as the definition of a disease's natural history. The circumscription, "The natural history of a disease describes the expected course followed by the given disease over time, its characteristic pattern, and its time-inten-sity gradient," depicts the disease-specific behavior more precisely.

E-mail address: alex.straumann@hin.ch

1052-5157/08/$ - see front matter © 2008 Elsevier Inc. All rights reserved.
doi:10.1016/j.giec.2007.09.009   *giendo.theclinics.com*

Importance of knowing the natural history of a disease

A PubMed literature search with the key word "natural history" (not specifically of EE) revealed that in 1 single year, 2006, 1651 articles were published on this topic. There are at least three reasons for this proliferation of publications:

1. Research purposes: In the development of any novel medical or surgical strategy, the natural history of the disorder is the benchmark against which the efficacy and safety of all new therapeutic measures are compared.
2. Patient care purposes: Newly confronted with a disease, patients and family members are eager to learn precise information about the disease and its prognosis. Specifically, survival, risk of disability, inability to work, and the impact of the disease on quality of life are topics anxiously explored in the search for information about the disease's natural history. For treating physicians, knowing the particular disease behavior establishes the cornerstone on which counseling and patient care is based.
3. Socioeconomic purposes: For health care institutions, epidemiology services, social institutions, and health and life insurances, knowledge of the natural course of a disease is crucial in planning appropriate measures and in estimating the burden of disease, including direct and indirect costs.

Particularities of natural history studies

The primary objective of a natural history study is to monitor, as punctiliously as possible, the unaltered course of a specific disease. One could even consider such a study as a clinical trial that has the particularity that no drug is under investigation. Nevertheless, this small difference from therapeutic clinical trials presents relevant practical consequences for executing and evaluating natural history studies.

The main difference between natural history studies and therapeutic clinical trials is the risk for the study participants. Whereas in a therapeutic trial the side effects of the study medication are the main safety concern, in a natural history study a "wait and watch" attitude poses the main risk for participants. If the natural course of a disorder is associated with relevant disturbances, or if the disease has a risk for complications or even for a fatal outcome, ethical considerations prohibit performing such observational studies if an approved treatment is available. Further differences between these two types of study are that the planning and execution of natural history studies are not as rigidly defined or supervised by regulatory authorities as therapeutic trials; fundraising may be difficult because of the lack of commercial interests; and, methodologically, the established study designs have different rankings for their level of evidence [8].

Designs for natural history studies

In general, natural history studies can be performed with study designs that are identical to those for therapeutic clinical trials. In natural history studies, however, the levels of evidence in well-established study designs are different from those seen in clinical trials. The ideal natural history study assesses, in a prospective and controlled fashion, all relevant disease-specific aspects, including survival, factors interfering with the quality of life (eg, pain, dysphagia, diarrhea), general and disease-specific complications, hospitalizations, surgical procedures, absenteeism, and direct and indirect costs. The study should have a disease-adjusted time frame and should include an appropriate number of affected individuals as well as a representative, nonaffected control population. Following increasing levels of evidence, each study design discussed here can be used to assess the natural history of a given disease [8].

Case reports

Especially for novel diseases, case reports—single-spot observations—may be of importance in drawing attention to a previously unrecognized aspect of a particular disease. Their level of evidence, however, is limited by the risk that the case actually may report a phenomenon not related to, or not even representative of, the particular disease. This study type thus has the lowest level of evidence. Conclusions fashioned from case reports always require confirmation by more robust ascertainments.

Case series

The pooling of observations in case series allows a more precise description of a phenomenon than that provided by a single case report. The weakness of case series is that the documentation of the cases does not follow a previously defined protocol and thus may differ among the study participants. Additionally, case series have an inherent risk of a selection bias with consecutive misinterpretations.

Database analyses

In general, in a database, the information is collected continuously without a predefined goal. Databases therefore contain large amounts of data but pose a difficulty in performing an analysis that focuses on a particular issue. Nevertheless, databases are good instruments for recruiting participants for cohort studies.

Placebo-group analyses

Placebo-controlled trials are well established for assessing the efficacy and safety of new medications. The placebo groups from randomized, double-blind trials are well-defined groups of patients who are followed in accordance with predefined protocols. The analysis of a placebo group therefore provides a comprehensive description of the natural history of a given disorder. A placebo-group analysis is the only type of interventional study that can be used to assess the natural history of a disease; all other methods are observational studies. The value of the evidence from this type of study for natural history investigations is not as high as for therapeutic trials, however, because in a particular trial the application of a placebo and the follow-up examinations are interventions that themselves may interfere with the natural course of a disease. Furthermore, clinical trials normally cover only a limited follow-up period, and this period may not be long enough to assess the course of chronic, long-standing diseases.

Cohort studies

Observational cohort studies are considered the reference standard for natural history studies. In a cohort study, a group of individuals is followed over time, following a previously defined protocol. If therapeutic interventions cannot be avoided during the follow-up period, all medications, hospitalizations, and endoscopic and surgical procedures are recorded. In a classic cohort study, the participants are included in the cohort before the end point of interest (eg, the appearance of EE) occurs. The natural history cohort is an exception to this rule, because all individuals included in the cohort are affected with the given disease. This difference creates the limitation that the description of the natural course lacks a comparison. To eliminate this drawback, a control population of healthy individuals is included, according to a case-control technique. This controlled-cohort type of study has the highest level of evidence among natural history studies. Because these studies are time-consuming, expensive, and limited by ethical considerations, only few natural history studies follow this design.

Natural history of eosinophilic esophagitis

Which data characterize the natural history of eosinophilic esophagitis?

In reading this article, it is important to keep in mind that, to date, only one prospective study describing the natural history of EE has been published [9]. Except for one analysis of a placebo group from the only randomized, double-blind, placebo-controlled therapeutic trial in children [10], all data cited in this article have been gathered from analyses of case series and case reports. To supplement this limited information and to illustrate specific points, the author has included a few unpublished observations from the EE clinic at the Kantonsspital Olten, which has provided care for more than 200 adult patients who had EE referred from throughout Switzerland.

Which parameters reflect the activity of eosinophilic esophagitis?

Clinicopathologically, EE is characterized by esophageal symptoms and a dense esophageal eosinophilia, both of which persist despite prolonged treatment with proton-pump inhibitors or in the face of normal pH monitoring of the distal esophagus [4,11]. Of note, EE cannot be defined using endoscopic findings: the diagnostic value of endoscopy is limited because eosinophilic inflammation evokes a variety of mucosal abnormalities, not a single cardinal sign or characteristic pattern [12,13]. (See the article by Fox, elsewhere in this issue.)

The clinical part of the EE definition is reflected by esophageal symptoms that vary according to the age of the patient. In adolescents and adults, dysphagia for solid food, starting as an unpleasant feeling during swallowing and escalating to food impaction, is the leading manifestation of EE [1–3,14]. In addition, a considerable subset of patients suffers from retrosternal pain that is independent of the swallowing act. This pain sometimes is induced by imbibing alcoholic beverages, white wine in particular. Pediatric patients who have EE show a broader spectrum of symptoms, including vomiting, abdominal pain, chest pain, dysphagia, food impaction, failure to thrive, and symptoms mimicking gastroesophageal reflux disease (GERD) [4,15]. (See the article by Putnam, elsewhere in this issue.)

The previously published (and subsequently slightly modified) grading score (Box 1) has proven to be a useful instrument in assessing the severity of the clinical aspects of EE in both practice and research [9]. Because patients who have EE naturally adapt their eating habits to avoid difficulty in swallowing, they must be instructed to answer the questions as if they exercised completely "normal" eating habits, without any restrictions or precautions. The severity of the dysphagia attacks also may vary within any individual patient. Patients thus should be instructed to list their "typical" attack, one which corresponds to their most common and frequently occurring attack. This grading score is of limited value in pediatric settings, because children present a wider spectrum of EE symptoms [15,16] and cannot express their discomfort as discernibly as adolescents or adults. (See the article by Putnam, elsewhere in this issue.)

The pathology part of the EE characterization is reflected by distinct histopathologic alterations. (See the article by Collins, elsewhere in this issue.)

What is known about the natural history of eosinophilic esophagitis?

Eosinophilic esophagitis is a chronic disease

Even the initial comprehensive descriptions of EE intimated the chronicity of this disorder; indeed, patients often recounted a history of dysphagia that had lasted for years before the diagnosis of EE was finally established [1,3]. As illustration, in the author and colleagues' first case series from 1994, patients had suffered from swallowing disturbances for an average of 4.3 years (range, 1–13 years) before receiving the diagnosis of EE [3]. A second indicator of the chronic nature of EE was the observation that relapses in symptoms and eosinophilic inflammation frequently occurred after the cessation of therapy. In one therapeutic study from Australia, 14 of 19 patients (74%) experienced a relapse within 3 months after cessation of successful topical corticosteroid

---

Box 1. Grading score for symptoms of eosinophilic esophagitis in adults

Frequency of dysphagia events
No dysphagia events
Once per month
Once per week
Several times per week
Once per day
Several times daily

Duration of dysphagia events
None
Less than 10 seconds
More than 10 seconds to 1 minute
More than 1 to 10 minutes
More than 10 to 60 minutes
More than 60 minutes

Intensity of dysphagia events
Swallowing unhindered without pain
Spontaneous passage with a slight feeling of retrosternal
  resistance (food passage without delay)
Spontaneous passage with a feeling of retching (food passage
  with a short delay)
Forced anterograde passage (short periods of obstruction,
  necessitating intervention, such as drinking)
Forced retrograde removal (complete obstruction, removable
  only by vomiting or retching)
Necessity for endoscopic intervention (continuous obstruction,
  not removable by patient)

Presence of retrosternal pain not related to swallowing
(occurring spontaneously or alcohol-induced)
No pain
Once per month
Once per week
Several times per week
Once per day
Several times daily

---

treatment [14]. Additional evidence that EE is a chronic disease was furnished by one study that focused primarily on the natural history in which 30 adults were followed for an average of 7 years [9]. The vast majority of the patients had persistent dysphagia over years, with a significant impact on the quality of life. This analysis further demonstrated that the eosinophilic infiltration persisted in all symptomatic patients.

Nevertheless, one important uncertainty remains, and that is whether children who have EE grow up to become adults who have EE or whether this chronic inflammation can be outgrown. Unfortunately the natural history of EE has not been followed in children, but several observations indicate that the pediatric form of EE is clinically and histologically like the adult form, a chronic disease. For instance, it is common for children who have EE to have a parent with a long-standing history of dysphagia or even with documented esophageal strictures. In some cases, examination of esophageal biopsy slides from the parent reveals evidence of long-standing esophageal eosinophilia [17]. In addition, the phenomenon of symptom and inflammation relapse after cessation of successful treatment is as common in children as it is in adults [16] EE thus is currently considered a chronic disorder and harbors, if untreated, the potential and yet unmeasured risks of uncontrolled and persistent inflammatory process.

The activity of eosinophilic esophagitis may fluctuate spontaneously

In general, a chronic disease has the potential to follow several courses. (1) It may resolve spontaneously after a certain time with permanent resolution. (2) It may enter a temporary remission with subsequent relapse. (3) It may progress to a fixed stable state (burned out, but still abnormal). (4) It may follow a relentless progression.

Based on clinical observations, patients who have EE have a waxing and waning course that can occur independent of any therapeutic intervention. The analysis of the placebo group from a therapeutic trial investigating the efficacy of fluticasone propionate in pediatric patients who had EE provides evidence of the spontaneously occurring fluctuations in disease activity [10]. Fifteen children who had active EE, defined as having a peak infiltration of 24 or more eosinophils per high-power field (HPF) in the esophageal mucosa, were assigned randomly to receive placebo and served as untreated controls for the fluticasone group. At study end, 11 placebo patients could be analyzed. Among these 11 patients inhaling placebo, 1 (9%) achieved histologic remission, and 3 (27%) experienced resolution of vomiting during the 3-month study period. This trial thus demonstrates that, in children, EE may resolve spontaneously, at least for a limited time. Fig. 1 demonstrates that fluctuation in the disease activity occurs in adults as well.

The activity of eosinophilic esophagitis may fluctuate depending on exogenous allergens

In contrast to the established experience that the natural course of EE is independent of exogenous factors, at least one environmental factor may influence the activity of EE. Fogg and coworkers [18] reported a 21-year-old female patient who had EE and concomitant allergic asthma and rhinitis,

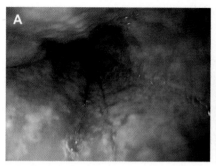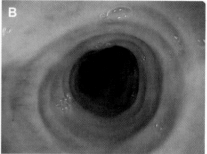

Fig. 1. Spontaneous fluctuation in eosinophilic esophagitis activity. Endoscopic pictures from a 45-year-old man who had a history of dysphagia commencing in 1998 and a diagnosis of EE in 2000. (*A*) An endoscopy performed during a symptomatic relapse revealed a severely inflamed esophageal mucosa covered with white exudates and more than 150 eosinophils per HPF. The patient was screened for a therapeutic trial and received no treatment. The dysphagia then disappeared spontaneously. (*B*) The examination performed 3 months later, during pollen season, revealed that the mucosa had resolution of the acute exudates and the presence of several corrugated rings. Histology revealed a peak infiltration of 12 eosinophils per HPF, a level that did not fulfill the established diagnostic criteria of EE.

with a worsening of symptoms during the pollen season. They further documented that the eosinophilic infiltration in the esophageal tissue paralleled the clinical course: symptoms and eosinophils were almost absent during the winter season, but both symptoms and inflammation relapsed during the pollen season. This case, together with a report of seasonal variation in EE incidence, with the lowest diagnostic rate during the winter period when the levels of outdoor allergens are low [19], indicates that inhalant allergens may play a pathogenic role in the development of EE.

Eosinophilic esophagitis does not seem to limit life expectancy

When one is confronted with a new disease, the first crucial question usually focuses on life expectancy and, in particular, on the risk of a fatal outcome. In the 11.5-year follow-up study by the author and colleagues [9], all 30 adults survived in good health and with stable nutrition. Furthermore, in their database of more than 200 adolescents or adult patients during the last 17 years, no EE-related death has been registered. This information concurs with the current literature that reports no fatal outcomes for patients who have EE. Nevertheless, the observation period for EE is still too short to make definitive statements regarding long-term survival.

Eosinophilic esophagitis impairs the quality of life

Eating and drinking replenish nutrients and also constitute fundamental pleasures in life. Esophageal disorders therefore may impinge substantially on the quality of life. In their study investigating the potential impact that

EE exerted on social and professional activities (ie, on the quality of life), the author and colleagues [9] used a structured interview format. In half of the patients, the dysphagia led to minor lifestyle changes, such as influencing menu choices with respect to food texture, consistently avoiding ingestion of solid foods without simultaneously imbibing liquids, or eschewing eating in restaurants. One of the 30 study participants (3%), a traveling engineer with many customer contacts who needed to eat frequently in restaurants, described how the disease exerted such a major impact on his life that he ultimately had to change jobs. For the remaining 14 patients (47%), the dysphagia exerted no impact on lifestyle.

In summary, EE substantially influences the quality of life in many adults, but most patients learn to cope with their symptoms. For children, no solid data specifically investigating this subject are available, but it can be speculated that, because of their more severe symptoms, the often imposed dietary restrictions, and the ensuing social consequences, the negative impact on quality of life probably is much greater in children than in adults [16,20].

Eosinophilic esophagitis is a disease restricted to the esophagus

To date, almost all reported patients who have EE suffer from an isolated esophageal disease, and esophageal involvement (eg, as is seen with eosinophilic gastroenteritis) tends to be the exception rather than the rule [2,21,22]. It has been shown, however, that in patients who have well-documented EE restricted to the esophagus, peripheral blood eosinophils are able to produce and release functional interleukin-13, and EE must be considered as being, at least in part, a systemic disorder [23]. This consideration prompted the author and colleagues to examine whether a spread from the esophagus-limited EE to eosinophilic gastroenteritis or to an idiopathic hypereosinophilic syndrome could occur and whether EE might be the beginning of a gastrointestinal or even systemic eosinophilic disorder. Endoscopically and histologically, these investigators found no signs of an eosinophilic gastritis or duodenitis. The laboratory tests revealed no abnormalities with respect to hepatic or pancreatic inflammation, and none of the patients developed a persistent, severe eosinophilia in the peripheral blood or an expansion of abnormal T-cell clones. In the ensuing follow-up period, the eosinophilic inflammation has remained limited to the esophagus in all patients [9]. Based on clinical experience and the literature to date, EE is a disease that does not transition to eosinophilic gastroenteritis or other diseases but remains limited to the esophagus. If new symptoms develop, or mucosal eosinophilia is identified in other parts of the gastrointestinal tract, alternative diagnostic possibilities should be reconsidered.

Eosinophilic esophagitis may lead to a remodeling of the esophagus

From other disorders, such as asthma, it is well known that chronic and persistent eosinophilic inflammation can induce irreversible structural changes in the affected organ [24]. In asthma, this so-called "remodeling" refers to structural changes that include subepithelial fibrosis and angiogenesis, leading finally to a loss of function [24]. Transforming growth factor beta 1 (TGF-β1) plays a crucial role in this process, because patients who have asthma have elevated levels of this profibrotic molecule, and an inhibition of TGF-β1 expression reduces the development of remodeling signs [25]. (See the article by Chehade, elsewhere in this issue.)

Murine and translational studies support a role for eosinophils in the development of structural abnormalities observed in the esophageal mucosa [26]. In patients who have EE, the histologic analysis of the subepithelial compartments in the esophagus is hampered because biopsy samples contain almost exclusively epithelial structures. Nonetheless, the author and colleagues obtained adequate subepithelial tissue to permit a representative qualitative analysis in 7 of the 30 patients (23%). In the subepithelial compartments of 6 of these 7 patients (86%), the investigators measured increased fibrous tissue, with thickening and alteration in the subepithelial architecture [9]. This observation has been supported by several later studies that also detected esophageal fibrosis in subepithelial layers [27–29]. For instance, Aceves and colleagues [30] recently identified subepithelial structural alterations in the esophagi of children who had EE. The investigators examined seven children who had a healthy esophagus, seven children who had reflux esophagitis, and seven children who had EE. They found an esophageal mucosa with significantly increased fibrosis, vascularity, and vascular activation in the subepithelial compartment of all patients who had EE. These alterations were not observed in patients who had reflux esophagitis [30]. In contrast to the patients who had GERD and to normal controls, children who had EE demonstrated increased TGF-β1 expression in their esophageal mucosa. It is interesting to speculate that these findings may correspond to endosonographic findings, demonstrating thickened mucosal, submucosal, and muscularis propria layers in the esophagus of patients who have EE [31].

In summary, the chronic eosinophilic inflammation in EE leads to an irreversible remodeling of the esophagus that probably is responsible for several disease-inherent complications. Whether this process develops in all patients who have EE or whether it occurs in only a subset of patients is not clear, however. It also remains to be determined whether this remodeling is dependent on the activity of the underlying inflammation and whether it can be prevented with therapeutic measures.

Eosinophilic esophagitis has not been associated with increased risk of premalignant or malignant conditions

Many immune-mediated, chronic, inflammatory diseases of the gastrointestinal tract (eg, chronic-atrophic gastritis and ulcerative colitis) carry an increased risk of developing local malignancies. Furthermore, patients who have chronic eosinophilic disorders are characterized by abnormal

T-cell clones and increased risk for lymphoproliferative disorders [32,33]. In the natural history study by the author and colleagues [9], all patients were examined thoroughly for malignant and premalignant conditions at the site of the inflammation and in the peripheral blood. No malignant tumors or dysplasias were detected in the esophagus, either endoscopically or histologically. Additionally, the flow cytometric analysis of the peripheral lymphocytes did not reveal any evidence of T-cell clones or lymphoproliferative diseases. After 15 years of collective follow-up of 200 patients, no local or systemic premalignant or malignant condition related to EE has been identified, and no case series have been yet reported. The author and colleagues therefore consider the risk for developing malignancies in EE as low, but extended observation is needed before this possibility can be excluded irrefutably.

Predictive factors for clinical course of patients who have eosinophilic esophagitis

Two predictive factors have been identified to date. One concerns the natural course, and the other concerns the response to therapy. For adult patients, those who have a peripheral eosinophilia experience more dysphagia attacks during the course of the disease than do those who have normal peripheral blood counts [9]. Children who have IgE-mediated forms of EE do not respond as well to treatment with corticosteroids as do those who have nonallergic forms [10]. It still is too early, however, to define the significance of other potential predictive factors, such as age at presentation, gender, phenotype, or response to treatment.

Complications of eosinophilic esophagitis

The complications EE can be divided into two categories: complications that are direct sequelae of the uninfluenced (non-intervened) ongoing inflammation and therefore are related to the natural history of EE and complications related to medical or endoscopic interventions.

Disease-inherent complications

For many chronic inflammatory disorders (eg, asthma) and noninflammatory disorders (eg, diabetes), the underlying process itself, uninfluenced by intervention, may lead to long-term complications. Because EE is a typical representative of a chronic inflammatory disease, it is not surprising that the inflammation may result in local complications.

Eosinophilic esophagitis may lead to food impaction
Acute food impaction—a primary manifestation of dysphagia—is a leading and common complication of EE in children [15] as well as in adults

[14,27]. For example, 17 of 31 adult patients (60%) referred for a diagnostic work-up for food impaction received the diagnosis of EE [5]. This complication may occur at any stage of the disease, as an initial manifestation or after many years of EE duration. The risk of impaction primarily depends on the consistency of the food; particularly problematic are dry rice and fibrous meat (eg, chicken and beef). The first indication is a feeling of retrosternal resistance with a delayed passage of the bolus, precisely at the niveau of the impacted food, immediately followed by hypersalivation. Complete obstruction may resolve spontaneously or persist for hours. If the bolus is impacted in the proximal part of the esophagus, the patient occasionally can remove the food particle with forced regurgitation. This extremely disagreeable and frightening form of dysphagia is a sword of Damocles hanging permanently over almost all patients who have EE. It substantially impairs the quality of life and may affect the patient's lifestyle, profession, and social contacts. The best way to prevent food impaction is to treat the underlying inflammation and to dilate relevant strictures. In contrast, there is no established medical treatment for the management of an acute blockade. Calcium-channel blockers, nitroglycerin, and spasmolytic analgesics have no proven value. If the blockade persists for more than 1 hour, the chance of self-resolution is small, and the patient should be referred to an emergency gastroenterology service. The impacted bolus must be removed with a flexible endoscope. (See the article by Aceves and colleagues, elsewhere in this issue.) Rigid esophagoscopy is strongly discouraged in patients who have EE because of the potential increased relevant risk of perforation, as discussed in the later section in this article on procedure-related complications and in the article by Aceves and colleagues, elsewhere in this issue.

Short-segment esophageal narrowing

Short-segment stenoses or so-called "esophageal strictures" are a further well-known and frequently observed complication of EE in both children [15] and in adults [2,12,28,34]. One radiographic study documented strictures in 10 of 13 patients who had EE (77%) [2], and another endoscopic analysis identified strictures in 17 of 31 (57%) adult patients who had EE [12]. Endoscopy generally is considered more sensitive than radiography in detecting short-segment narrowing [27]. Despite the assumption that stricture formation represents a long-term sequela of EE, an analysis of one pediatric series demonstrates that strictures can occur even early in the course of EE [15]. The risk of stricture formation may be much lower in children than in adults, because in a barium contrast study in a large series of 381 pediatric patients, Liacouras and colleagues [16] found esophageal narrowing in only 24 patients (~ 6%). EE-associated strictures may have the appearance of a solitary ring, of a short ringed segment, of a short homogenous narrowed segment, or of normal-appearing mucosa that resist endoscope passage (Fig. 2) [35].

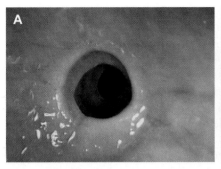 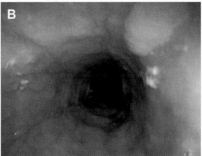

Fig. 2. Eosinophilic esophagitis with strictures of different sizes and types. (*A*) Endoscopic picture from a 27-year-old man who had EE and a 7-year history of dysphagia. The two neighboring rings in the proximal esophagus led to severe obstruction, impassable even with a small-caliber pediatric endoscope. (*B*) Endoscopic picture from a 54-year-old man who had EE and an 8-year history of dysphagia. The narrow mid-esophageal segment shows a cobble-stone- and ring-like structure not passable with a standard endoscope before therapy.

An analysis of 10 patients who had steroid-refractory strictures revealed that narrowed segments appear solitary or multiple and may involve the proximal, the middle, and/or the distal esophagus without any predilection [36]. The degree of the stenosis may vary from a mild form, found incidentally, to severe stenosis evoking severe swallowing disturbances and impairing endoscope passage.

If strictures lead to symptoms, treatment is indicated. As a first step, the author and colleagues recommend that several biopsies be taken from the strictured segment to distinguish inflammatory from fibrotic strictures to exclude a malignant stenosis. If endoscopy and histology indicate an inflammatory stricture, the author and colleagues recommend a course of topical corticosteroids (eg, 2 mg oral fluticasone, daily, for at least 4 weeks) as a first-line therapy. To assess the efficacy of the treatment, a clinical and endoscopic/histologic follow-up examination is recommended. For strictures refractory to this medication or for fibrotic strictures, gentle dilation is indicated. This procedure can be performed safely and usually leads to prompt symptom relief for up to 1 year. The underlying inflammation is not influenced by dilation, however. The role of anti-inflammatory drugs in primary and secondary prevention of stricture formation requires further clarification. (See the articles by Liacouras, and Aceves and colleagues, elsewhere in this issue.)

Long-segment esophageal narrowing

In EE, the narrowing also may encompass the full length of the esophagus. To date, this is the most severe disease-inherent complication of long-standing EE. Two different forms of long-segment stenoses have been reported. The literature refers to the first form as "trachealization" [37], "corrugated ringed esophagus" [38], "multiple-concentric ringed esophagus" [39], or "feline esophagus" [40]. All these terms describe an esophagus that has multiple, concentric, trachea-like and sometimes subtle and inconstant rings. The second form is described as "small-caliber esophagus" [41] and "congenital too small esophagi" [42]. These descriptions refer to a diffuse, non-ringed, long-segment esophageal stenosis. It has not yet clear why the narrowing process in EE may differ in size and type. This second form may be more apparent on an esophagram when the physiologic contractions that normally are visible are lost because of the severe underlying inflammation and remodeling. The therapeutic strategy for patients who have a long-segment stenosis is comparable to that discussed previously for short-segment stenoses. In accordance with the literature, the author and colleagues also recommend medical therapy first be undertaken for long-segment stenoses and that dilation be considered only in patients who do not respond to anti-inflammatory treatment [40]. (See the article by Aceves and colleagues, elsewhere in this issue.)

Eosinophilic esophagitis may lead to secondary gastroesophageal reflux disease

In addition to the leading symptom of dysphagia, up to 30% of patients who have EE experience retrosternal pain that is not associated with the act of swallowing [27,43]. Clinically, it may be difficult to distinguish between pain resulting from the eosinophilic inflammation and pain resulting from a coexisting reflux disease (eg, GERD). The definition of EE therefore includes the proviso that the symptoms must persist despite a prolonged therapy with proton-pump inhibitors [4]. In addition, reflux often is excluded by pH-monitoring studies before a diagnosis of EE finally is established [44]. It is common, however, to find that typical reflux symptoms that do respond to acid-suppressive medication appear during the long-term course of EE. In their case series, Remedios and colleagues [14] found that among 26 adult patients who had EE, 10 had coexisting reflux disease that had been confirmed by pH monitoring. Furthermore, based on motility studies, the authors found that 8 of the 10 patients who had coexisting reflux also had a dysfunction of the lower esophageal sphincter with reduced pressure. In contrast, endoscopically, no typical signs of a reflux disease, such as hiatal hernia, were reported. (See the article by Fox, elsewhere in this issue.) In summary, clinical observations and the findings from the study by Remedios and colleagues [14] suggest that, in EE, the chronic inflammation can lead to a dysfunction of the lower esophageal sphincter and thus to a clinically relevant, secondary reflux disease.

Eosinophilic esophagitis may predispose a patient to esophageal infections

On endoscopic or histologic examination it common to encounter *Candida albicans* infection in patients who have EE. Fungal infections are a well-known complication of therapy with topical corticosteroids, but, as illustrated in Fig. 3, esophageal candidiasis also can occur spontaneously in patients who have EE.

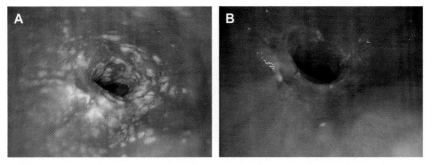

Fig. 3. Eosinophilic esophagitis with Candida superinfection. (*A*) Endoscopic picture of a 23-year-old man who had EE and a history of allergic rhinitis and dysphagia of 9 years' duration. The endoscopically noted inflamed mucosa from the distal third of the esophagus was covered by white membranes. Histology confirmed a *Candida albicans* infection that was treated with a topical antifungal medication and led to improvement of dysphagia. (*B*) Six weeks later, endoscopy revealed a mild stenosis with a few white exudates. Biopsies from this segment showed the typical sings of EE, with a peak infiltration of 38 eosinophils per HPF, thereby confirming the diagnosis of EE for which topical corticosteroids were administered.

In addition, EE also may lead to viral infections of the esophagus, as demonstrated in Fig. 4.

These two cases illustrate that, in pre-existing EE, fungal and viral infections may occur even in the absence of risk factors such as therapy with topical corticosteroids or immunosuppressive conditions.

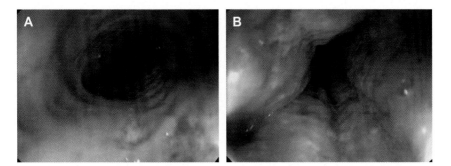

Fig. 4. Eosinophilic esophagitis with Herpes simplex superinfection. (*A*) Endoscopic pictures from a 25-year-old woman with a 9-year history of EE. After being almost completely symptom-free without any therapy for several years, the patient experienced acute severe odynophagia, fever, and malaise, almost preventing the ingestion even of liquids. An emergency upper endoscopy showed a homogenously severely inflamed esophageal mucosa with deep, ring-shaped ulcers. Histology revealed an acute, severe inflammation with a pure neutrophilic infiltration. Serologic analyses revealed a high antibody titer for Herpes simplex virus type 1 IgM. Herpes esophagitis was diagnosed, and antiviral medication commenced. Symptoms disappeared over the next few days. (*B*) Endoscopic control 5 weeks later showed an irregular surface of the esophageal mucosa but also the typical sings of EE in the form of extensive white exudates and some red furrows. Histologically, a dense eosinophilic infiltration of the esophageal epithelium with microabscesses was found.

Eosinophilic esophagitis may lead to spontaneous esophageal rupture
(Boerhaave's syndrome)

To date, three cases have been reported in which patients who had EE experienced a spontaneously occurring transmural esophageal rupture [45–47]. Two patients experienced the rupture during an acute episode with nausea and repeated vomiting, probably caused by a gastrointestinal infection. In the third patient the rupture occurred during repeated retching caused by an impacted food bolus. All patients had suffered from pre-existing dysphagia for years, but the diagnosis of EE had not been made before the esophageal rupture occurred. These three cases broaden the clinical spectrum and extend the risk profile of EE. Patients who have long-standing EE therefore are at risk for retching-induced esophageal rupture. Although their underlying diagnosis has not been identified, all three patients were treated surgically in accordance with established guidelines for esophageal perforations [48] and recovered well. EE-associated esophageal rupture therefore can be managed according to established standards and does not require a special procedure. Because Boerhaave's syndrome may be the first presentation of EE, the author and colleagues recommend that, after the patient has recovered from this life-threatening event, an upper endoscopy should be performed with biopsy sampling from the proximal and the distal esophagus to assess for mucosal inflammation that may benefit from medical or nutritional treatments

Procedure-related complications

Procedure-related complications also are discussed in the article by Aceves and colleagues, elsewhere in this issue.

Peri- and postprocedural pain

It is frequently observed that, in contrast to other patients, patients who have EE experience retrosternal pain during or even after a completely uneventful endoscopy [35] or during biopsy sampling. Furthermore, it is well known that after dilation of EE-related esophageal stenoses, patients may suffer from severe retrosternal pain, mostly associated with swallowing, for several days. This experience contrasts with the retrosternal pain unassociated with swallowing, which is a prevalent EE symptom. An analysis of efficacy and risks associated with the dilation of corticosteroid-refractory EE stenosis found that 6 of 10 patients suffered from severe odynophagia for an average of 2 days (range, 1–3 days) [36]. Peri- and postprocedural retrosternal pain therefore is a common and almost EE-specific problem.

This abnormal behavior of the EE esophagi must be taken into account if invasive examinations (eg, endoscopies, endoscopic ultrasound examinations, and manometric studies) and endoscopic therapies are planned. This behavior has the following practical consequences:

1. All procedures must be performed extremely gently.
2. Procedures should be performed under sedation.

3. The patient must be informed about this potential complication before the procedure is performed.

Procedure-related esophageal perforation

The esophagus is a hidden organ, and invasive procedures, such as upper endoscopy, frequently are required for diagnostic or surveillance purposes that are usually accompanied by a small risk of perforation. In contrast, patients who have EE often require therapeutic procedures, including removal of impacted food or dilation of strictures, and have a substantially increased risk of mucosal renting or even perforation [40]. This particularity is caused by a remodeling process [30] that results in an extremely fragile, inelastic, and rigid esophageal wall structure that tears easily [49]. To date, four esophageal perforations have been reported. One occurred after simple passage of the endoscope [40], one occurred after dilation [50], and two developed during an attempt to remove impacted food by rigid endoscopy [47]. All patients had intense chest pain immediately after the procedure, and the clinically suspected perforation was confirmed by CT scan, which revealed either a frank perforation with pneumomediastinum and pneumoperitoneum or a sealed perforation with intramural air in the esophagus. All four patients were treated conservatively and recovered completely without any further complications. Fig. 5 illustrates this life-threatening complication in a patient in whom a procedure-related perforation occurred during an ear, nose, and throat surgeon's attempt to remove impacted food with rigid esophagoscopy.

In summary, at least four procedure-related esophageal perforations have been reported. Half of these life-threatening complications occurred during a rigid esophagoscopy for removing impacted food. Intense retrosternal and upper abdominal pain after a diagnostic or therapeutic procedure is performed should raise the suspicion of perforation. All four cases were

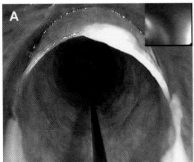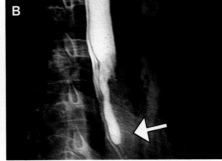

Fig. 5. Eosinophilic esophagitis with esophageal dissection. (*A*) Flexible endoscopy in a 37-year-old woman who had a 20-year history of dysphagia, performed immediately after an ear, nose, and throat surgeon's attempt to remove an impacted bolus using rigid esophagoscopy. A complete and circular dissection of the esophageal wall can be seen. (*B*) Esophagography of the same patient showing a huge dissection channel (*white arrow*) with a compression of the remaining esophageal lumen.

manageable without surgery. Close monitoring under ICU conditions, naso-gastric intubation, total parenteral nutrition, and parenteral application of antibiotics may be necessary. Of note, rigid esophagoscopy seems to be impose increased risks of perforation than flexible endoscopy and should be strongly discouraged in patients who have EE.

Summary

Based on the information available, it is clear that EE is a chronic and persisting or a chronic and relapsing disease that, left untreated, probably leads to irreversible structural alterations of the esophagus. Nevertheless, the knowledge of the natural history of EE and of the underlying mechanisms leading to the perpetuation of this inflammation [11] is still limited, and many aspects and complications may still be unknown. To learn more about the course and the complications of this recently described disorder, vigorous efforts are needed to carry out properly designed, long-term natural history studies in pediatric and adult patients.

Acknowledgments

The author and his colleagues would like to thank their Swiss gastroenterology colleagues for referring patients to our EE clinic in Olten. The author also thanks Dr. Stephan Bucher for his critical review and comments regarding the section on study design, Kathleen Bucher for her competent editorial work, and Drs. Christian Bussmann and Hanspeter Spichtin for their excellent pathology contribution.

References

[1] Attwood SE, Smyrk TC, Demeester TR, et al. Esophageal eosinophilia with dysphagia. A distinct clinicopathologic syndrome. Dig Dis Sci 1993;38:109–16.
[2] Vitellas KM, Bennett WF, Bova JG, et al. Idiopathic eosinophilic esophagitis. Radiology 1993;186:789–93.
[3] Straumann A, Spichtin HP, Bernoulli R, et al. [Idiopathic eosinophilic esophagitis: a frequently overlooked disease with typical clinical aspects and discrete endoscopic findings] [in German with English abstract]. Schweiz Med Wochenschr 1994;124:1419–29.
[4] Furuta GT, Straumann A. The pathogenesis and management of eosinophilic oesophagitis. Aliment Pharmacol Ther 2006;24:173–82.
[5] Desai TK, Stecevic V, Chang CH, et al. Association of eosinophilic inflammation with esophageal food impaction in adults. Gastrointest Endosc 2005;61:795–801.
[6] Noel RJ, Putnam PE, Rothenberg ME. Eosinophilic esophagitis. N Engl J Med 2004;351: 940–1.
[7] Kim DJ, Lifschitz CH, Bonis PA. Eosinophilic esophagitis. In: UpToDate in gastroenterology and hepatology. 2006;vol. 10/06.
[8] Hulley SB, Cummings SR, Browner WS, et al. Designing clinical research. 3rd edition. Philadelphia Baltimore, New York, London, Buenos Aires, Hong Kong, Sidney, Tokyo: Lippincott Wiliams & Wilkins, Wolters Kluwer; 2007. p. 97–106.

[9] Straumann A, Spichtin HP, Grize L, et al. Natural history of primary eosinophilic esophagitis: a follow-up of 30 adult patients for up to 11.5 years. Gastroenterology 2003;125:1660–9.

[10] Konikoff MR, Noel RJ, Blanchard C. A randomized, double-blind, placebo-controlled trial of fluticasone propionate for pediatric eosinophilic esophagitis. Gastroenterology 2006;131: 1381–91.

[11] Furuta GT, Liacouras CA, Collins MH, et al. Eosinophilic esophagitis in children and adults: a systematic review and consensus recommendations for diagnosis and treatment. Gastroenterology 2007;133:1342–63.

[12] Croese J, Fairley SK, Masson JW, et al. Clinical and endoscopic features of eosinophilic esophagitis in adults. Gastrointest Endosc 2003;58:516–22.

[13] Straumann A, Spichtin HP, Bucher KA, et al. Eosinophilic esophagitis: red on microscopy, white on endoscopy. Digestion 2004;70:109–16.

[14] Remedios M, Campbell C, Jones DM, et al. Eosinophilic esophagitis in adults: clinical, endoscopic, histologic findings, and response to treatment with fluticasone propionate. Gastrointest Endosc 2006;63:3–12.

[15] Khan S, Orenstein SR, Di Lorenzo C, et al. Eosinophilic esophagitis: strictures, impactions, dysphagia. Dig Dis Sci 2003;48:22–9.

[16] Liacouras CA, Spergel JM, Ruchelli E, et al. Eosinophilic esophagitis: a 10-year experience in 381 children. Clin Gastroenterol Hepatol 2005;3:1198–206.

[17] Rothenberg ME. Eosinophilic gastrointestinal disorders (EGID). J Allergy Clin Immunol 2004;113:11–28.

[18] Fogg MI, Ruchelli E, Spergel JM. Pollen and eosinophilic esophagitis [Letter]. J Allergy Clin Immunol 2003;112:796–7.

[19] Wang FY, Gupta SK, Fitzgerald JF. Is there a seasonal variation in the incidence or intensity of allergic eosinophilic esophagitis in newly diagnosed children? J Clin Gastroenterol 2007; 41:451–3.

[20] Walsh SV, Antonioli DA, Goldman H, et al. Allergic esophagitis in children: a clinicopathological entity. Am J Surg Pathol 1999;23:390–6.

[21] Dobbins JW, Sheahan DG. Behar J. Eosinophilic gastroenteritis with esophageal involvement. Gastroenterology 1977;72:1312–6.

[22] Mahajan L, Wyllie R, Petras R, et al. Idiopathic eosinophilic esophagitis with stricture formation in a patient with long-standing eosinophilic gastroenteritis. Gastrointest Endosc 1997;46:557–60.

[23] Schmid-Grendelmeier P, Altznauer F, Fischer B, et al. Eosinophils express functional IL-13 in eosinophilic inflammatory diseases. J Immunol 2002;169:1021–7.

[24] Reed CE. The natural history of asthma in adults: the problem of irreversibility. J Allergy Clin Immunol 1999;103:539–47.

[25] Cho JY, Miller M, Baik KJ, et al. Immunostimulatory DNA inhibits transforming growth factor-beta expression and airway remodeling. Am J Respir Cell Mol Biol 2004; 30:651–61.

[26] Mishra A, Hogan SP, Brandt EB, et al. An etiological role for aeroallergens and eosinophils in experimental esophagitis. J Clin Invest 2001;107:83–90.

[27] Potter JW, Saeian K, Staff D, et al. Eosinophilic esophagitis in adults: an emerging problem with unique esophageal features. Gastrointest Endosc 2004;59:355–61.

[28] Parfitt JR, Gregor JC, Suskin NG, et al. Eosinophilic esophagitis in adults: distinguishing features from gastroesophageal reflux disease: a study of 41 patients. Mod Pathol 2006;19:90–6.

[29] Mueller S, Aigner T, Neureiter D, et al. Eosinophil infiltration and degranulation in oesophageal mucosa from adult patients with eosinophilic oesophagitis: a retrospective and comparative study on pathological biopsy. J Clin Pathol 2006;59:1175–80.

[30] Aceves SS, Newbury RO, Dohil R, et al. Esophageal remodeling in pediatric eosinophilic esophagitis. J Allergy Clin Immunol 2007;119:206–12.

[31] Fox VL, Nurko S, Teitelbaum, et al. High-resolution EUS in children with eosinophilic "allergic" esophagitis. Gastrointest Endosc 2003;57:30–6.

[32] Bauer S, Schaub N, Dommann-Scherrer CC, et al. Long-term outcome of idiopathic hypereosinophilic syndrome — transition to eosinophilic gastroenteritis and clonal expansion of T-cells. Eur J Gastroenterol Hepatol 1996;8:181–5.

[33] Simon HU, Plötz SG, Dummer R, et al. Abnormal clones of T cells producing interleukin-5 in idiopathic eosinophilia. N Engl J Med 1999;341:1112–20.

[34] Feczko PJ, Halpert RD, Zonca M. Radiographic abnormalities in eosinophilic esophagitis. Gastrointest Radiol 1985;10:321–4.

[35] Van Rosendaal GM, Anderson MA, Diamant NE. Eosinophilic esophagitis: case report and clinical perspective. Am J Gastroenterol 1997;92:1054–6.

[36] Schoepfer AM, Gschossmann J, Scheurer U, et al. Esophageal strictures in eosinophilic esophagitis: dilation is an effective and safe therapeutic alternative after failure of topical corticosteroids. Endoscopy 2007, in press.

[37] Langdon DE. "Congenital" esophageal stenosis, corrugated ringed esophagus, and eosinophilic esophagitis. Am J Gastroenterol 2000;95:2123–4.

[38] Langdon DE. Corrugated ringed esophagus. Am J Gastroenterol 1993;88:1461.

[39] Siafakas CG, Ryan CK, Brown MR, et al. Multiple esophageal rings: an association with eosinophilic esophagitis: case report and review of the literature. Am J Gastroenterol 2000;95:1572–5.

[40] Kaplan M, Mutlu EA, Jakate S, et al. Endoscopy in eosinophilic esophagitis: "feline" esophagus and perforation risk. Clin Gastroenterol Hepatol 2003;1:433–7.

[41] Vasilopoulos S, Murphy P, Auerbach A, et al. The small-caliber esophagus: an unappreciated cause of dysphagia for solids in patients with eosinophilic esophagitis. Gastrointest Endosc 2002;55:99–106.

[42] Langdon DE. Corrugated ringed and too small esophagi. Am J Gastroenterol 1999;94:542–3.

[43] Orenstein SR, Shalaby TM, DiLorenzo C, et al. The spectrum of pediatric eosinophilic esophagitis beyond infancy: a clinical series of 30 children. Am J Gastroenterol 2000;95:1422–30.

[44] Kelly KJ, Lazenby AJ, Rowe PC, et al. Eosinophilic esophagitis attributed to gastroesophageal reflux: improvement with an amino acid-based formula. Gastroenterology 1995;109:1503–12.

[45] Riou PJ, Nicholson AG, Pastorino U. Esophageal rupture in a patient with idiopathic eosinophilic esophagitis. Ann Thorac Surg 1996;62:1854–6.

[46] Cohen MS, Kaufmann AB, Palazzo JP, et al. An audit of endoscopic complications in adult eosinophilic esophagitis. Clin Gastroenterol Hepatol 2007;5:1149–53.

[47] Straumann A, Bussmann C, Zuber M, et al. Eosinophilic Esophagitis: Analysis of food impaction and perforation in 251 adult patients. Clin Gastroenterol Hepatol 2007 [under review].

[48] Tilanus HW, Bossuyt P, Schattenkerk ME, et al. Treatment of oesophageal perforation: a multivariate analysis. Br J Surg 1991;78:582–5.

[49] Straumann A, Rossi L, Simon HU, et al. Fragility of the esophageal mucosa: a pathognomonic endoscopic sign of primary eosinophilic eesophagitis? Gastrointest Endosc 2003;57:407–12.

[50] Eisenbach C, Merle U, Schirmacher P. Perforation of the esophagus after dilation treatment of dysphagia in a patient with eosinophilic esophagitis. Endoscopy 2006;38:E43–4.

ELSEVIER
SAUNDERS

Gastrointest Endoscopy Clin N Am
18 (2008) 119–132

GASTROINTESTINAL
ENDOSCOPY CLINICS
OF NORTH AMERICA

Eosinophilic Esophagitis: Association with Allergic Disorders

Amal Assa'ad, MD

*Division of Allergy and Immunology, Cincinnati Children's Hospital Medical Center,
3333 Burnet Avenue, MLC 2000, Cincinnati, OH 45229, USA*

When diagnosed with eosinophilic esophagitis (EE) based on the pathology results of a biopsy of the esophagus obtained at an esophago-gastroduodenoscopy, most patients or their parents verbalize their understanding of the biopsy results as: 'the esophagus is filled with allergy cells'. Given the known association of eosinophils with allergic disorders, it is quite intuitive that an allergic etiology for the disorder of EE is sought; with a hope for a cure if the allergen, expected to be a food allergen due to the gut localization of the eosinophilia, is identified and removed. The goal of this article is to unravel any source of bias that may lead to a preconceived conclusion and examine the clinical evidence for a true association of atopy with EE. The article will also examine the suitability of the current diagnostic methods to establish an association of EE with food allergy, and the significance of this association to the therapy and outcome of EE.

Sources of bias in linking atopy and eosinophilic esophagitis

*Allergic diseases and eosinophilic esophagitis are prevalent
in the pediatric population*

The atopic march [1] is known to start almost at birth with atopic dermatitis and food allergy and progresses to allergic rhinitis and asthma by 5 years of age. Although the age at diagnosis of EE is broad, with new literature now defining adult patients who have EE, most of the literature reports patients in the pediatric age range. Because there is a delay in the diagnosis, the onset of symptoms is believed to precede diagnosis by almost 2 years, giving a possibly even younger age of onset of the disorder than the published mean ages [2].

E-mail addresses: amal.assa'ad@cchmc.org; assaa0@cchmc.org

1052-5157/08/$ - see front matter © 2008 Elsevier Inc. All rights reserved.
doi:10.1016/j.giec.2007.09.001

*The symptoms of early childhood atopy and eosinophilic
esophagitis overlap*

Infants and toddlers who have food allergy often present with vague
symptoms of fussiness, abdominal pain and infantile colic, and formula intolerance ranging from spitting up to recurrent vomiting, leading to frequent
changes in the protein basis of the formula [3]. The presenting symptoms of
EE are abdominal pain, feeding intolerance, and food refusal [2]. The same
early management with frequent formula changes has been noted. Although
not studied systematically, the persistence of the symptoms, rather than the
type of symptoms, is the driving factor in pursuing a further diagnosis of EE
beyond food allergy [2].

*An increase in the number of eosinophils in the blood stream
or in the tissues has been a hallmark of atopic disorders*

Eosinophils are increased in the airway of subjects who have asthma, in
the nasal mucosa of subjects who have allergic rhinitis, and in the skin of
subjects who have atopic dermatitis [4]. In light of this eosinophilia observed
in tissue and secretions from patients who have allergic diseases, and the histologic finding of epithelial eosinophilia in EE, an allergic cause for EE has
been entertained. In this regard, the prevalent belief is that, although exposure to the allergen, whether food or environmental, does not lead to immediate symptoms, it is either the cumulative exposure or a delayed reaction
mechanism that results in the accumulation of eosinophils in the esophagus.

The converse hypothesis, which has not been pursued to the same degree,
could be true. Would some or most subjects who have atopy have a degree
of eosinophilic infiltration of the esophagus? Would that degree of eosinophilic infiltration of the esophagus amount to the level that would be diagnostic of EE? Would the symptoms of food allergy (eg, abdominal pain,
fussiness, or feeding intolerance) or of asthma (eg, cough) be attributable
to undiagnosed EE?

**Difficulties in establishing link between food allergies and eosinophilic
esophagitis**

The attempt to distinguish the role of food allergy in EE is complex because sensitization to environmental and food allergens is prevalent, particularly in the atopic population, and testing for food allergies is limited to
testing for IgE-mediated food allergic diseases. Sensitization refers to the
subject having produced IgE antibodies to the environmental or food
allergen. The IgE that circulates in the bloodstream can be measured with
the radioallergosorbent test (RAST) or similar laboratory techniques
(eg, the ImmunoCAP®, Madison, New Jersey) and the IgE that is attached
to the skin mast cells is detected by skin prick test (SPT). Food allergy is the

term reserved for clinical signs and symptoms occurring in a timely relation to the ingestion of a food.

Allergic sensitization

IgE-mediated sensitization

Because many of the data on the association of food and environmental allergens with EE have relied on demonstration of sensitization to the allergens, we need to first examine the background prevalence of this sensitization. One of the larger population-based studies that reported on prevalence of sensitization to environmental and food allergens is the Isle of Wight study, in which a birth cohort of 1456 Anglo-Saxon white children had allergy assessments with SPT to food and inhalant allergens at 4 and 10 years of age [5]. Any reaction with mean wheal diameter at least 3 mm greater than negative control was regarded positive. Of the 832 children who had skin tests at both ages, never-atopics, who had negative SPT on both occasions, constituted 68% of the group. Of the 32% atopics, 4% were early childhood atopics (ie, had positive SPT only at 4 years), 11% were delayed childhood atopics (ie, had positive SPT only at 10 years), and 17% were chronic childhood atopics (ie, had positive SPT both times). Children were assessed at 4 and 10 years of age with SPT to milk, hen eggs, soy, cod, and peanut. Overall, 47 (5.7%) had positive SPT to foods, with 33 having the positive tests at 4 years and an additional 14 developing new positive SPT to foods at 10 years. Food allergy was defined as vomiting, diarrhea, colic, or rash within 4 hours of ingesting a particular food on at least two occasions. The prevalence (18.6%) of food allergy, as defined by the previous historical clinical symptoms, was higher than the prevalence (5.7%) of positive SPT to foods, although the study does not clearly indicate the extent of the overlap between the 47 children who had positive skin tests to foods and the 69 atopic children who had historical clinical symptoms of food allergy. Clinical food allergy occurred in 13.9% of the never-atopic children (Fig. 1).

Although IgE attached to the skin mast cells is usually detected by using the SPT, only subjects who demonstrate clinical symptoms when exposed to the environmental allergen or when they ingest the food allergen are labeled as allergic. The amount of IgE and the dose of allergen that produce a clinical reaction vary by the allergen and by the individual, so that establishing diagnostic levels of IgE or diagnostic amounts of allergen applicable to all individuals has proved extremely difficult. Nasal provocation challenges have been used primarily in research protocols to determine allergic rhinitis, inhalation challenges have been used to determine airway reactivity to inhaled allergens, and oral food challenges have been used to determine clinical allergy to foods. Oral food challenges are the gold standard for identifying food allergens; these tests require the skills of a well-trained allergist.

Oral food challenges provide two important pieces of data. The first is that the clinical reactions are mostly immediate, with a range of a few

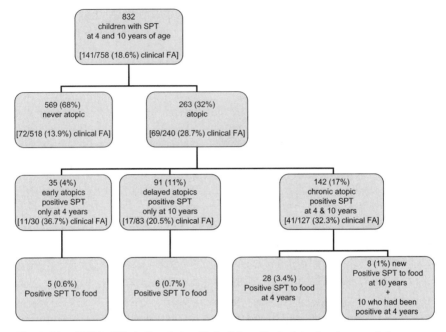

Fig. 1. Isle of Wight Whole Population Birth Cohort Study data showing population prevalence of sensitization, sensitization to foods and environmental allergens, and prevalence of clinical food allergy. 47/832 (5.7%) had positive skin prick tests to foods while 141/758 (18.6%) had clinical food allergy. (*Data from* Kurukulaaratchy RJ, Matthews S, Arshad SH. Defining childhood atopic phenotypes to investigate the association of atopic sensitization with allergic disease. Allergy 2005;60(10):1280–6.)

minutes to up to 2 hours and rarely extending to 4 to 6 hours after the challenge. The second is that even in the presence of large amounts of IgE, SPT of up to 8-mm diameter wheal, or peanut RAST of up to15 KU/L, clinical reactions may be absent. For some foods (eg, soy) no RAST level could be associated with clinical reactivity [6].

A few foods have emerged as the most common food allergens in the pediatric age group. Most of the skin test and RAST reports have included these foods, referred to as the top or big eight. These include cow milk, hen eggs, peanut, soy, tree nuts, fish, shellfish, and wheat. Consequently only these foods have been studied systematically. The prevalence of sensitization or clinical allergy to only a few other food allergens that have a regional predilection or that cross-react with plant pollen causing the oral allergy syndrome has been studied.

So how do food sensitization and clinically relevant food allergic diseases correlate with the disease EE? We studied 89 children who had EE who were similar to the Isle of Wight population in ethnic origin, being 94.4% white [2]. The EE patients were skewed in the distribution of gender with a higher preponderance of the male sex (78%) that is different from the almost equal distribution of genders in the general population. The age of patients in our study was a 6.6 ± 4.8 years (mean ± SD), 4.9 years median. Further subanalysis of the prevalence of positive skin tests by gender or by age showed no statistical difference, however. The striking difference in the results of SPT for environmental and food allergens is the much higher prevalence of positive SPT in the EE population, with 84.6% of the patients who had EE having positive SPT to environmental allergens compared with 32% in the general population and 77% having positive SPT to food allergens compared with 5.7% in the general atopic population (Fig. 2). The environmental allergens tested in both studies were equivalent, but the food allergens tested in the EE population were more extensive. If we only consider equivalent allergens, the percent of children in the Isle of Wight study who had positive SPT to the common food allergens peanut, milk, eggs, soy, and wheat were all less than 10%, whereas in the patients who had EE the percent with positive SPT to egg and peanut were 39% each, soy 34%, and cow milk 29%. Although there are no available age-, gender-, race-, year of testing-, or geographic location–matched controlled studies of the prevalence of atopy with sensitization to environmental and food allergens, the above comparison indicates that patients who have EE have a true higher prevalence of sensitization than the general population.

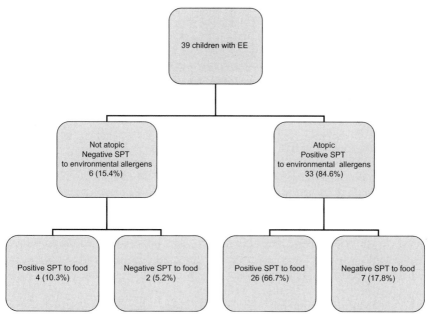

Fig. 2. Prevalence of sensitization to foods and environmental allergens in pediatric patients who have eosinophilic esophagitis. 30/39 (77%) had positive skin prick tests to foods. (*Data from* Assa'ad AH, Putnam PE, Collins MH, et al. Pediatric patients with eosinophilic esophagitis: an 8-year follow-up. J Allergy Clin Immunol 2007;119(3):731–8.)

Although the list of foods reported to cause a clinical reaction includes most edible plants and animal meats, reports are mostly individual clinical case reports. In the emerging literature that examined the association of EE with food allergy, testing has included longer lists of foods and patterns of sensitization and cross-sensitization have emerged. For example, Fiocchi and colleagues [7] determined that the prevalence of sensitization to beef in the general population is 6.5%, whereas a survey of perception of food allergy in Europe found a perception among parents of their children's food allergy to meat to range from approximately 4% to 15% depending on the country [8]. In the EE population, positive SPT to beef were found in 25% of patients tested, once again higher than the prevalence in the general population [3]. Beef has several allergens, but the most common positive SPT is to bovine serum albumin, which is also found in cow milk [9], hence the potential for cross-sensitization, a phenomenon seen commonly in SPT in the EE population. In the author's experience, when skin testing to large panels of food allergens, the positive SPT cluster in groups of cross-reacting allergens: peanuts and tree nuts to which sensitization is known to coexist; peanuts, peas, and beans, which are legumes; wheat, barley, and oats, which are grains; and beef, pork, and lamb, which are animal meats. Often, subjects who are sensitized to plant pollens, trees, grasses, and weeds are cosensitized to fruits and vegetables and present with clinical reactivity that has been termed the oral allergy syndrome because of the preponderance of mouth itching and tongue tingling [10,11].

Delayed IgE-mediated and non–IgE-mediated sensitization

In a quest for an association between food allergy and EE, and with the idea that EE is a manifestation of delayed reactions to foods or a non–IgE-mediated immunologic reaction, other methods of testing have emerged, namely the atopy patch test (APT). The APT had been used by various groups, primarily in Europe, to predict clinical reactivity to foods in two different situations. The first is the clinical situation in which IgE to a food is detectable by either SPT or RAST but the clinical reactivity is not immediate, rather it is delayed for 24 hours or more. The second situation occurs when clinical reactivity to a food can be documented by a food challenge, but no evidence of the presence of IgE to the food can be elicited by either SPT or RAST tests. Before the use of APT in patients who have EE, most of the published studies on its use in food allergy have examined its usefulness in patients who have atopic dermatitis; these studies have tested only a few common food allergens, including cow milk, hen eggs, wheat, and occasional other grains. Because of the lack of standardization of these tests and the lack of commercial extracts for them, the European Task Force on Atopic Dermatitis developed guidelines and proceeded with a large multicenter to test the correlation of the procedure with history of atopic dermatitis [12]. In the study, 314 patients (age range 1.6–80 years; 177 female: mean age 22.6 ± 14.3 years [median 22.09]; 137 male: mean age 22.9 ±

17.3 years [median 21.63]) who had atopic eczema in actual remission (ie, in a stable phase without acute flares of eczema) were enrolled. The group included 76 (24%) children (<10 years of age). The food extracts tested included egg white (740 µg/mL), wheat flour (158 µg/mL), and celery (44 µg/mL). Milk as a relevant food allergen in children could not be produced in a standardized APT preparation for the study. Grading of positive APT reactions was similar to the criteria used in conventional contact allergy patch testing (International Contact Dermatitis Research Group rules) with the modifications of the European Task Force on Atopic Dermatitis Consensus Meetings [13]; (ie, −, negative result; ?, only erythema, questionable; +, erythema, infiltration; ++, erythema, few papules [up to three]; +++, erythema, papules from four to < many; ++++, erythema, many or spreading papules; +++++, erythema, vesicles. A patch test with the pure vehicle served as negative control. Ten non-atopic subjects were used as controls. With these stringent methods, the study found that of 76 children only 11%, 15%, and 12% of patients had a positive patch test to eggs, wheat, and celery, respectively. A positive APT without SPT or IgE for the respective allergen was seen in 17% of the whole population of patients.

APT in subjects who had EE was pioneered by Spergel and colleagues with two studies where they have provided data supporting the validity of APT with a diagnostic power for identification of "offending foods" and pursuing dietary interventions [14–16]. Reporting on 146 patients who had EE, they found that 85% of the patients had at least one positive result on APT. Despite the high rate of sensitization detected by SPT and APT methods per patient, sensitization detected to the same food by both testing methods concomitantly was low, with only 7% of food test results found to be positive by both SPT and APT. In the 146 patients, the list of foods giving a positive APT and the frequency distribution in descending order was: corn (35, 24%), soy (26, 18%), wheat (25, 17%), milk (22, 15%), rice and chicken (21 each, 14%), beef and potato (20 each, 13.7%), egg (18, 12%), peas (9, 6%), and peanut (1, 0.7%). The peanut results may reflect fewer subjects tested by the APT because of large wheal and flare to skin tests [15]. The only other large series published on the results of APT in patients who had EE is the one from our center, in which patch tests were placed on a subset of 38 of 89 patients [2]. Fourteen (37%) had a positive APT. Of these patients, 5 (36%), 5 (36%), 2 (14%), 1 (7%), and 1 (7%) had 1, 2, 3, 5, and 10 positive foods, respectively. APT identified as atopic only an additional 5 (13%) patients who were SPT-negative but APT–positive. The foods giving positive APT were beef (5, 36%); lamb, oat, rye, soy, and wheat (4 each, 28%); corn, egg, ham, pear, and veal (2 each, 14%); and chicken, peach, tomato, turkey, and potato (1, 7% each). The absence of cow milk and peanuts from our list is explained by the high prevalence of positive skin tests to these foods in our population, which precluded putting an APT to them. Of both studies lists, the only food APT that can be compared with the European prevalence study are those to egg and wheat, and in both instances the EE population in the Spergel and Assa'ad studies had a slightly higher prevalence of positive APT compared with the atopic dermatitis population (egg: 12% and 14%, respectively, versus 11%; wheat: 17% and 28% versus 15%, for the pediatric age subset in the atopic dermatitis population). The prevalence of patients who have positive APT is also higher in the Spergel and Assa'ad studies than the atopic dermatitis population (85% and 37%, respectively, versus 10%). Given the above results of the European Task Force on Atopic Dermatitis, further work to standardize the reagents used in APT and the interpretation of the tests is clearly needed.

Atopic disorders

Case reports and case series on EE have reported that atopic disorders, allergic rhinitis, asthma, atopic dermatitis, and food allergy are common among patients who have EE. The true prevalence of atopic disorders, and particularly of a combination of several disorders, varies with the date of the study and with the population studied. Because food allergy is the disorder that has been proposed to have pathogenetic implications in EE, we first need to establish what is known about the prevalence of food allergy. Keeping in mind that food allergy is a term that is frequently used loosely to denote any adverse reaction to a food and is only infrequently confirmed by an oral food challenge, the prevalence of food allergy is often obtained through telephone surveys. A recent meta-analysis found self-reported prevalence of food allergy varied from 1.2% to 17% for milk, 0.2% to 7% for egg, 0% to 2% for peanuts and fish, 0% to 10% for shellfish, and 3% to 35% for any food [17], whereas a recent survey limited to children in Europe found a prevalence of parentally perceived food allergy in children of 4.7%. The most affected group was 2- to 3-year-olds with a prevalence of 7.2% [8].

Determination of link between atopy and eosinophilic esophagitis

In an attempt to further identify the link between EE and atopic disorders, a comprehensive review of the English language publications between 1976 and 2007 (inclusive) was performed using the term "eosinophilic esophagitis." Some 257 articles were retrieved and when these were further narrowed with the terms "human" and "atopy" or "allergy" or "skin test" a total of 69 articles were identified. Of these, 32 publications were reviews or editorials [18–49], one was a meta-analyses [50] and an additional 9 had no patient characteristics with regard to skin tests, RAST tests, or history of atopy [51–59]. In total, 28 articles were reviewed and tabulated for patient characteristics regarding coexisting atopic disorders and sensitization by skin tests or RAST to food and environmental allergens [2,14,15,60–83].

Articles reporting atopic characteristics in patients who had EE included a total of 1037 subjects, with 18 subjects reported as individual case reports and 1019 reported in case series; reporting on the same series of subjects from the same center in consecutive publications could not be ruled out. The geographic distribution of the reports covered many states in the United States (Ohio, Pennsylvania, Minnesota, Massachusetts, and California) and a few countries around the world, including Canada, Switzerland, Italy and Spain. Cumulatively, 179 subjects were tested for food allergens by SPT, of whom 127 (70%) and 101 (56%) were reported positive to foods and environmental allergens tested, respectively. The number tested with RAST was much lower, except for 2 case series, composed of 102 and 30 subjects, of whom 40 and 24 were reported positive by RAST, respectively [62,80]. Studies that reported on history of atopy included 709 subjects; 288 (41%) had a history of atopy that included one or more of the following disorders: asthma, allergic rhinitis, eczema, urticaria, or food allergy. When subjects were divided according to their atopic status, Bullock and colleagues found a cytokine profile discriminating between atopic and non-atopic individuals who had EE [65]. In a similar study, Noel and colleagues found that response to steroids applied topically to the esophagus was decreased in the atopic individuals [84].

Usefulness of food allergy testing in the diagnosis and management of eosinophilic esophagitis

The above discussion provides strong evidence that atopy is a marker of subjects who have EE, and plays a role in the pathogenesis of the disorder. The question arises: how can this information be used for better diagnosis and treatment? We have shown that there is an almost 2-year delay from the onset of symptoms to the diagnostic endoscopy [2]. A clinical scenario can be entertained in which children who present with the gastrointestinal complaints consistent with those of EE would receive SPTs to foods and environmental allergens. For those who would have positive responses consistent with the ones seen in the EE population, or in whom an obvious cause for their GI complaints is not identified (anatomic malformation, lactose intolerance, and so forth), an endoscopy would be recommended.

Regarding treatment, there is still a continuous debate in the literature about the influence of dietary manipulations on the symptoms and pathology of EE. The published studies in the pediatric population with a large patient series are all analyses of retrospectively collected data [2,15,24,49,74,77,84,85]. The dietary interventions varied from feeding only a non–protein-based elemental diet, specific food elimination based on the results of SPT and APT, and specific food elimination based on known common food allergens, namely cow milk protein, egg, soy, wheat, peanut, and seafood. Spergel and colleagues [22], analyzing specific food-elimination diets, have eventually produced a list of causative foods that includes common food allergens (cow milk, egg, soy, wheat, and peanut) in addition to uncommon food allergens, including animal proteins (beef and chicken) and plant proteins (corn, rice, oat, barley, and potato). In an analysis of 94 patients who had evidence of response, either by improvement or by worsening of EE, based on a single food eliminated or reintroduced at a time, Spergel and colleagues found the number of patients and the number of causative foods for each patient to be: 18, 30, 22, 14, 5, and 1 patients had 1, 2, 3, 4, 5, 6, and 7 foods, respectively (Jonathan M. Spergel, MD, PhD, personal communication, 2007). The only prospective placebo controlled and randomized trial of specific food eliminations was conducted in 6 adults who had EE who were sensitized to wheat and rye by serum-specific IgE measurements, and who were not sensitized to the common food allergens [79]. The patients did not experience any immediate EE symptoms on a blinded oral challenge with the food, and did not experience histologic resolution of EE after a complete elimination of wheat and rye.

Comparing a six common foods–elimination diet and an elemental diet, the elemental diet produced better resolution of EE, as indicated by the number of responders and the decrease in the number of eosinophils on pathology specimens of the esophagus [85]. Our retrospective analysis comparing various therapeutic interventions, again including elemental diets or selective elimination diets, showed that the selective elimination diet had a statically significant association with nonresolution of EE [2]. Liacouras and colleagues [74] also found that elemental diet was associated with the highest rate of resolution of EE and persistence of resolution for at least 6 months. Taken together the data and experience suggest an association of EE with diet, although distinctly identifying a list of foods in each patient, even using SPT and APT, is a tedious, long process, and generalizations are not yet possible. Although a large-scale prospective blinded placebo-controlled trial would be difficult to design because of the long list of implicated foods and the chronicity of the disorder, such a study is utterly needed.

No intervention studies have shown that environmental allergen avoidance is effective in resolution of EE. In clinical practice, most subjects who have environmental allergens sensitization (ie, with allergic rhinitis) receive either medical or immunotherapy treatment of the allergic rhinitis but nevertheless present with EE that is chronic despite continuation of the allergic rhinitis therapy.

The atopic status was predictive of less responsiveness to the medical therapies of EE [84]. Children who had atopy and EE had a distinctive cytokine profile and genetic signature that distinguished them from children who had other gastrointestinal disorders and from children who had EE but not atopy [64,65]. This finding led to seeking other therapies that address the atopic pathogenesis. Studies are underway using biologic modalities, including anti–IL-5 [81] and anti-IgE in the disorder [86].

In summary, atopy is more prevalent in subjects who have EE than in the general population. The diagnostic tools for atopy and their interpretation need to be examined constantly to improve on their predictive value in this patient population. Using the atopic characteristics in this patient population may improve diagnosis and provide further treatment modalities [86].

References

[1] Kjellman NI, Nilsson L. From food allergy and atopic dermatitis to respiratory allergy. Pediatr Allergy Immunol 1998;9(11 Suppl):13–7.

[2] Assa'ad AH, Putnam PE, Collins MH, et al. Pediatric patients with eosinophilic esophagitis: an 8-year follow-up. J Allergy Clin Immunol 2007;119(3):731–8.

[3] Assa'ad AH. Gastrointestinal food allergy and intolerance. Pediatr Ann 2006;35(10): 718–26.

[4] Rosenberg HF, Phipps S, Foster PS. Eosinophil trafficking in allergy and asthma. J Allergy Clin Immunol 2007;119(6):1303–10; quiz 1302–1311.

[5] Kurukulaaratchy RJ, Matthews S, Arshad SH. Defining childhood atopic phenotypes to investigate the association of atopic sensitization with allergic disease. Allergy 2005; 60(10):1280–6.

[6] Sampson HA, Ho DG. Relationship between food-specific IgE concentrations and the risk of positive food challenges in children and adolescents. J Allergy Clin Immunol 1997;100(4): 444–51.

[7] Fiocchi A, Bouygue GR, Restani P, et al. Accuracy of skin prick tests in IgE-mediated adverse reactions to bovine proteins. Ann Allergy Asthma Immunol 2002;89(6 Suppl 1):26–32.

[8] Steinke M, Fiocchi A, Kirchlechner V, et al. Perceived food allergy in children in 10 European nations. A randomised telephone survey. Int Arch Allergy Immunol 2007;143(4): 290–5.

[9] Restani P, Beretta B, Fiocchi A, et al. Cross-reactivity between mammalian proteins. Ann Allergy Asthma Immunol 2002;89(6 Suppl 1):11–5.

[10] Amlot PL, Kemeny DM, Zachary C, et al. Oral allergy syndrome (OAS): symptoms of IgE-mediated hypersensitivity to foods. Clin Allergy 1987;17(1):33–42.

[11] Ortolani C, Ispano M, Pastorello E, et al. The oral allergy syndrome. Ann Allergy 1988; 61(6 Pt 2):47–52.

[12] Darsow U, Laifaoui J, Kerschenlohr K, et al. The prevalence of positive reactions in the atopy patch test with aeroallergens and food allergens in subjects with atopic eczema: a European multicenter study. Allergy 2004;59(12):1318–25.

[13] Kunz B, Oranje AP, Labreze L, et al. Clinical validation and guidelines for the SCORAD index: consensus report of the European Task Force on Atopic Dermatitis. Dermatology 1997;195(1):10–9.

[14] Spergel JM, Beausoleil JL, Mascarenhas M, et al. The use of skin prick tests and patch tests to identify causative foods in eosinophilic esophagitis. J Allergy Clin Immunol Feb 2002; 109(2):363–8.

[15] Spergel JM, Andrews T, Brown-Whitehorn TF, et al. Treatment of eosinophilic esophagitis with specific food elimination diet directed by a combination of skin prick and patch tests. Ann Allergy Asthma Immunol Oct 2005;95(4):336–43.

[16] Spergel JM, Brown-Whitehorn T, Beausoleil JL, et al. Predictive values for skin prick test and atopy patch test for eosinophilic esophagitis. J Allergy Clin Immunol Feb 2007; 119(2):509–11.

[17] Rona RJ, Keil T, Summers C, et al. The prevalence of food allergy: A meta-analysis. J Allergy Clin Immunol Sep 2007;120:638–46.

[18] Zeiter DK, Hyams JS. Gastroesophageal reflux: pathogenesis, diagnosis, and treatment. Allergy Asthma Proc Jan-Feb 1999;20(1):45–9.

[19] Yan BM, Shaffer EA. Eosinophilic esophagitis: a newly established cause of dysphagia. World J Gastroenterol Apr 21 2006;12(15):2328–34.

[20] Wagelie-Steffen A, Aceves SS. Eosinophilic disorders in children. Curr Allergy Asthma Rep Nov 2006;6(6):475–82.

[21] Straumann A, Simon HU. The physiological and pathophysiological roles of eosinophils in the gastrointestinal tract. Allergy Jan 2004;59(1):15–25.

[22] Spergel JM, Brown-Whitehorn T. The use of patch testing in the diagnosis of food allergy. Curr Allergy Asthma Rep Jan 2005;5(1):86–90.

[23] Spergel JM. Eosinophilic oesophagitis and pollen. Clin Exp Allergy Nov 2005;35(11):1421–2.

[24] Spergel JM, Beausoleil J, Brown-Whitehorn T, et al. Authors' response to detection of causative foods by skin prick and atopy patch tests in patients with eosinophilic esophagitis: things are not what they seem. Ann Allergy Asthma Immunol Feb 2006;96(2):376–8.

[25] Spergel JM. Eosinophilic esophagitis in adults and children: evidence for a food allergy component in many patients. Curr Opin Allergy Clin Immunol Jun 2007;7(3):274–8.

[26] Sicherer SH, Leung DY. Advances in allergic skin disease, anaphylaxis, and hypersensitivity reactions to foods, drugs, and insects. J Allergy Clin Immunol Jun 2007;119(6):1462–9.

[27] Sicherer SH. Clinical aspects of gastrointestinal food allergy in childhood. Pediatrics Jun 2003;111(6 Pt 3):1609–16.

[28] Sgouros SN, Bergele C, Mantides A. Eosinophilic esophagitis in adults: what is the clinical significance? Endoscopy May 2006;38(5):515–20.

[29] Seibold F. Food-induced immune responses as origin of bowel disease? Digestion 2005;71(4):251–60.

[30] Salvatore S, Vandenplas Y. Gastro-oesophageal reflux disease and motility disorders. Best Pract Res Clin Gastroenterol Apr 2003;17(2):163–79.

[31] Rothenberg ME, Mishra A, Collins MH, et al. Pathogenesis and clinical features of eosinophilic esophagitis. J Allergy Clin Immunol Dec 2001;108(6):891–4.

[32] Rothenberg ME. Eosinophilic gastrointestinal disorders (EGID). J Allergy Clin Immunol Jan 2004;113(1):11–28; quiz 29.

[33] Nelson HS. Advances in upper airway diseases and allergen immunotherapy. J Allergy Clin Immunol Apr 2004;113(4):635–42.

[34] Murch SH. Clinical manifestations of food allergy: the old and the new. Eur J Gastroenterol Hepatol Dec 2005;17(12):1287–91.

[35] Mishra A, Hogan SP, Brandt EB, et al. An etiological role for aeroallergens and eosinophils in experimental esophagitis. J Clin Invest Jan 2001;107(1):83–90.

[36] Liacouras CA, Ruchelli E. Eosinophilic esophagitis. Curr Opin Pediatr Oct 2004;16(5):560–6.

[37] Liacouras CA, Markowitz JE. Eosinophilic esophagitis: A subset of eosinophilic gastroenteritis. Curr Gastroenterol Rep Jun 1999;1(3):253–8.

[38] Liacouras CA. Eosinophilic esophagitis: treatment in 2005. Curr Opin Gastroenterol Mar 2006;22(2):147–52.

[39] Katzka DA. Eosinophilic esophagitis. Curr Opin Gastroenterol Jul 2006;22(4):429–32.

[40] Hogan SP, Rothenberg ME. Eosinophil Function in Eosinophil-associated Gastrointestinal Disorders. Curr Allergy Asthma Rep Feb 2006;6(1):65–71.

[41] Hogan SP, Rothenberg ME. Review article: The eosinophil as a therapeutic target in gastrointestinal disease. Aliment Pharmacol Ther Dec 2004;20(11-12):1231–40.

[42] Heine RG. Pathophysiology, diagnosis and treatment of food protein-induced gastrointestinal diseases. Curr Opin Allergy Clin Immunol Jun 2004;4(3):221–9.

[43] Garcia-Careaga M Jr, Kerner JA Jr. Gastrointestinal manifestations of food allergies in pediatric patients. Nutr Clin Pract Oct 2005;20(5):526–35.

[44] Furuta GT. Eosinophilic esophagitis: an emerging clinicopathologic entity. Curr Allergy Asthma Rep Jan 2002;2(1):67–72.

[45] Foroughi S, Prussin C. Clinical management of eosinophilic gastrointestinal disorders. Curr Allergy Asthma Rep Jul 2005;5(4):259–61.

[46] Chehade M. IgE and non-IgE-mediated food allergy: treatment in 2007. Curr Opin Allergy Clin Immunol Jun 2007;7(3):264–8.
[47] Blanchard C, Wang N, Rothenberg ME. Eosinophilic esophagitis: pathogenesis, genetics, and therapy. J Allergy Clin Immunol Nov 2006;118(5):1054–9.
[48] Bischoff SC. Food allergies. Curr Gastroenterol Rep Oct 2006;8(5):374–82.
[49] Assa'ad A. Detection of causative foods by skin prick and atopy patch tests in patients with eosinophilic esophagitis: things are not what they seem. Ann Allergy Asthma Immunol Oct 2005;95(4):309–11.
[50] Norvell JM, Venarske D, Hummell DS. Eosinophilic esophagitis: an allergist's approach. Ann Allergy Asthma Immunol Mar 2007;98(3):207–14; quiz 207–214, 238.
[51] Fujiwara H, Morita A, Kobayashi H, et al. Infiltrating eosinophils and eotaxin: their association with idiopathic eosinophilic esophagitis. Ann Allergy Asthma Immunol Oct 2002; 89(4):429–32.
[52] Kelly KJ, Lazenby AJ, Rowe PC, et al. Eosinophilic esophagitis attributed to gastroesophageal reflux: improvement with an amino acid-based formula. Gastroenterology Nov 1995; 109(5):1503–12.
[53] Kokkonen J, Ruuska T, Karttunen TJ, et al. Mucosal pathology of the foregut associated with food allergy and recurrent abdominal pains in children. Acta Paediatr Jan 2001; 90(1):16–21.
[54] Nicholson AG, Li D, Pastorino U, et al. Full thickness eosinophilia in oesophageal leiomyomatosis and idiopathic eosinophilic oesophagitis. A common allergic inflammatory profile? J Pathol Oct 1997;183(2):233–6.
[55] Pentiuk SP, Miller CK, Kaul A. Eosinophilic esophagitis in infants and toddlers. Dysphagia Jan 2007;22(1):44–8.
[56] Plaza-Martin AM, Jimenez-Feijoo R, Andaluz C, et al. Polysensitization to aeroallergens and food in eosinophilic esophagitis in a pediatric population. Allergol Immunopathol (Madr) Jan-Feb 2007;35(1):35–7.
[57] Straumann A, Bauer M, Fischer B, et al. Idiopathic eosinophilic esophagitis is associated with a T(H)2-type allergic inflammatory response. J Allergy Clin Immunol Dec 2001; 108(6):954–61.
[58] Straumann A, Simon HU. Eosinophilic esophagitis: escalating epidemiology? J Allergy Clin Immunol Feb 2005;115(2):418–9.
[59] Taminiau JA. Gastro-oesophageal reflux in children. Scand J Gastroenterol Suppl 1997;223: 18–20.
[60] Aceves SS, Dohil R, Newbury RO, et al. Topical viscous budesonide suspension for treatment of eosinophilic esophagitis. J Allergy Clin Immunol Sep 2005;116(3):705–6.
[61] Aceves SS, Newbury RO, Dohil R, et al. Esophageal remodeling in pediatric eosinophilic esophagitis. J Allergy Clin Immunol Jan 2007;119(1):206–12.
[62] Aceves SS, Newbury RO, Dohil R, et al. Distinguishing eosinophilic esophagitis in pediatric patients: clinical, endoscopic, and histologic features of an emerging disorder. J Clin Gastroenterol Mar 2007;41(3):252–6.
[63] Anton Remirez J, Escudero R, Caceres O, et al. Eosinophilic esophagitis. Allergol Immunopathol (Madr) Mar-Apr 2006;34(2):79–81.
[64] Blanchard C, Wang N, Stringer KF, et al. Eotaxin-3 and a uniquely conserved gene-expression profile in eosinophilic esophagitis. J Clin Invest Feb 2006;116(2):536–47.
[65] Bullock JZ, Villanueva JM, Blanchard C, et al. Interplay of adaptive th2 immunity with eotaxin-3/c-C chemokine receptor 3 in eosinophilic esophagitis. J Pediatr Gastroenterol Nutr Jul 2007;45(1):22–31.
[66] Cheung KM, Oliver MR, Cameron DJ, et al. Esophageal eosinophilia in children with dysphagia. J Pediatr Gastroenterol Nutr Oct 2003;37(4):498–503.
[67] Dauer EH, Freese DK, El-Youssef M, et al. Clinical characteristics of eosinophilic esophagitis in children. Ann Otol Rhinol Laryngol Nov 2005;114(11):827–33.

[68] Dauer EH, Ponikau JU, Smyrk TC, et al. Airway manifestations of pediatric eosinophilic esophagitis: a clinical and histopathologic report of an emerging association. Ann Otol Rhinol Laryngol Jul 2006;115(7):507–17.

[69] De Angelis P, Markowitz JE, Torroni F, et al. Paediatric eosinophilic oesophagitis: towards early diagnosis and best treatment. Dig Liver Dis Apr 2006;38(4):245–51.

[70] Feczko PJ, Halpert RD, Zonca M. Radiographic abnormalities in eosinophilic esophagitis. Gastrointest Radiol 1985;10(4):321–4.

[71] Fogg MI, Ruchelli E, Spergel JM. Pollen and eosinophilic esophagitis. J Allergy Clin Immunol Oct 2003;112(4):796–7.

[72] Garrett JK, Jameson SC, Thomson B, et al. Anti-interleukin-5 (mepolizumab) therapy for hypereosinophilic syndromes. J Allergy Clin Immunol Jan 2004;113(1):115–9.

[73] Khan S, Orenstein SR, Di Lorenzo C, et al. Eosinophilic esophagitis: strictures, impactions, dysphagia. Dig Dis Sci Jan 2003;48(1):22–9.

[74] Liacouras CA, Spergel JM, Ruchelli E, et al. Eosinophilic esophagitis: a 10-year experience in 381 children. Clin Gastroenterol Hepatol Dec 2005;3(12):1198–206.

[75] Luis AL, Rinon C, Encinas JL, et al. Non stenotic food impaction due to eosinophilic esophagitis: a potential surgical emergency. Eur J Pediatr Surg Dec 2006;16(6):399–402.

[76] Martin-Munoz MF, Lucendo AJ, Navarro M, et al. Food allergies and eosinophilic esophagitis–two case studies. Digestion 2006;74(1):49–54.

[77] Orenstein SR, Shalaby TM, Di Lorenzo C, et al. The spectrum of pediatric eosinophilic esophagitis beyond infancy: a clinical series of 30 children. Am J Gastroenterol Jun 2000; 95(6):1422–30.

[78] Potter JW, Saeian K, Staff D, et al. Eosinophilic esophagitis in adults: an emerging problem with unique esophageal features. Gastrointest Endosc Mar 2004;59(3):355–61.

[79] Simon D, Straumann A, Wenk A, et al. Eosinophilic esophagitis in adults–no clinical relevance of wheat and rye sensitizations. Allergy Dec 2006;61(12):1480–3.

[80] Simon D, Marti H, Heer P, et al. Eosinophilic esophagitis is frequently associated with IgE-mediated allergic airway diseases. J Allergy Clin Immunol May 2005;115(5):1090–2.

[81] Stein ML, Collins MH, Villanueva JM, et al. Anti-IL-5 (mepolizumab) therapy for eosinophilic esophagitis. J Allergy Clin Immunol Dec 2006;118(6):1312–9.

[82] Teitelbaum JE, Fox VL, Twarog FJ, et al. Eosinophilic esophagitis in children: immunopathological analysis and response to fluticasone propionate. Gastroenterology May 2002; 122(5):1216–25.

[83] Yan BM, Shaffer EA. Eosinophilic esophagitis: an overlooked entity in chronic dysphagia. Nat Clin Pract Gastroenterol Hepatol May 2006;3(5):285–9.

[84] Noel RJ, Putnam PE, Collins MH, et al. Clinical and immunopathologic effects of swallowed fluticasone for eosinophilic esophagitis. Clin Gastroenterol Hepatol Jul 2004;2(7):568–75.

[85] Kagalwalla AF, Sentongo TA, Ritz S, et al. Effect of six-food elimination diet on clinical and histologic outcomes in eosinophilic esophagitis. Clin Gastroenterol Hepatol Sep 2006;4(9): 1097–102.

[86] Foroughi S, Foster B, Kim N, et al. Anti-IgE treatment of eosinophil-associated gastrointestinal disorders. J Allergy Clin Immunol Sep 2007;120(3):594–601.

ELSEVIER
SAUNDERS

Gastrointest Endoscopy Clin N Am
18 (2008) 133–143

GASTROINTESTINAL
ENDOSCOPY CLINICS
OF NORTH AMERICA

Basic Pathogenesis of Eosinophilic Esophagitis

Carine Blanchard, PhD[a,b],
Marc E. Rothenberg, MD, PhD[a,b,*]

[a]Division of Allergy and Immunology, Cincinnati Children's Hospital Medical Center,
3333 Burnet Avenue, Cincinnati, OH 45229, USA
[b]Department of Pediatrics, University of Cincinnati College of Medicine,
3333 Burnet Avenue, Cincinnati, OH 45229, USA

Eosinophilic esophagitis (EE) is characterized by a marked accumulation of eosinophils in the esophageal mucosa, suggesting a Th2 disease. In addition to "guilt by association," experimental models in mice implicate eosinophils in disease pathogenesis. However, eosinophils may neither be the first nor the only critical contributor in EE. Environmental exposure, allergen sensitization, eosinophils and other cells, molecules released, and genetic predisposition, all interplay in EE pathogenesis.

Environmental pathogenesis: a Th2 disease

Epidemiologic studies provided the first indirect information about the pathogenesis of EE. The allergic component of EE was apparent from the strong association of EE with allergic diseases (Fig. 1). About 70% of EE patients have current or past allergic diseases, or a positive skin prick test, especially to a variety of foods [1]. Of note, only a minority of EE patients present with food anaphylaxis, indicating distinct mechanisms compared with classical-IgE-mediated mast cell and basophil activation

This work was funded in part by the NIH #AI070235 and #AI45898 (M.E. Rothenberg), the Food Allergy and Anaphylaxis Network (FAAN) (M.E. Rothenberg), Campaign Urging Research for Eosinophil Disorders (CURED), the Buckeye Foundation (M.E. Rothenberg), The Food Allergy Project (M.E. Rothenberg), The American Heart Association #0,625,296B (C. Blanchard) and The Thrasher Research Fund NR-0014 (C. Blanchard).

* Corresponding author. Division of Allergy and Immunology, Cincinnati Children's Hospital Medical Center, 3333 Burnet Avenue, MLC 7028, Cincinnati, OH 45229.

E-mail address: rothenberg@cchmc.org (M.E. Rothenberg).

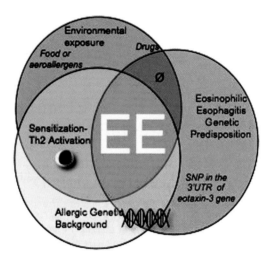

Fig. 1. Etiologic factors involved in EE development. More then 500 gene polymorphisms has been shown to be associated to allergic diseases, and the genetic context generated by the presence of these polymorphisms predispose individuals to asthma, atopic dermatitis, and food allergy, among other diseases. Although allergic diseases are common in the population, all allergic patients do not develop EE, suggesting that a specific genetic predisposition for EE might be required to develop EE. As such, a complex interplay between single nucleotide polymorphisms increases the risk of a Th2 inflammation in the esophagus. To date, only one single nucleotide polymorphism (SNP) has been associated with EE. This SNP is located in the 3'UTR of the eotaxin-3 gene (T/G +2496). All together, this complex genetic background and the environmental exposures (food and aeroallergens) contribute to the development of EE.

[1,2]. As such, a local esophageal population of allergen-specific IgE-producing B cells is possible. Indeed, EE patients without allergic disease still respond to an elemental diet [3,4]. Recently, EE has been found in two patients with anticonvulsant hypersensitivity syndrome [5]. Notably, withdrawal of carbamazepine completely restored the endoscopic appearance of the esophagus, suggesting that oral agents (in addition to food) could have an etiologic involvement in EE. Like EE, anticonvulsant hypersensitivity syndrome has a male predominance [5].

Patients with EE sometimes report seasonal variations in their symptoms and changes in their esophageal eosinophil levels [6,7], suggesting a role for aeroallergens. This was indeed recently supported by the study of Yamazaki and colleagues [8], wherein common food and environmental allergens induced cytokine production by peripheral blood mononuclear cells (PBMCs) in adult patients with EE. Production of interleukin (IL)-5 and IL-13 production by PBMCs in EE patients was increased, compared with healthy individuals, after stimulation with aero or food allergens. Thus, the immune responses in EE are characterized by enhanced production of Th2-associated cytokines in response to both food and environmental allergens. Finally, in a recent study examining intracellular staining of PBMC cytokines and cytokine production after stimulation in EE patients, the systemic parameters of EE patients were highly similar to atopic non-EE patients [9].

Treatment, such as food avoidance or elemental diet, has also reinforced the link between EE and the allergic etiology [3,10–12]. In several studies, allergen avoidance has been shown to completely restore normal esophageal pathology [3,4,10–15]. Food allergen and aeroallergen have been shown to be involved in EE pathogenesis, suggesting that direct contact of the allergen with the esophagus may not be required. Additionally, topical or systemic glucocorticoid treatment, used in allergic diseases such as asthma or atopic dermatitis, has been proven to be efficient in the treatment of EE, particularly in nonallergic EE patients [16–18].

Animal models have linked EE and allergic diseases and assess the sensitization pathways that could occur in human EE. Experimental models of EE can be induced in mice by allergen sensitization and exposure, as well as by administration or overexpression of Th2 cytokines [19,20]. A strong link has been established between EE and lung inflammation in mice. Most published models so far have shown an association between lung and esophageal eosinophilia. Two recent studies have shown that skin sensitization primes for EE [21,22]. EE and atopic dermatitis (AD) share common features, including eosinophil infiltration, eosinophil degranulation, and squamous epithelial cell hyperplasia, suggesting that common pathogenetic mechanisms may be operational. Epicutaneous exposure to the allergens ovalbumin or *Aspergillus fumigatus* alone induces AD-like skin inflammation, but eosinophils do not migrate into the esophagus despite a strong systemic Th2 response, chronic cutaneous antigen exposure, and accelerated bone marrow eosinophilopoiesis and circulating eosinophilia. However, when epicutaneously sensitized mice are subsequently exposed only once to intranasal antigen, esophageal eosinophilia (and lung inflammation) is powerfully induced [21,22]. In these studies, mice genetically deficient in signal transducer and activator of transcription 6 (STAT6), IL-13, IL-4, and IL-5 have impaired induction of esophageal eosinophilia in response to allergen [21,22]. It is interesting to note that all murine models of EE had an inflammation of another organ, such as the lungs, and that the instillation of intratracheal IL-13 in mice induces both airway and esophageal eosinophilia [23,24], suggesting that the direct contact of the allergen with the esophagus or gastrointestinal tract is not required for development of EE. Collectively, these experimental systems demonstrate an intimate connection between the development of eosinophilic inflammation in the respiratory tract, the skin, and the esophagus not only in response to external allergic triggers, but also to intrinsic Th2 cytokines.

Genetic predisposition

As already described in other Th2 diseases, EE pathogenesis is likely to be associated with allergen sensitization in predisposed individuals (see Fig. 1).

EE has a strong familial pattern based on the growing clinical literature and the authors' own patient data. Among pediatric patients with EE, approximately 8% have at least one sibling or parent with EE as well [1]. In addition, Patel and Falchuk [25] have recently reported three adult brothers with dysphagia who were found to have EE. Taken together, EE appears to demonstrate a strong familial pattern with a much higher prevalence in siblings.

Gender predisposition and familial clustering emphasize the genetic predisposition of this disease. In both pediatric and adult patients, EE exhibits a remarkable male predilection: about 70% of the patients are male [1]. One explanation for such a high prevalence in males may in part be a result of the presence of a mutation on the sexual chromosome X that would not be corrected by the Y chromosome genes in males, leading to increased susceptibility in males that have only one copy of the affected gene. Of note, two chains for the IL-13 receptor, IL-13 Rα 1 and IL-13 Rα 2, are on the X chromosomes in position Xq13.1-q28.

Both population-based case-control comparison and family-based transmission disequilibrium tests have shown an association between the allele G of the SNP (rs2302009) locates at the 3'UTR of the eotaxin-3 gene in EE disease [24]. One can hypothesize that the position of this SNP in the 3'UTR might indeed contribute to eotaxin-3 mRNA stability; however, at the present time, the mechanism by which this SNP contributes to EE is unclear. Although only one SNP has been associated so far with EE, the authors predict that multiple other genetic components will be involved [26].

Molecular pathogenesis

Substantial evidence is accumulating that EE is associated with a Th2 type immune response and local or systemic Th2 cytokine overproduction. IL-5 is a cytokine involved in eosinophil production, survival, and activation. IL-5 mRNA is increased in the biopsies of EE patients compared with normal (NL) patients ([27–29] and unpublished data). Peripheral CD4 + T cells show an increase in intracellular IL-5 in the blood of EE patients, compared with nonatopic non-EE patients [9]. Determining the role of IL-5 in EE is of importance because two independent studies have shown an improvement in the clinical and pathologic symptoms of EE after anti-IL-5 treatment [30–32]. IL-5 is known to increase proliferation and survival of eosinophils and facilitate their migration from the bone marrow to the blood [19,33]. As IL-5 can be expressed by eosinophils, it is important to elucidate if IL-5, increased in EE biopsies, has a local role in the esophageal eosinophils of EE patients. One can hypothesize that anti-IL-5 therapy may thus have a systemic action on eosinophil trafficking and survival and a local effect in the esophagus.

Using microarray expression profile analysis, an EE transcript signature remarkably conserved across allergic and nonallergic EE patient phenotypes has been identified [24]. This demonstrates that the effector phase of the disease is conserved between individuals, despite the driving trigger of the inflammation. This EE signature is characterized by 574 dysregulated genes in EE patients compared with normal individuals. Of the entire dysregulated genome, the gene with the greatest overexpression was eotaxin-3, induced approximately 50-fold, compared with control individuals and highly correlated with eosinophil number in the biopsies [24]. While eotaxin-3 was highly up-regulated in EE patients, eotaxin-1 and -2 were not significantly up-regulated [24]. The literature describes the eotaxin family as IL-13-induced molecules in several tissues and cell types. The authors recently demonstrated that in skin keratinocytes, IL-13 selectively induces eotaxin-3 but not eotaxin-1 and -2 in primary keratinocytes (Fig. 2). This phenomenon is most likely, mainly transcriptional and dependent upon the transcription factor STAT6 [34]. The authors also demonstrated that IL-13 mRNA (but not IL-4) is in indeed induced in EE patients compared with NL individuals [34]. It is also interesting to note that murine models have demonstrated that IL-13 and STAT6 are required to develop esophageal eosinophilia in mice [21,22]. Taken together, these results suggest that IL-13 induces eotaxin-3 expression in epithelial cells of the esophagus through a STAT6 phenomenon in EE.

Cellular pathogenesis

While absent in the normal esophagus, eosinophils markedly accumulate in the esophagus of EE patients. A minimum of 15 eosinophils per high power field is now used as clinical diagnostic criteria for EE [35–37]. Analysis of the EE transcriptome reveals that the strong accumulation of esophageal eosinophils is not accompanied by an increase in eosinophil specific transcripts [24]. Recently, Locksley's group demonstrated that eosinophil granule protein mRNAs were detectable in the early development of eosinophils, but not once eosinophils infiltrate into the tissue [38]. Although not actively transcribed in the esophagus, granule proteins are present in the esophageal eosinophils, and major basic protein (MBP) deposition was detected by immunohistochemistry in EE patient esophageal biopsies. As such, granule proteins may influence disease via their cytotoxic activity. Eosinophil granules contain a crystalloid core composed of MBP-1 and MBP-2, and a matrix composed of eosinophil cationic protein (ECP), eosinophil-derived neurotoxin (EDN), and eosinophil peroxidase (EPO) [39]. These cationic proteins share certain proinflammatory properties but differ in other ways. For example, MBP, EPO, and ECP have cytotoxic effects on epithelium in concentrations similar to those found in biologic fluids from patients with eosinophilia. Additionally, ECP and EDN belong to the ribonuclease A superfamily and possess antiviral and ribonuclease activity [40–42]. ECP can insert voltage insensitive, ion-nonselective toxic pores into the membranes of target cells, and these pores may facilitate the entry of other toxic molecules [43]. MBP directly increases smooth muscle

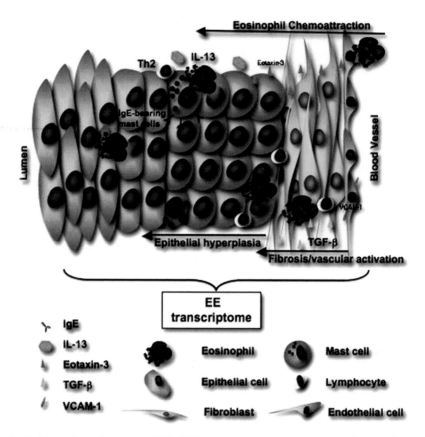

Fig. 2. Molecular pathogenesis of EE. EE involves the complex interaction of genetic factors and environmental exposures leading to a Th2-associated disease, localized in the esophagus of predisposed patients. Such processes involve increased expression of Th2 cytokines, chemokines, and chemokine receptors by PBMC (IL-4, IL-13, IL-5) and eosinophils (IL-13, IL-5, CCR3). In the esophagus, increased expression of IL-13 and TGF-β likely contributes to eotaxin-3 release by epithelial cells, as well as increased collagen production (fibrosis) and vascular activation (VCAM-1 expression). Finally, IgE, systematically or locally synthesized by B cells, is detected on the surface of mast cells and likely contributes to mast cell activation by food antigens.

reactivity by causing dysfunction of vagal muscarinic M2 receptors [44]. MBP also triggers degranulation of mast cells and basophils [45]. Triggering of eosinophils by engagement of receptors for cytokines, immunoglobulins, and complement can lead to the generation of a wide range of inflammatory cytokines including IL-1, IL-3, IL-4, IL-5, IL-13, granulocyte-macrophage colony-stimulating factor, transforming growth factor-β (TGF-β), tumor necrosis factor-α, regulated upon activation, normal T cell expressed and secreted (RANTES), macrophage inflammatory protein-1α, and eotaxin-1, indicating that they have the potential to modulate multiple aspects of the immune response [46,47].

Additionally, eosinophils can directly activate T cells by antigen presentation, which has been demonstrated in vitro and in vivo [48,49]. Further eosinophil-mediated damage is caused by toxic hydrogen peroxide and halide acids generated by EPO, and by superoxide, generated by the respiratory burst oxidase enzyme pathway in eosinophils. Eosinophils also generate large amounts of the cysteinyl leukotriene C_4 (LTC4) that is metabolized to LTD_4 and LTE_4 [50]. These three lipid mediators increase vascular permeability and mucus secretion, and are potent stimulators of smooth muscle contraction [50]. Indeed, leukotriene modifiers appear to improve clinical symptoms in EE patients [51]. Notably, dysregulated expression of the mRNA for numerous enzymes involved in arachidonic acid metabolism is present in the esophagus of EE patients [24].

While eosinophil genes are not well represented in the EE transcriptome, mast cell gene expression (such as tryptase or carboxypeptidase 3) is highly increased in EE [24]. Several studies have shown that mast cells, present in the normal esophagus, have an increased density in esophageal biopsies of EE patients [24,28,52–54]. In other tissues, activated mast cells are known to release mediators (such as cytokines, histamine, proteases) able to modify physiologic parameters, such as smooth muscle contraction phenomenon that may occur in EE [55]. Indeed, a recent study demonstrated that esophageal mast cells (as well as eosinophils) are activated in EE patients (see Fig. 2), compared with gastroesophageal reflux disease (GERD) patients, and were likely to be IgE-bearing cells [53,54]. These findings implicate the presence of a sufficient local Th2 response to activate IgE production by B cells.

Several studies have shown an increase in lymphocytes in pediatric and adult EE patients [18,24,28,53,54], but only one study so far has described the presence of B cells in EE [54]. Using anti-CD20 immunohistochemistry, the investigators described the presence of B cells in EE esophageal biopsies. In the same study, immunoreactivity for CD3+, CD8+ and CD4+ cells was demonstrated to be at higher levels in EE biopsies [54]. A critical role for T cells in disease induction has been demonstrated in recent murine modeling studies [56].

While infiltrated cells are likely to be involved in EE pathogenesis, the resident cells of the esophageal mucosa are likely to be one of the first effector cells responsible for the chemoattraction of hematopoietic cells. Notably, the esophagus contains CD1a+ dendritic cells that may link innate and adaptive immunity in the esophagus [54]. In addition, the esophageal epithelium is likely to contribute to disease induction and propagation, as eotaxin-3 is chiefly produced by esophageal epithelial cells.

The epithelium of the esophagus is a squamous epithelium. In contrast to the skin, the human esophagus is generally not keratinized and thus keratinocytes are in direct contact with the esophageal content. As such, the permeability, the elasticity, and the integrity of the esophagus may contribute to EE disease pathogenesis. Epithelial cells are highly hyperplastic in EE patients [57]. Several external factors are known to increase basal cell expansion, such as gastric acid content in GERD disease. But the basal layer expansion observed in EE patients is more extensive than in GERD patients [57], suggesting that other etiologic factors influence EE disease pathogenesis. The authors have, for example, demonstrated that the epithelium is the main source of the eotaxin-3 chemokine [24], certainly responsible for the chemoattraction of eosinophils. Lymphocytes, eosinophils, and mast cells infiltrated into the esophagus may release soluble mediators able to activate the transcription of epithelial cell genes; for example, Th2 cell-derived IL-13 may act directly on epithelial cells to induce the release of eotaxin-3 (see Fig. 2).

In a recent pediatric EE population, remodeling of the esophageal mucosa, and especially the lamina propria, has been described [58]. In this study, patients with EE had an increased esophageal fibrosis, vascularity, and vascular activation. The investigators also described an increased expression of TGF-β1 (see Fig. 2) and its signaling molecule phosphorylated SMAD2/3 (phospho-SMAD2/3). Additionally, esophageal biopsies in patients with EE demonstrate an increased vascular density and an increased expression of the vascular endothelial adhesion molecule, VCAM-1. In addition to its role in fibrosis, TGF-β is known to increase smooth muscle cell hyperplasia and all together these results suggest an implication of TGF-β, VCAM-1, and SAMAD2/3 in the formation of strictures and in the loss of elasticity of the esophageal wall [58].

Summary and future direction

EE has a complex pathogenesis, in which multiple etiologic factors interact. The environmental factors and a predisposed genetic background certainly interplay in EE onset and pathogenesis. A gene polymorphism, eotaxin-3, has been shown to be associated with EE [24], and we predict that EE, like most Th2 diseases, is a polygenic disorder with multiple environmental factors strongly contributing to disease expression (see Fig. 1). Although advances have been made in the understanding of human pathogenesis, the next challenge will be to understand the molecular mechanisms involved in EE disease development. The overlap with other Th2 diseases tends to complicate the study and interpretation of the results on systemic parameters. The inclusion of the appropriate controls, atopic non-EE and nonatopic individuals, is necessary to fully advance the understanding of disease specific pathogenesis. It will thus be of interest to investigate whether the genetics that underlie atopy and EE are partly similar. The authors hope that from these studies new biomarkers, able to differentiate EE disease from GERD and other atopic diseases, will emerge.

Although some treatments are effective in EE, the molecular mechanisms involved in the remission have still not been established. The development of in vitro and in vivo models may help to dissect the molecular mechanisms involved in remission or resistance to therapy; the overall goal is to be able to molecularly classify patients as a function of their predicted response to treatment. Our current knowledge suggests that targeting the IL-13/eotaxin-3/ CCR3 axis may be a promising therapeutic strategy for EE.

References

[1] Noel RJ, Putnam PE, Rothenberg ME. Eosinophilic esophagitis. N Engl J Med 2004;351(9): 940–1.
[2] Garcia-Careaga M Jr, Kerner JA Jr. Gastrointestinal manifestations of food allergies in pediatric patients. Nutr Clin Pract 2005;20(5):526–35.
[3] Spergel JM. Eosinophilic esophagitis in adults and children: evidence for a food allergy component in many patients. Curr Opin Allergy Clin Immunol 2007;7(3):274–8.
[4] Markowitz JE, Spergel JM, Ruchelli E, et al. Elemental diet is an effective treatment for eosinophilic esophagitis in children and adolescents. Am J Gastroenterol 2003;98(4): 777–82.
[5] Balatsinou C, Milano A, Caldarella MP, et al. Eosinophilic esophagitis is a component of the anticonvulsant hypersensitivity syndrome: description of two cases. Dig Liver Dis 2007; in press.
[6] Fogg MI, Ruchelli E, Spergel JM. Pollen and eosinophilic esophagitis. J Allergy Clin Immunol 2003;112(4):796–7.
[7] Wang FY, Gupta SK, Fitzgerald JF. Is there a seasonal variation in the incidence or intensity of allergic eosinophilic esophagitis in newly diagnosed children? J Clin Gastroenterol 2007; 41(5):451–3.
[8] Yamazaki K, Murray JA, Arora AS, et al. Allergen-specific in vitro cytokine production in adult patients with eosinophilic esophagitis. Dig Dis Sci 2006;51(11):1934–41.
[9] Bullock JZ, Villanueva JM, Blanchard C, et al. Interplay of adaptative Th2 immunity with eotaxin-3 C-C chemokine receptor 3 in eosinophilc esophagitis. J Pediatr Gastroenterol Nutr 2007;45(1):22–31.
[10] Spergel JM, Andrews T, Brown-Whitehorn TF, et al. Treatment of eosinophilic esophagitis with specific food elimination diet directed by a combination of skin prick and patch tests. Ann Allergy Asthma Immunol 2005;95(4):336–43.
[11] Ngo P, Furuta GT. Treatment of eosinophilic esophagitis in children. Curr Treat Options Gastroenterol 2005;8(5):397–403.
[12] Kagalwalla AF, Sentongo TA, Ritz S, et al. Effect of six-food elimination diet on clinical and histologic outcomes in eosinophilic esophagitis. Clin Gastroenterol Hepatol 2006;4(9): 1097–102.
[13] Kelly KJ, Lazenby AJ, Rowe PC, et al. Eosinophilic esophagitis attributed to gastroesophageal reflux: improvement with an amino acid-based formula. Gastroenterology 1995; 109(5):1503–12.
[14] Simon D, Straumann A, Wenk A, et al. Eosinophilic esophagitis in adults—no clinical relevance of wheat and rye sensitizations. Allergy 2006;61(12):1480–3.
[15] Pentiuk SP, Miller CK, Kaul A. Eosinophilic esophagitis in infants and toddlers. Dysphagia 2007;22(1):44–8.
[16] Noel RJ, Putnam PE, Collins MH, et al. Clinical and immunopathologic effects of swallowed fluticasone for eosinophilic esophagitis. Clin Gastroenterol Hepatol 2004;2(7):568–75.
[17] Teitelbaum JE, Fox VL, Twarog FJ, et al. Eosinophilic esophagitis in children: immunopathological analysis and response to fluticasone propionate. Gastroenterology 2002; 122(5):1216–25.
[18] Konikoff MR, Noel RJ, Blanchard C, et al. A randomized, double-blind, placebo-controlled trial of fluticasone propionate for pediatric eosinophilic esophagitis. Gastroenterology 2006; 131(5):1381–91.

[19] Mishra A, Hogan SP, Brandt EB, et al. IL-5 promotes eosinophil trafficking to the esophagus. J Immunol 2002;168(5):2464–9.

[20] Mishra A, Hogan SP, Brandt EB, et al. An etiological role for aeroallergens and eosinophils in experimental esophagitis. J Clin Invest 2001;107(1):83–90.

[21] Akei HS, Mishra A, Blanchard C, et al. Epicutaneous antigen exposure primes for experimental eosinophilic esophagitis in mice. Gastroenterology 2005;129(3):985–94.

[22] Akei HS, Brandt EB, Mishra A, et al. Epicutaneous aeroallergen exposure induces systemic TH2 immunity that predisposes to allergic nasal responses. J Allergy Clin Immunol 2006; 118(1):62–9.

[23] Mishra A, Rothenberg ME. Intratracheal IL-13 induces eosinophilic esophagitis by an IL-5, eotaxin-1, and STAT6-dependent mechanism. Gastroenterology 2003;125(5):1419–27.

[24] Blanchard C, Wang N, Stringer KF, et al. Eotaxin-3 and a uniquely conserved gene-expression profile in eosinophilic esophagitis. J Clin Invest 2006;116(2):536–47.

[25] Patel SM, Falchuk KR. Three brothers with dysphagia caused by eosinophilic esophagitis. Gastrointest Endosc 2005;61(1):165–7.

[26] Blanchard C, Wang N, Rothenberg ME. Eosinophilic esophagitis: pathogenesis, genetics, and therapy. J Allergy Clin Immunol 2006;118(5):1054–9.

[27] Mishra A, Wang M, Pemmaraju VR, et al. Esophageal remodeling develops as a consequence of tissue specific IL-5-induced eosinophilia. Gastroenterology 2007; in press.

[28] Straumann A, Bauer M, Fischer B, et al. Idiopathic eosinophilic esophagitis is associated with a T(H)2-type allergic inflammatory response. J Allergy Clin Immunol 2001;108(6): 954–61.

[29] Straumann A, Kristl J, Conus S, et al. Cytokine expression in healthy and inflamed mucosa: probing the role of eosinophils in the digestive tract. Inflamm Bowel Dis 2005; 11(8):720–6.

[30] Garrett JK, Jameson SC, Thomson B, et al. Anti-interleukin-5 (mepolizumab) therapy for hypereosinophilic syndromes. J Allergy Clin Immunol 2004;113(1):115–9.

[31] Stein ML, Collins MH, Villanueva JM, et al. Anti-IL-5 (mepolizumab) therapy for eosinophilic esophagitis. J Allergy Clin Immunol 2006;118(6):1312–9.

[32] Simon D, Braathen LR, Simon HU. Anti-interleukin-5 antibody therapy in eosinophilic diseases. Pathobiology 2005;72(6):287–92.

[33] Rothenberg ME. Eosinophilic gastrointestinal disorders (EGID). J Allergy Clin Immunol 2004;113(1):11–28.

[34] Blanchard C, Mingler MK, Vicario M, et al. Interleukin-13 involvement in EE: transcriptome analysis and reversibility with glucocorticoids. J Allergy Clin Immunol 2007; In press.

[35] Lim JR, Gupta SK, Croffie JM, et al. White specks in the esophageal mucosa: an endoscopic manifestation of non-reflux eosinophilic esophagitis in children. Gastrointest Endosc 2004; 59(7):835–8.

[36] Potter JW, Saeian K, Staff D, et al. Eosinophilic esophagitis in adults: an emerging problem with unique esophageal features. Gastrointest Endosc 2004;59(3):355–61.

[37] Gonsalves N, Policarpio-Nicolas M, Zhang Q, et al. Histopathologic variability and endoscopic correlates in adults with eosinophilic esophagitis. Gastrointest Endosc 2006;64(3): 313–9.

[38] Voehringer D, van Rooijen N, Locksley RM. Eosinophils develop in distinct stages and are recruited to peripheral sites by alternatively activated macrophages. J Leukoc Biol 2007; 81(6):1434–44.

[39] Gleich GJ, Adolphson CR. The eosinophilic leukocyte: structure and function. Adv Immunol 1986;39:177–253.

[40] Rosenberg HF, Dyer KD. Eosinophil cationic protein and eosinophil-derived neurotoxin. Evolution of novel function in a primate ribonuclease gene family. J Biolumin Chemilumin 1995;270(37):21539–44.

[41] Rosenberg HF, Dyer KD, Tiffany HL, et al. Rapid evolution of a unique family of primate ribonuclease genes. Nat Genet 1995;10(2):219–23.

[42] Slifman NR, Loegering DA, McKean DJ, et al. Ribonuclease activity associated with human eosinophil-derived neurotoxin and eosinophil cationic protein. J Immunol 1986;137(9): 2913–7.

[43] Young JD, Peterson CG, Venge P, et al. Mechanism of membrane damage mediated by human eosinophil cationic protein. Nature 1986;321(6070):613–6.

[44] Jacoby DB, Gleich GJ, Fryer AD. Human eosinophil major basic protein is an endogenous allosteric antagonist at the inhibitory muscarinic M2 receptor. J Clin Invest 1993;91(4): 1314–8.

[45] O'Donnell MC, Ackerman SJ, Gleich GJ, et al. Activation of basophil and mast cell histamine release by eosinophil granule major basic protein. J Exp Med 1983;157(6):1981–91.

[46] Kita H. The eosinophil: a cytokine-producing cell? J Allergy Clin Immunol 1996;97(4): 889–92.

[47] Shinkai K, Mohrs M, Locksley RM. Helper T cells regulate type-2 innate immunity in vivo. Nature 2002;420(6917):825–9.

[48] Shi HZ, Humbles A, Gerard C, et al. Lymph node trafficking and antigen presentation by endobronchial eosinophils. J Clin Invest 2000;105(7):945–53.

[49] Mattes J, Yang M, Mahalingam S, et al. Intrinsic defect in T cell production of interleukin (IL)-13 in the absence of both IL-5 and eotaxin precludes the development of eosinophilia and airways hyperreactivity in experimental asthma. J Exp Med 2002;195(11):1433–44.

[50] Lewis RA, Austen KF, Soberman RJ. Leukotrienes and other products of the 5-lipoxygenase pathway. Biochemistry and relation to pathobiology in human diseases. N Engl J Med 1990;323(10):645–55.

[51] Attwood SE, Lewis CJ, Bronder CS, et al. Eosinophilic oesophagitis: a novel treatment using Montelukast. Gut 2003;52(2):181–5.

[52] Nicholson AG, Li D, Pastorino U, et al. Full thickness eosinophilia in oesophageal leiomyomatosis and idiopathic eosinophilic oesophagitis. A common allergic inflammatory profile? J Pathol 1997;183(2):233–6.

[53] Kirsch R, Bokhary R, Marcon MA, et al. Activated mucosal mast cells differentiate eosinophilic (allergic) esophagitis from gastroesophageal reflux disease. J Pediatr Gastroenterol Nutr 2007;44(1):20–6.

[54] Lucendo AJ, Navarro M, Comas C, et al. Immunophenotypic characterization and quantification of the epithelial inflammatory infiltrate in eosinophilic esophagitis through stereology: an analysis of the cellular mechanisms of the disease and the immunologic capacity of the esophagus. Am J Surg Pathol 2007;31(4):598–606.

[55] Mann NS, Leung JW. Pathogenesis of esophageal rings in eosinophilic esophagitis. Med Hypotheses 2005;64(3):520–3.

[56] Mishra A, Schlotman J, Wang M, et al. Critical role for adaptive T cell immunity in experimental eosinophilic esophagitis in mice. J Leukoc Biol 2007;81(4):916–24.

[57] Sant'Anna AM, Rolland S, Fournet JC, et al. Eosinophilic esophagitis in children: Symptoms, histology and pH probe results. J Pediatr Gastroenterol Nutr 2004;39(4):373–7.

[58] Aceves SS, Newbury RO, Dohil R, et al. Esophageal remodeling in pediatric eosinophilic esophagitis. J Allergy Clin Immunol 2007;119(1):206–12.

ELSEVIER
SAUNDERS

Gastrointest Endoscopy Clin N Am
18 (2008) 145–156

GASTROINTESTINAL
ENDOSCOPY CLINICS
OF NORTH AMERICA

Translational Research on the Pathogenesis of Eosinophilic Esophagitis

Mirna Chehade, MD

Pediatric Gastroenterology and Nutrition, Pediatric Allergy and Immunology,
Mount Sinai School of Medicine, New York, NY 10029, USA

Eosinophilic esophagitis (EE) is an inflammatory disease of the esophagus characterized by eosinophilic infiltration of the esophageal epithelium. EE is a relatively new disease from clinical and research standpoints. A recent surge in basic and translational studies has emerged to understand its pathogenesis since its recognition as a separate entity from acid-induced gastroesophageal reflux disease in 1995 [1]. Our understanding of this disease is still limited, however. In this article, available evidence from translational studies on EE is discussed, focusing on the allergic nature of the disease and highlighting the role of various inflammatory cells found in the esophagus of patients who have EE. Esophageal remodeling in EE is also discussed.

The esophagus as an immunologic organ

The normal esophagus is a hollow, highly distensible, muscular tube that extends from the epiglottis in the pharynx at the level of the C6 vertebra to the gastroesophageal junction at the level of the T11 or T12 vertebra [2]. (See also the article by Collins, elsewhere in this issue.) Its length increases from 10 to 11 cm in the newborn to 25 cm in the adult. The wall of the esophagus consists of a mucosa, submucosa, muscularis propria, and adventitia, reflecting the general structural organization of the gastrointestinal tract except for the lack of a serosal coat [2].

The mucosa is composed of three parts: a nonkeratinizing stratified squamous epithelial layer, lamina propria, and muscularis mucosa. The epithelial layer has mature squamous cells overlying basal cells with great proliferative

Pediatrics, Box 1198, Mount Sinai School of Medicine, One Gustave L. Levy Place, New York, NY 10029.
E-mail address: mirna.chehade@mssm.edu

1052-5157/08/$ - see front matter © 2008 Elsevier Inc. All rights reserved.
doi:10.1016/j.giec.2007.09.013   *giendo.theclinics.com*

potential. Basal cells occupy 10% to 15% of the thickness of the epithelial layer. Various immune cells are present in the deeper portion of the epithelial layer, including dendritic cells, a few T lymphocytes, and rare mast cells [3–6]. Other immune cells, such as eosinophils, are absent [6,7]. The lamina propria is the nonepithelial portion of the mucosa, above the muscularis mucosa. It consists of loose areolar connective tissue, vascular structures, and leukocytes, the latter being poorly characterized. The muscularis mucosa consists of longitudinally oriented smooth muscle bundles.

Deep to the mucosa is the submucosa, consisting of loose connective tissue containing blood vessels and a rich network of lymphatics, some leukocytes, occasional lymphoid follicles, nerve fibers, and submucosal glands. Submucosal glands connect to the lumen by way of squamous epithelium-lined ducts, and secrete mucin-containing fluid that lubricates the esophagus [2]. The muscularis propria consists of an inner circular and an outer longitudinal coat of smooth muscle with an intervening myenteric plexus.

Esophageal peristalsis results in passage of a wide range of luminal contents from the pharynx to the stomach (see the article by Nerko, elsewhere in this issue). The combination of esophageal peristalsis, the presence of a lower esophageal sphincter at the esophagogastric junction, squamous epithelial barrier, salivary and submucosal gland products, and immune cells in the esophagus contributes to esophageal defense against injury [8]. The function of the various immune cells residing in the esophagus has not been well studied, although their function in immune tolerance and disease has been well studied in other organ systems. Their presence in the esophagus suggests a possible role in defense, similar to the rest of the gastrointestinal tract, because some of these cells increase in various inflammatory diseases of the esophagus, including EE.

Because of the limitation in depth of endoscopically obtained esophageal biopsies, many of the translational studies involving esophageal tissue are limited to the epithelial layer of the mucosa. Few esophageal biopsies are deep enough to include a portion of the subepithelial lamina propria [5]. With few exceptions, therefore, only the immune cells residing in the epithelial layers or those obtained from the peripheral circulation have been studied in EE.

Eosinophilic esophagitis is an allergic disease

Histopathologically, similar to other allergic diseases, EE is characterized by an inflammatory infiltrate in the epithelial layer of the esophagus, consisting of increased numbers of T lymphocytes, dendritic cells, mast cells, and eosinophils [6,9,10]. Eosinophils serve as the histologic hallmark for EE (see the article by Collins, elsewhere in this issue). Finding up to 15 to 24 eosinophils per high power field on microscopic examination of esophageal mucosal biopsies is considered diagnostic in the proper clinical context [11–13]. The various immune cells residing in the esophagus seem to be activated, contributing to the allergic phenotype of EE. Increased numbers of mast cells, IgE-positive cells, and a cytokine profile consistent with a T-helper type 2 phenotype suggest its allergic etiology [6,10] (see the article by Blanchard and Rothenberg, elsewhere in this issue). Furthermore, EE was found to be strongly associated with other allergic disorders in children and adults [14,15] (see the articles by Assa'ad, and Spergel and Shuker, elsewhere in this issue). Multiple food allergens and possibly aeroallergens have been implicated [1,16,17].

The role of food allergens in eosinophilic esophagitis

The pathogenesis of EE is poorly understood. Substantial evidence from short-term clinical studies implicates dietary food antigens, however (see the articles by Assa'ad, and Spergel and Shuker, elsewhere in this issue). Various clinical trials of food eliminations resulted in various extents of clinical response and esophageal histologic improvement in EE. These trials included amino acid–based formula therapy, elimination of suspected allergens based on skin testing, and empiric elimination of several foods suspected to be highly allergenic [1,16,18,19]. Reintroduction of the foods resulted in reoccurrence of EE symptoms [1], proving the causative relationship of EE with dietary antigens.

The immunologic reaction to foods is believed to be a mix of IgE-mediated allergic reactions and non-IgE, cell-mediated allergic reactions. This finding was first evidenced by Kelly and colleagues [1] who found symptom recurrence in patients who had EE on reintroduction of foods following an elimination diet, despite having negative skin prick tests to these foods. Skin prick tests reflect IgE-mediated allergic reactions to antigens. Spergel and colleagues [16] further demonstrated this phenomenon by performing a combination of skin prick and patch tests on children who had EE. Although skin prick tests reflect IgE-mediated sensitization, patch tests reflect delayed, non-IgE, cell-mediated allergic reactions. Removal of foods that tested positive by both tests from the diet of children who had EE resulted in a 70% success rate. Different allergenic foods were identified on skin prick versus patch tests [16] (see the article by Spergel and Shuker, elsewhere in this issue).

The following discussion provides a brief overview of the immunology of EE, focusing on the role of different inflammatory cells in this disease.

The role of lymphocytes in eosinophilic esophagitis

T lymphocytes are increased in the esophagus in eosinophilic esophagitis

Rare intraepithelial lymphocytes are normally present in the esophageal mucosa of healthy individuals, whether children or adults [6,20,21] (see the article by Collins, elsewhere in this issue). These cells were historically referred to as squiggle cells by histopathologists, because of their irregular nuclear contours seen on microscopic examination of hematoxylin and eosin–stained sections of the esophagus, caused by their tight intermingling with esophageal epithelial cells [21]. Squiggle cells were shown to be T lymphocytes [20,21], with a predominance of the T-suppressor (CD8 positive) subset over the T-helper (CD4 positive) subset in the esophageal epithelium [4,6]. In the subepithelial lamina propria of the normal esophagus, T helper cells seem to constitute the predominant subset of T lymphocytes [4].

In EE, esophageal intraepithelial T lymphocytes were shown to be increased compared with healthy controls, as demonstrated by immunohistochemical staining of these cells for the marker CD3 [6,9,10]. T lymphocytes tend to be distributed in the deeper epithelial layers, creating a cell density the closer they are to the regenerative epithelial layers [6]. Both CD4 and CD8 subsets of T lymphocytes were found to increase in the esophageal epithelium (Fig. 1) [6,9], with a maintenance of CD8 predominance over CD4 cells [6]. This finding is in contrast to other allergic diseases, such as atopic dermatitis, in which CD4 cells constitute the predominant T-cell population [22]. The significance of this finding is not clear. All immunopathologic studies of the esophagus in EE have been limited, however, to the epithelium. Whether this CD8 predominance is also true in the deeper, subepithelial lamina propria layer of the esophagus is unknown.

Pathways of T-lymphocyte trafficking and recruitment into the esophagus of patients who have EE and the exact role these cells play in EE have not been studied. Both CD4 and CD8 subsets of T lymphocytes decrease in number following successful treatment of patients who have EE with topical corticosteroids [6,9].

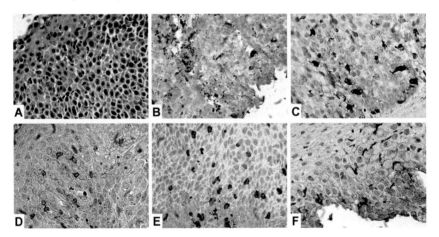

Fig. 1. Sections from esophageal biopsies of patients who have eosinophilic esophagitis showing various immune cells infiltrating the esophageal epithelium (original magnification ×400): (*A*) eosinophils (hematoxylin and eosin stain), (*B*) eosinophils with extensive degranulation (immunoperoxidase stain for MBP), (*C*) mast cells (immunoperoxidase stain for tryptase), (*D*) CD4 lymphocytes (immunoperoxidase stain for CD4), (*E*) CD8 lymphocytes (immunoperoxidase stain for CD8), and (*F*) dendritic cells (immunoperoxidase stain for CD1a).

T lymphocytes in eosinophilic esophagitis carry an allergic phenotype

The T-lymphocyte reaction in EE is believed to be of a T helper type 2 (Th2) phenotype in response to a food protein, consistent with an allergic mechanism. Evidence for this allergic phenotype stems from various studies of T cells in the esophagus and in the peripheral blood of patients who had EE, although it is not definitive.

Straumann and colleagues [10] studied cytokine production by peripheral blood mononuclear cells (PBMCs) in the peripheral circulation after in vitro stimulation with phytohemagglutinin, a nonspecific cell stimulant. Increased release of the Th2 cytokine IL-13 was found in 40% of the patients studied. Yamazaki and colleagues [23] later conducted similar experiments, however, using specific allergens. PBMCs from 15 adult patients who had EE were incubated in vitro with nine different food allergen extracts or aeroallergen extracts. Food extracts consisted of milk, egg, soy, wheat, and peanut. Compared with healthy controls, PBMCs from patients who had EE secreted significantly more of the Th2 cytokines IL-5 or IL-13 in response to various allergens, even in the absence of clear-cut sensitization to the allergens when serum levels of allergen-specific IgE were measured. Whether the Th2 response is secondary to the concomitant atopic features of the patients remains unknown, because 73% of the patients in the study who had EE had concurrent allergic disease, a finding common to patients who have EE, whether children or adults [14,15]. A study comparing patients who had EE with non-EE allergic controls is needed to confirm these findings.

In the esophagus, increased levels of the Th2 cytokine IL-5 in biopsies of patients who had EE was found, whether assayed at the messenger (mRNA) level by real-time polymerase chain reaction (RT-PCR) or at the protein level using immunohistochemical staining of esophageal sections [10,24], although further identification of the specific inflammatory cells producing this cytokine was not done. Other Th2 cytokines, such as IL-4 and IL-13, were not found to be globally elevated in esophageal tissue when assayed as a whole by gene microarray or when mRNA levels for these cytokines were measured [24,25]. When esophageal eosinophils were specifically examined for Th2 cytokine expression by immunostaining of esophageal sections of patients who had EE, 60% of these cells were found to express IL-4 and IL-13 [26].

B lymphocytes are slightly increased in the esophagus in eosinophilic esophagitis

Although B lymphocytes are absent from the esophageal epithelium of healthy individuals [6], they were shown to be present in the subepithelial lamina propria, along with T helper cells [4]. In EE, B lymphocytes were found to infiltrate the esophageal epithelial layer, as demonstrated by immunohistochemical staining for the B-cell marker CD20, albeit in small numbers [6]. It is not known whether these B lymphocytes bear IgE, hence contributing to the pool of IgE-positive cells found in the esophagus of patients who have EE, most of which are believed to be mast cells [6,10]. In addition, B lymphocytes are capable of holding antigens to their surface for recognition by specific T lymphocytes along with MHC class II molecules [27]. The potential role of B cells in antigen presentation in EE remains to be tested.

The role of eosinophils in eosinophilic esophagitis

Eosinophils are increased in the esophagus in eosinophilic esophagitis

Eosinophils have received the most attention by researchers because they constitute the diagnostic hallmark of EE. Eosinophils are significantly increased in number in the esophageal epithelium of patients who have EE compared with those who have acid-induced gastroesophageal reflux disease [18] or healthy controls, the latter individuals having no esophageal intraepithelial eosinophils [6,7]. Finding 15 or more eosinophils per high power field on microscopic examination of the esophageal epithelium has been accepted as a histologic criterion for EE (see Fig. 1) [11–13]. Intraepithelial eosinophils significantly decrease in number following successful treatment of patients who have EE with dietary restriction or corticosteroids [1,9,11,18].

In the circulation, eosinophils are increased only in about 50% of patients who have EE [9,28]. In adults who had EE and dysphagia, persistent peripheral eosinophilia correlated with persistent dysphagia [29].

Pathways of eosinophil recruitment into the esophagus in eosinophilic esophagitis

Eosinophils are recruited into tissues by way of several inflammatory mediators. In a murine model of esophageal eosinophilia, the cytokine IL-5 and the chemokine eotaxin were shown to be important in eosinophil recruitment into the esophagus following intranasal challenge with an antigen [30]. In eotaxin-deficient mice, eosinophil recruitment into the esophagus in response to allergen challenge was attenuated compared with wild-type mice. In IL-5 gene targeted mice with resultant absence of IL-5, eosinophil accumulation in the esophagus was completely ablated in response to aeroallergen stimulation. In a subsequent murine study using antigen challenge by way of the oral route, the Th2 cytokine IL-5 was again demonstrated as necessary and sufficient for the induction of eosinophil trafficking to the esophagus [31]. IL-13, another Th2 cytokine, was also demonstrated to be important in induction of esophageal eosinophilia in mice by an IL-5, eotaxin-1, and STAT6-dependent mechanism. STAT6 is known as a signal transducer and activator of transcription important in regulating allergen-induced eosinophilia in the lung [32].

Similar to murine studies, the role of eotaxin in eosinophil trafficking to the esophagus was demonstrated in human EE by the same investigators.

Esophageal tissues obtained by endoscopic biopsies from children who had EE were analyzed by genome-wide microarray expression analysis. The gene encoding eotaxin-3 was found to be the most highly induced gene in these patients compared with healthy individuals [25]. These findings were confirmed by assaying esophageal tissue from patients who had EE for eotaxin-3 mRNA by RT-PCR and for eotaxin-3 protein by Western blot. Because eotaxin-3 is known to regulate CCR3-expressing cells in vitro, including eosinophils and mast cells, eotaxin-3 mRNA and protein levels in esophageal tissue of patients who had EE strongly correlated with the extent of esophageal eosinophil and mast cell infiltration. The above results implicate eotaxin-3 as an important chemoattractant for eosinophils in human EE. The potential role for IL-5 in eosinophil recruitment to the esophagus in human EE may be as important as that of eotaxin-3, as demonstrated by a significant decrease in number in circulating and esophageal eosinophils when an antibody to IL-5 was administered to patients who had the disease in an open-label phase I/II clinical trial [33].

Functional role of eosinophils in eosinophilic esophagitis

Eosinophils are present in an activated state in EE, as demonstrated by eosinophilic degranulation and release of major basic protein (MBP), an eosinophil mediator normally present in its cytoplasmic granules. On immunohistochemical staining of esophageal tissues of children who had EE for MBP, this mediator was found not only in the cytoplasm of infiltrating eosinophils but also free in the vicinity of the cells, indicating degranulation (see Fig. 1) [5]. Eosinophil activation is not universal to all patients who have EE however, as demonstrated by finding various extents of eosinophil degranulation in the esophagus of children who had EE [5] and finding variable expression of the surface activation marker CD25 and the Th2 cytokines IL-4, IL-5, and IL-13 in esophageal eosinophils of adults who had EE when these were evaluated by immunohistochemical staining of esophageal tissue [26]. The extent of eosinophil degranulation was not related to the number of esophageal intraepithelial eosinophils [5], and expression of CD25 and the Th2 cytokines was variable even in the same patient. This finding indicates a possible dichotomy with respect to the extent of eosinophilic infiltration and eosinophilic activation in the esophagus. The potential clinical significance for this variability in activation has been examined in relation to a well-described complication of EE, that of esophageal subepithelial lamina propria fibrosis. In children who had EE, esophageal fibrosis correlated with the extent of intraepithelial eosinophil activation rather than the number of intraepithelial eosinophils [5]. Esophageal fibrosis is a histologic hallmark for esophageal remodeling, and likely a predictor of development of dysphagia in children who have EE [5,34].

Eosinophil activation is likely not restricted to the esophagus, as shown by elevated serum levels of various eosinophil activation markers, including eosinophil cationic protein and eosinophil-derived neurotoxin in some children who have EE despite having normal peripheral blood eosinophil counts [35]. Furthermore, increased expression of the Th2 cytokine IL-13 was found in peripheral blood eosinophils and in duodenal eosinophils of patients who had EE compared with controls, despite having histologically normal duodenum [26,36]. The latter finding points to the possibility that IL-13 expression in EE eosinophils is induced before tissue infiltration. Evidence suggests that expression of IL-13 by eosinophils is a cytokine-derived process in response to inflammatory conditions, as shown by generation of IL-13 by peripheral blood eosinophils from healthy individuals when stimulated with GM-CSF or IL-5 in vitro [36]. In addition, stimulation of blood eosinophils containing IL-13 by eotaxin results in rapid release of this cytokine. IL-13 is a Th2 cytokine important in IgE and IgG4 class switching in B cells. The specific effect of eosinophil-derived IL-13 in the immunopathogenesis of EE has not been studied in humans, although it was demonstrated to have an important role in induction of esophageal eosinophilia in mice [32].

The role of mast cells in eosinophilic esophagitis

Mast cells are increased in the esophagus in eosinophilic esophagitis

Although present in small numbers in the esophageal epithelium of healthy individuals, mast cells were increased in the esophageal epithelium of patients who had EE, whether children or adults (see Fig. 1) [5,6]. In contrast to eosinophils, mast cells were mostly located in the deeper layers of the esophageal epithelium, close to lymphocytes and dendritic cells [37]. Their number correlated with that of intraepithelial eosinophils [5,25] and was found to decrease significantly following successful therapy of EE [6].

Functional role of mast cells in eosinophilic esophagitis

Similar to eosinophils, mast cells were found to be present in an activated state in the esophageal epithelium of patients who had EE, as evidenced by degranulation and release of tryptase, a mast cell mediator, into the esophageal mucosa on immunohistochemical staining of esophageal tissue for tryptase [37] and by electron microscopic examination of esophageal mast cells in this disease demonstrating features of degranulation [38]. It is possible that cross-talk between mast cells and eosinophils is an important contributor to the pathogenesis of EE in humans. Activated intestinal mast cells were shown to be a potent source of IL-5 in patients who had intestinal inflammatory diseases [39], a cytokine important in eosinophilic recruitment. The mast cell mediator tryptase was also shown to stimulate the selective release of interleukin-8 [40], a cytokine that participates in eosinophilic migration [41]. Using mast cell–depleted mice, Das and colleagues [42] also demonstrated a role for mast cells in eotaxin-induced eosinophil accumulation after allergen sensitization. These studies suggest a possible role for mast cells in the pathogenesis of eosinophilic gastrointestinal diseases, including EE.

The role of dendritic cells in eosinophilic esophagitis

Dendritic cells are potent antigen-presenting cells. They express major histocompatibility complex (MHC) class II antigens on their surface, through which they can present the antigen to T-helper lymphocytes, leading to their antigen-specific activation. Dendritic cells of the esophagus, also referred to as Langerhans cells, are normally located deep in the basal and suprabasal layers of the esophageal epithelium, where T lymphocytes also reside [3], indicating possible interaction with T lymphocytes in the pathogenesis of EE.

Langerhans cells stain positive for CD1a, which has been used for their identification by immunohistochemical staining of the esophagus (see Fig. 1F) [3]. Although their number does not seem to be significantly higher in EE compared with healthy controls, they were shown to decrease in response to steroid therapy in children but not adults who had EE [6,9]. In vitro experiments testing the functional role of these cells in taking up food allergens are needed, especially to help elucidate the site of antigen uptake in the gastrointestinal tract of patients who have EE.

Esophageal fibrosis in eosinophilic esophagitis

Dysphagia and food impactions necessitating urgent endoscopic removal are common presenting symptoms in adults and children who have EE [43,44]. Narrowing, strictures, and thickening of the esophageal wall have been found in some patients who have EE by endoscopic and radiologic studies [29,45,46]. Esophageal subepithelial lamina propria fibrosis was found in patients who had these strictures, both adults and children [29,34]. Some children who had dysphagia and food impactions but not esophageal strictures were also found to have fibrosis [5,34], indicating that fibrosis may be causing esophageal dysmotility. In fact, abnormal esophageal motility was found in 40% of adult patients who had EE [47]. When children who had EE were examined for subepithelial lamina propria fibrosis regardless of their symptoms, fibrosis was found in 57% of these children [5]. Forty-two percent of these patients had dysphagia, 80% of whom had esophageal food impactions. These symptoms were present only in patients who had esophageal fibrosis. This finding may indicate that fibrosis is a prelude for future complications, such as dysmotility and strictures, with resultant dysphagia and food impactions.

Factors involved in triggering esophageal fibroblast proliferation and collagen deposition have not yet been studied in detail. Activated eosinophils may be playing an important role in fibrosis formation. In children who have EE, fibrosis was found to be related to the extent of esophageal eosinophilic activation rather than esophageal numbers [5]. MBP may be an important eosinophilic mediator in fibrosis, because extracellular degranulation products of eosinophils stained strongly for MBP in these patients [5]. MBP was previously demonstrated to be released in other inflammatory fibrotic lesions, such as idiopathic retroperitoneal fibrosis, sclerosing cholangitis, and pulmonary fibrosis [48]. In addition, the profibrotic cytokine TGF-β may be contributing to esophageal fibrosis in EE. TGF-β was found to be increased in the esophageal lamina propria of children who had fibrosis. Eosinophils were the main immune cells expressing this cytokine [34]. Other cytokines, such as IL-4 and IL-13, were not studied in patients who had EE and fibrosis, although they may be potential candidates, because esophageal eosinophils express variable degrees of these cytokines [26], and these cytokines have been implicated in sustained airway remodeling in asthma in murine studies [49]. The long-term natural history of esophageal fibrosis and its potential reversibility with therapy for EE remain to be studied.

Summary

EE is an emerging disease with significant health impact in children and adults alike. Attempts to understand its pathogenesis in individuals affected by this disease continue. Despite limited data available so far, largely composed of descriptive studies, it is becoming clear that EE is caused by an immune dysregulation secondary to the presence of food allergens and possibly aeroallergens. Various inflammatory cells, including T lymphocytes, mast cells, and eosinophils and their mediators, play a role in its pathogenesis. The relative importance of each inflammatory cell and its mediators and the interactions between these cells still need to be elucidated in individuals who have EE. More translational research studies are eagerly awaited for further understanding of the mechanism of disease in EE, possibly leading to targeted, more efficient therapies.

References

[1] Kelly KJ, Lazenby AJ, Rowe PC, et al. Eosinophilic esophagitis attributed to gastroesophageal reflux: improvement with an amino acid-based formula. Gastroenterology 1995;109: 1503–12.
[2] Liu C, Crawford JM. The gastrointestinal tract. In: Kumar V, Abbas AK, Fausto N, editors. Robbins and Cotran pathologic basis of disease. 7th edition. Philadelphia, PA: Elsevier; 2005. p. 797–875.
[3] Terris B, Potet F. Structure and role of Langerhans' cells in the human oesophageal epithelium. Digestion 1995;56(Suppl 1):9–14.
[4] Geboes K, De Wolf-Peeters C, Rutgeerts P, et al. Lymphocytes and Langerhans cells in the human oesophageal epithelium. Virchows Arch A Pathol Anat Histopathol 1983;401:45–55.
[5] Chehade M, Sampson HA, Morotti RA, et al. Esophageal subepithelial fibrosis in children with eosinophilic esophagitis. J Pediatr Gastroenterol Nutr 2007;45:319–28.

[6] Lucendo AJ, Navarro M, Comas C, et al. Immunophenotypic characterization and quanti-fication of the epithelial inflammatory infiltrate in eosinophilic esophagitis through stereol-ogy: an analysis of the cellular mechanisms of the disease and the immunologic capacity of the esophagus. Am J Surg Pathol 2007;31:598–606.

[7] Winter HS, Madara JL, Stafford RJ, et al. Intraepithelial eosinophils: a new diagnostic criterion for reflux esophagitis. Gastroenterology 1982;83:818–23.

[8] Furuta GT. Clinicopathologic features of esophagitis in children. Gastrointest Endosc Clin N Am 2001;11:683–715.

[9] Teitelbaum JE, Fox VL, Twarog FJ, et al. Eosinophilic esophagitis in children: immuno-pathological analysis and response to fluticasone propionate. Gastroenterology 2002;122: 1216–25.

[10] Straumann A, Bauer M, Fischer B, et al. Idiopathic eosinophilic esophagitis is associated with a T(H)2-type allergic inflammatory response. J Allergy Clin Immunol 2001;108:954–61.

[11] Liacouras CA, Wenner WJ, Brown K, et al. Primary eosinophilic esophagitis in children: successful treatment with oral corticosteroids. J Pediatr Gastroenterol Nutr 1998;26:380–5.

[12] Rothenberg ME, Mishra A, Collins MH, et al. Pathogenesis and clinical features of eosino-philic esophagitis. J Allergy Clin Immunol 2001;108:891–4.

[13] Furuta GT, Liacouras CA, Collins MH, et al. Eosinophilic esophagitis in children and adults: a systematic review and consensus recommendations for diagnosis and treatment. Gastroenterology 2007;133:1342–63.

[14] Simon D, Marti H, Heer P, et al. Eosinophilic esophagitis is frequently associated with IgE-mediated allergic airway diseases. J Allergy Clin Immunol 2005;115:1090–2.

[15] Liacouras CA, Spergel JM, Ruchelli E, et al. Eosinophilic esophagitis: a 10-year experience in 381 children. Clin Gastroenterol Hepatol 2005;3:1198–206.

[16] Spergel JM, Beausoleil JL, Mascarenhas M, et al. The use of skin prick tests and patch tests to identify causative foods in eosinophilic esophagitis. J Allergy Clin Immunol 2002;109:363–8.

[17] Fogg MI, Ruchelli E, Spergel JM. Pollen and eosinophilic esophagitis. J Allergy Clin Immu-nol 2003;112:796–7.

[18] Markowitz JE, Spergel JM, Ruchelli E, et al. Elemental diet is an effective treatment for eosinophilic esophagitis in children and adolescents. Am J Gastroenterol 2003;98:777–82.

[19] Kagalwalla AF, Sentongo TA, Ritz S, et al. Effect of six-food elimination diet on clinical and histologic outcomes in eosinophilic esophagitis. Clin Gastroenterol Hepatol 2006;4: 1097–102.

[20] Mangano MM, Antonioli DA, Schnitt SJ, et al. Nature and significance of cells with irregular nuclear contours in esophageal mucosal biopsies. Mod Pathol 1992;5:191–6.

[21] Cucchiara S, D'Armiento F, Alfieri E, et al. Intraepithelial cells with irregular nuclear contours as a marker of esophagitis in children with gastroesophageal reflux disease. Dig Dis Sci 1995;40:2305–11.

[22] Leung DY, Bieber T. Atopic dermatitis. Lancet 2003;361:151–60.

[23] Yamazaki K, Murray JA, Arora AS, et al. Allergen-specific in vitro cytokine production in adult patients with eosinophilic esophagitis. Dig Dis Sci 2006;51:1934–41.

[24] Gupta SK, Fitzgerald JF, Kondratyuk T, et al. Cytokine expression in normal and inflamed esophageal mucosa: a study into the pathogenesis of allergic eosinophilic esophagitis. J Pediatr Gastroenterol Nutr 2006;42:22–6.

[25] Blanchard C, Wang N, Stringer KF, et al. Eotaxin-3 and a uniquely conserved gene-expression profile in eosinophilic esophagitis. J Clin Invest 2006;116:536–47.

[26] Straumann A, Kristl J, Conus S, et al. Cytokine expression in healthy and inflamed mucosa: probing the role of eosinophils in the digestive tract. Inflamm Bowel Dis 2005;11:720–6.

[27] Pierce SK, Morris JF, Grusby MJ, et al. Antigen-presenting function of B lymphocytes. Immunol Rev 1988;106:149–80.

[28] Orenstein SR, Shalaby TM, Di Lorenzo C, et al. The spectrum of pediatric eosinophilic esophagitis beyond infancy: a clinical series of 30 children. Am J Gastroenterol 2000;95: 1422–30.

[29] Straumann A, Spichtin HP, Grize L, et al. Natural history of primary eosinophilic esophagitis: a follow-up of 30 adult patients for up to 11.5 years. Gastroenterology 2003;125: 1660–9.

[30] Mishra A, Hogan SP, Brandt EB, et al. An etiological role for aeroallergens and eosinophils in experimental esophagitis. J Clin Invest 2001;107:83–90.

[31] Mishra A, Hogan SP, Brandt EB, et al. IL-5 promotes eosinophil trafficking to the esophagus. J Immunol 2002;168:2464–9.

[32] Mishra A, Rothenberg ME. Intratracheal IL-13 induces eosinophilic esophagitis by an IL-5, eotaxin-1, and STAT6-dependent mechanism. Gastroenterology 2003;125:1419–27.

[33] Stein ML, Collins MH, Villanueva JM, et al. Anti-IL-5 (mepolizumab) therapy for eosinophilic esophagitis. J Allergy Clin Immunol 2006;118:1312–9.

[34] Aceves SS, Newbury RO, Dohil R, et al. Esophageal remodeling in pediatric eosinophilic esophagitis. J Allergy Clin Immunol 2007;119:206–12.

[35] Chehade M, Yershov O, Sampson HA. Serum eosinophil cationic protein and eosinophil derived neurotoxin are potential non-invasive biomarkers for eosinophilic esophagitis. Gastroenterology 2007;132:A6.

[36] Schmid-Grendelmeier P, Altznauer F, Fischer B, et al. Eosinophils express functional IL-13 in eosinophilic inflammatory diseases. J Immunol 2002;169:1021–7.

[37] Chehade M, Castro R, Magid M, et al. Tryptase is a potential diagnostic marker for eosinophilic esophagitis and eosinophilic gastroenteritis with esophageal involvement. J Pediatr Gastroenterol Nutr 2002;35:A105.

[38] Kirsch R, Bokhary R, Marcon MA, et al. Activated mucosal mast cells differentiate eosinophilic (allergic) esophagitis from gastroesophageal reflux disease. J Pediatr Gastroenterol Nutr 2007;44:20–6.

[39] Lorentz A, Schwengberg S, Mierke C, et al. Human intestinal mast cells produce IL-5 in vitro upon IgE receptor cross-linking and in vivo in the course of intestinal inflammatory disease. Eur J Immunol 1999;29:1496–503.

[40] Compton SJ, Cairns JA, Holgate ST, et al. The role of mast cell tryptase in regulating endothelial cell proliferation, cytokine release, and adhesion molecule expression: tryptase induces expression of mRNA for IL-1 beta and IL-8 and stimulates the selective release of IL-8 from human umbilical vein endothelial cells. J Immunol 1998;161:1939–46.

[41] Oliveira SH, Faccioli LH, Cunha FQ, et al. Participation of interleukin-5 and interleukin-8 in the eosinophil migration induced by a large volume of saline. Int Arch Allergy Immunol 1996;111:244–52.

[42] Das AM, Flower RJ, Perretti M. Resident mast cells are important for eotaxin-induced eosinophil accumulation in vivo. J Leukoc Biol 1998;64:156–62.

[43] Khan S, Orenstein SR, Di Lorenzo C, et al. Eosinophilic esophagitis: strictures, impactions, dysphagia. Dig Dis Sci 2003;48:22–9.

[44] Desai TK, Stecevic V, Chang CH, et al. Association of eosinophilic inflammation with esophageal food impaction in adults. Gastrointest Endosc 2005;61:795–801.

[45] Vasilopoulos S, Murphy P, Auerbach A, et al. The small-caliber esophagus: an unappreciated cause of dysphagia for solids in patients with eosinophilic esophagitis. Gastrointest Endosc 2002;55:99–106.

[46] Fox VL, Nurko S, Teitelbaum JE, et al. High-resolution EUS in children with eosinophilic "allergic" esophagitis. Gastrointest Endosc 2003;57:30–6.

[47] Sgouros SN, Bergele C, Mantides A. Eosinophilic esophagitis in adults: a systematic review. Eur J Gastroenterol Hepatol 2006;18:211–7.

[48] Noguchi H, Kephart GM, Colby TV, et al. Tissue eosinophilia and eosinophil degranulation in syndromes associated with fibrosis. Am J Pathol 1992;140:521–8.

[49] Leigh R, Ellis R, Wattie JN, et al. Type 2 cytokines in the pathogenesis of sustained airway dysfunction and airway remodeling in mice. Am J Respir Crit Care Med 2004;169:860–7.

ELSEVIER
SAUNDERS

Gastrointest Endoscopy Clin N Am
18 (2008) 157–167

GASTROINTESTINAL
ENDOSCOPY CLINICS
OF NORTH AMERICA

Noninvasive Markers of Eosinophilic Esophagitis

Sandeep K. Gupta, MD

*Indiana University School of Medicine, James Whitcomb Riley Hospital for Children,
702 Barnhill Drive, ROC 4210, Indianapolis, IN 46202, USA*

There has been an increasing awareness and recognition of eosinophilic esophagitis (EE) over the last decade. EE is a chronic condition with periods of exacerbation and remission. Currently, esophagogastroduodenoscopy (EGD) and histological examination of esophageal mucosal biopsies are required to establish the diagnosis, objectively assess response to therapy, document disease remission, and evaluate symptom recurrence [1]. Because of the invasiveness of EGD and the personal and financial costs associated with repeated procedures, there is an acute need to identify noninvasive biomarkers that correlate with disease presence, remission, severity, and response to therapy.

Biomarkers may be divided broadly into three groups (Table 1) [2]. Box 1 lists the characteristics of an ideal biomarker of EE. The most pressing need is identification of biomarkers of response.

Identifying a biomarker

It would be prudent to study the pathophysiology of EE to examine potential biomarker(s). Although there are gaps in the understanding of EE, it is thought to be a TH2 predominant inflammatory process that is interleukin (IL)-5- and IL-13-mediated and eotaxin-dependent [3]. Along with the pathophysiology of EE, the researcher should appreciate eosinophil physiology, including the various cytokines and chemokines that modulate eosinophil function, and the granular proteins contained within an eosinophil [4]. Several potentially toxic substances are released on eosinophil activation and subsequent degranulation, which then actively participate in the inflammatory cascade.

E-mail address: sgupta@iupui.edu

1052-5157/08/$ - see front matter © 2008 Elsevier Inc. All rights reserved.
doi:10.1016/j.giec.2007.09.004   *giendo.theclinics.com*

Table 1
Types of biomarkers

Exposure to external influences	Example: aflatoxin exposure and hepatocellular carcinoma risk
Susceptibility to disease	Example: α-1-antitrypsin phenotype and susceptibility to adult chronic lung disease
Response in disease	Example: tissue transglutaminase titer and compliance with gluten-free diet

The complex pathophysiology of EE and eosinophil physiology provide several candidate biomarkers (Fig. 1). These biomarkers could be studied on various non-invasively obtained body specimens, including sputum, breath, blood, stool, and urine. This article reviews several potential noninvasive biomarkers of eosinophilic diseases, specifically EE.

Mast cell products

Several reports have suggested a role for mast cells in the pathogenesis of EE, although the molecular events are defined poorly [5–7]. The exact role of mast cells in EE pathogenesis is unclear, as is which specific mast cell product(s) may participate (Fig. 2) [8]. Leukotrienes, a mast cell product, have been suggested as mediators of mast cell involvement in EE pathogenesis, with the thought that, if proven correct, leukotriene receptor antagonists (such as montelukast) could be used as therapeutic agents in patients who have EE. In a recent study, leukotriene protein levels were measured in esophageal mucosal biopsies of controls and children with EE, but found to be similar [9]. Interestingly, the levels were elevated in esophageal biopsies of patients with eosinophilic inflammation of the gastrointestinal (GI) tract that extended beyond the esophagus compared with controls. Thus, although leukotrienes may not be involved in the pathogenesis of EE, these

---

Box 1. Characteristics of an ideal biomarker for eosinophilic esophagitis

Correlate with EE state
Connect with EE severity
Reflect changes caused by therapy
Have high sensitivity
Carry high specificity
Dependably reproducible
Performed on specimens that are:
    Noninvasively obtained
    Relatively easy to collect
Simple methodology
Cost-effective

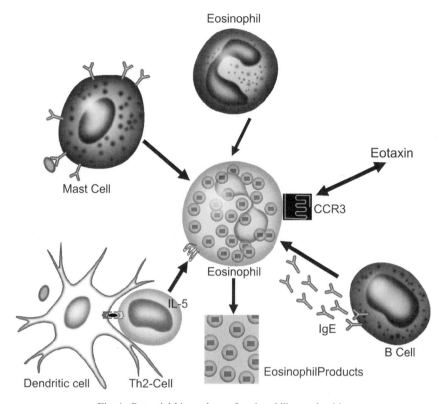

Fig. 1. Potential biomarkers of eosinophilic esophagitis.

mast cell proteins conceivably could serve as mediators of more extensive GI eosinophilic inflammation.

Another mast cell product to consider is histamine a stable metabolite of which, N-methylhistamine, can be measured in urine. This metabolite has been examined in patients who have inflammatory bowel disease but not in EE patients [10].

In summary, data generated over the last decade suggests that mast cells appear to play, although as yet undefined, a role in the pathogenesis of EE. Their role should be explored actively. Other mast cells products and regulators as shown in Fig. 2 could be targets of additional studies.

Peripheral blood eosinophilia (PBE)

Because of the intense tissue eosinophilic infiltration noted in patients who have EE, it is intriguing to study peripheral blood eosinophilia (PBE) in these patients. The reported incidence of PBE in patients who have EE varies between 10% and 100% depending on the particular study, age of patients, and what proportion of patients underwent this measurement. Overall, the reported incidence of PBE is higher in pediatric patients compared

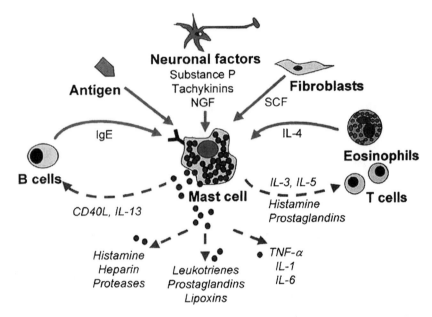

Fig. 2. Regulation of human mast cells. (*From* Bischoff SC, Mayer, JH, Manns MP. Allergy and the gut. Int Arch Allergy Immunol 2000;121:270–83; with permission.)

with adult studies (0% to 100% versus 5% to 50%) [9,11–27]. In the author's experience, PBE was documented in 67% of EE patients [26]. Interestingly, PBE also was noted in 35% of the author's patients who had mild (one to five eosinophils/high power field) and 50% of patients who had moderate (5 to 15 eosinophils/high power field) eosinophilic inflammation of the esophageal epithelium. Regardless, when present in patients who have EE, PBE is generally modest, with the percentage of eosinophils on peripheral smear being worse than absolute peripheral eosinophil count. There are very limited data correlating PBE with response to therapy [28].

In summary, PBE holds promise as a potential biomarker of EE, although several questions need answered as one moves forward in establishing the utility of this test as biomarker of EE. Research ideas on role of PBE as a biomarker include:

- Define and standardize a cut-off value for PBE
- Establish unit of measurement: percentage versus absolute count
- Study PBE in EE patients versus patients with no or mild esophageal eosinophilic inflammation
- PBE correlation with absence/presence of food allergies
- Effect(s) of concomitant atopic diseases on PBE
- Role of seasons on PBE
- Changes in PBE with disease modification/therapy
- Correlate PBE with eosinophil counts on esophageal mucosal biopsies

Serum IgE levels and CD23

IgE levels have been studied in GI allergic diseases; for example, luminal IgE has been isolated in patients with food allergies [29]. In addition, EE is a mixed allergic process with a part IgE component, and these reasons make IgE levels a potential biomarker worthy of further study (see article by Liacouras, elsewhere in this issue).

In addition to IgE levels, CD23 too is a potential biomarker. This low-affinity receptor for IgE is a membrane protein present on various cells including enterocytes, dendritic cells, eosinophils, and subpopulations of B cells, and T cells. CD23 expression is induced by cytokines associated with allergic responses, and CD23 could serve as a potential marker of GI allergy [30]. In a study by Hongxing and colleagues [31], CD23 was detected in the stools of patients who had food allergy(ies), but not in those of controls.

As with PBE, serum IgE levels have been measured in patients who have EE [9,12,15,18,19,22,23,25–27]. Elevated serum IgE levels have been reported in 4% to 69% of adults who have EE and in 33% to 71% of children who have EE. The data on serum IgE levels in children with no or milder esophageal eosinophilic inflammation are limited [26].

The utility of serum IgE levels and stool CD23 levels as markers of a mixed (IgE/non-IgE) allergic process, such as EE, is presently unclear. Potential questions on role of serum IgE level as a biomarker of EE include:

- Define and standardize a cut-off value for serum IgE level
- Study IgE levels in EE patients versus patients with no or mild esophageal eosinophilic inflammation
- Correlate serum IgE level with presence/absence of food allergies
- Effect(s) of concomitant atopic diseases on serum IgE levels
- Changes in serum IgE levels with disease status/therapy
- Effect(s) of seasons on serum IgE levels
- Compare serum IgE levels with esophageal mucosal histology

Additionally, Baxi and colleagues [26] suggest that the PBE and serum IgE levels are similar between EE patients with positive allergy testing and those with negative allergy tests. Future studies should also account for possible seasonal variation in EE. Wang and colleagues [32] reported a lower incidence of EE patients in the winter months compared with other seasons. Researchers need to be cognizant of age-specific normal values for serum IgE levels and also consider inter-lab variability.

Cytokines and chemokines

A multitude of cytokines and chemokines serve as inflammatory mediators. Some of these are specific to particular inflammatory states, while others are general mediators of inflammation. IL-5, an eosinophil specific cytokine, and eotaxin-3, an eosinophil chemoattractant, will be discussed further as these have been studied in noninvasively obtained specimens from EE patients. IL-5 is the lifeline of eosinophils, with several actions on eosinophils, including eosinophil differentiation and maturation in bone marrow, eosinophil mobilization from bone marrow, trafficking of eosinophils into tissue, and eosinophil survival [3]. (See article by Blanchard and Rothenberg, elsewhere in this issue.)

Eotaxins, from the C-C family of chemokines, are potent eosinophil chemoattractants and also promote eosinophil degranulation [33]. Of the three described eotaxins, eotaxin-1 (located on chromosome 17q21.1) is the most potent eosinophil chemoattractant. Eotaxin-2 and eotaxin-3 (located on chromosome 7q11.23) are described to have approximately 40% homology with eotaxin-1 [34]. Eotaxin mRNA is expressed constitutively in various parts of the GI tract, and eotaxins may be involved in the selective regulation of eosinophil homing into the GI tract. Eotaxins mediate their action by means of the CCR3 receptor, a seven transmembrane-spanning G protein-coupled receptor primarily expressed on eosinophils.

Several studies have examined eotaxin and IL-5 expression on esophageal biopsies of patients who have EE [35–37], but few have studied these in noninvasively-obtained specimens [28]. Briefly, eotaxin-3 gene, mRNA, and protein were up-regulated in esophageal biopsies of children with EE compared with controls [35]. In another study, IL-5 mRNA was measured to be higher on esophageal biopsies from children who had EE as compared with controls [36]. Konikoff and colleagues [28] recently published data on serum levels of IL-5 and eotaxin, and the results are presented later in this article. In a longitudinal study of 80 EE children conducted at the author's center, plasma IL-5 levels appear to correlate with disease activity (unpublished data).

In summary, the role of IL-5 and eotaxin, and other cytokines and chemokines, as potential biomarkers of EE is promising but needs further investigation. Targeted questions on cytokines and chemokines as biomarkers of EE include:

- Study various cytokines and chemokines
- Define significance of the differential expression of eotaxin subclasses in EE
- Study protein levels in addition to mRNA measurements in various noninvasively obtained specimens
- Examine and compare with reflux esophagitis and patients without upper GI tract inflammation
- Elucidate effects of therapy on these inflammatory mediators

Eosinophil-derived neurotoxin

Eosinophils contain cytoplasmic granules (Fig. 3) that degranulate on eosinophil stimulation and release various toxic mediators [34]. The crystalloid core of the granules is composed of major basic protein (MBP), and the

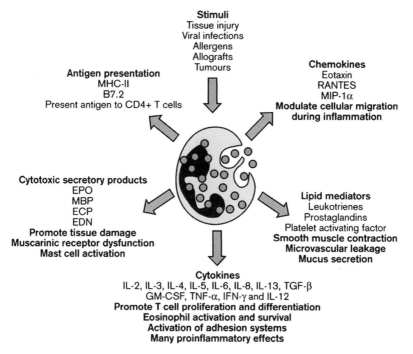

Fig. 3. Eosinophil secretory products and potential actions (bold) (*From* Hogan SP, Foster PS, Rothenberg ME. Experimental analysis of eosinophil-associated gastrointestinal diseases. Curr Opin Allergy Clin Immunol 2002;2:239–48; with permission.)

matrix contains eosinophil cationic protein (ECP), eosinophil peroxidase (EPO), and eosinophil-derived neurotoxin (EDN) [4]. Release of these cationic proteins is by regulated exocytosis and may be selective (eg, eosinophil activation by interferon (IFN)-γ mobilizes RANTES but not cationic proteins). EDN and ECP are members of the RNase A superfamily and have diverse biological functions. In addition to mediating tissue injury, EDN also may promote antigen uptake and processing by recruitment of dendritic cells to inflamed tissue, thereby helping sustain the inflammatory process [38]. In addition to eosinophils, EDN is expressed by neutrophils, macrophages, and monocytes [38].

Elevated levels of eosinophil granular proteins have been reported in the serum and urine of children who have asthma, and in the stool of children who have inflammatory bowel disease [28,39]. In a longitudinal study of children with EE, EDN levels in blood and stool significantly decreased at week 4 compared with baseline (week 0) following 4 weeks of corticosteroid therapy (Fig. 4) [40]. Chehade and colleagues [41] recently presented their preliminary data noting higher serum levels of ECP and EDN in children who had EE as compared with controls.

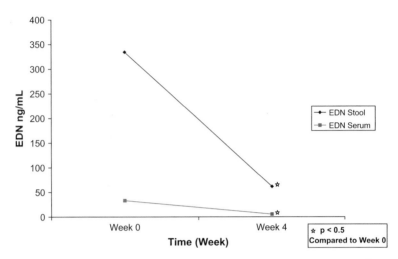

Fig. 4. Changes in stool and serum eosinophil-derived neurotoxin levels with corticosteroid therapy.

In summary, as with serum IgE levels, it might be worthwhile to examine EDN levels in various phenotypes of EE; EDN levels were reported to be higher in patients who had atopic dermatitis with allergic phenotype versus those who had nonallergic phenotype [42].

Biomarkers as a group

A recently published novel study examined a group of laboratory tests as markers of EE activity (Fig. 5) [28]. Children who had active EE, inactive EE, and controls were enrolled in this cross-sectional study. Plasma eosinophil counts, EDN levels, and eotaxin-3 levels were higher in active EE compared with controls. Levels of plasma IL-5, eotaxin-1 and eotaxin-2, and stool EDN were similar in active EE versus controls. Additional studies on this concept should be pursued, and be of longitudinal design.

Summary

There are several potential biomarkers of EE activity, and further studies are needed. I would pay special attention to mast cells (and their activation factors and products), EDN, IL-5, eotaxin family, and biomarker panel. As the field of EE matures, it behooves practitioners to study patients longitudinally, establish robust normal values, account for severity of concomitant atopic disease, and consider the effects of age, symptom profile, and gender on the results. Burdens to address with future research on biomarkers include:

• Study patients longitudinally
• Compare with esophageal biopsies (or symptoms alone??)

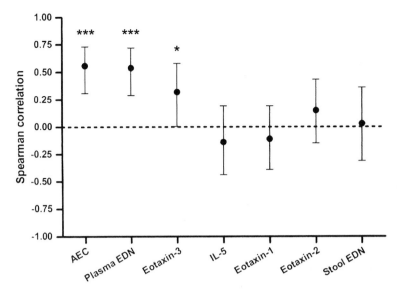

Fig. 5. Correlation of biomarker levels with mean esophageal eosinophil density in proximal and distal esophagus. * $P < .05$, *** $P < .001$. (*From* Konikoff MR, Blanchard C, Kirby C, et al. Potential of blood eosinophils, eosinophil-derived neurotoxin, and eotaxin-3 as biomarkers of eosinophilic esophagitis. Clin Gastroenterol Hepatol 2006;4:1328–36; with permission.)

- Establish robust normal values
- Consider effects of concomitant atopic diseases
- Examine effects of age, symptom profile, gender
- Investigate laboratory methods: valid methodology, quality assurance
- Explore cost-effectiveness in clinical practice

These parameters will need to be weighed against the associated costs, the practicality of methodology, and patient burdens associated with specimen collections.

Acknowledgments

I would like to thank Dr. Joseph and Mrs. Nell Fitzgerald for their guidance, mentoring, and nurturing over the last many years and for his contributions to the field of EE. I am grateful to my colleagues for assistance with clinical studies and indebted to my family for affording me the time for academic pursuits. Many thanks to Miriam Davis, BS, for help with EE studies, Dr. Girish Rao and Dr. Elizabeth Schaefer for illustrations and to Sharon McPheeters for expert secretarial assistance.

References

[1] Furuta GT, Liacouras CA, Collins MH, et al. Eosinophilic esophagitis in children and adults: a systematic review and consensus recommendations for diagnosis and treatment. Gastroenterology 2007;133:1342–63.

[2] Wielders PL, Dekhuijzen PN. Disease monitoring in chronic obstructive pulmonary disease: is there a role for biomarkers? Eur Respir J 1997;10:2443–5.

[3] Furuta GT, Straumann A. Review article: the pathogenesis and management of eosinophilic oesophagitis. Aliment Pharmacol Ther 2006;24:173–82.

[4] Rothenberg ME, Hogan SP. The eosinophil. Annu Rev Immunol 2006;24:147–74.

[5] Justinich CJ, Kalafus D, Esposito P, et al. Mucosal mast cells distinguish allergic from gastroesophageal reflux-induced esophagitis. J Pediatr Gastroenterol Nutr 1996;23:342.

[6] Vanderhoof JA, Young RJ, Hanner TL, et al. Montelukast use in pediatric patients with eosinophilic gastrointestinal disease. J Pediatr Gastroenterol Nutr 2003;36:293–4.

[7] Schwartz DA, Pardi DS, Murray JA. Use of montelukast as steroid-sparing agent for recurrent eosinophilic gastroenteritis. Dig Dis Sci 2001;46:1787–90.

[8] Bischoff SC, Mayer JH, Manns MP. Allergy and the gut. Int Arch Allergy Immunol 2000; 121:270–83.

[9] Gupta SK, Peters-Golden M, Fitzgerald JF, et al. Cysteinyl leukotrienes levels in esophageal mucosal biopsies of children with eosinophilic inflammation: are they all the same? Am J Gastroenterol 2006;101:1125–8.

[10] Winterkamp S, Weidenhiller M, Otte P, et al. Urinary excretion of N-methylhistamine as a marker of disease activity in inflammatory bowel disease. Am J Gastroenterol 2002;97: 3071–7.

[11] Parfitt JR, Gregor JC, Suskin NG, et al. Eosinophilic esophagitis in adults: distinguishing features from gastroesophageal reflux disease. A study of 41 patients. Mod Pathol 2006; 19:90–6.

[12] Straumann A, Spichtin H, Bucher KA, et al. Natural history of primary eosinophilic esophagitis: a follow-up of 30 adult patients for up to 11.5 years. Gastroenterology 2003;125: 1660–9.

[13] Arora AS, Perrault J, Smyrk TC. Topical corticosteroid treatment of dysphagia due to eosinophilic esophagitis in adults. Mayo Clin Proc 2003;78:830–5.

[14] Attwood SEA, Smyrk TC, Demeester TR, et al. Esophageal eosinophilia with dysphagia. A distinct clinicopathologic syndrome. Dig Dis Sci 1993;38:109–16.

[15] Straumann A, Kristl J, Conus S. Cytokine expression in healthy and inflamed mucosa: probing the role of eosinophils in the digestive tract. Inflamm Bowel Dis 2005;11:720–6.

[16] Zimmerman SL, Levine MS, Rubesin SE. Idiopathic eosinophilic esophagitis in adults: the ringed esophagus. Radiology 2005;236:159–65.

[17] Gonsalves N, Policarpio-Nicolas M, Zhang Q. Histopathologic variability and endoscopic correlates in adults with eosinophilic esophagitis. Gastrointest Endosc 2006;64:313–9.

[18] Croese J, Fairley SK, Masson JW, et al. Clinical and endoscopic features of eosinophilic esophagitis in adults. Gastrointest Endosc 2003;58:516–22.

[19] Remedios M, Campbell C, Jones, et al. Eosinophilic esophagitis in adults: clinical, endoscopic, histologic findings, and response to treatment with fluticasone propionate. Gastrointest Endosc 2006;63:3–12.

[20] Walsh SV, Antonioli DA, Goldman H, et al. Allergic esophagitis in children: a clinicopathological entity. Am J Surg Pathol 1999;23:390–6.

[21] Teitelbaum JE, Fox VL, Twarog FJ, et al. Eosinophilic esophagitis in children: immunopathological analysis and response to fluticasone proprionate. Gastroenterology 2002;122: 1216–25.

[22] Orenstein SR, Shalaby TM, Di Lorenzo C, et al. The spectrum of pediatric eosinophilic esophagitis beyond infancy: a clinical series of 30 children. Am J Gastroenterol 2000;95: 1422–30.

[23] Sant'Anna AM, Rolland S, Fournet JC, et al. Eosinophilic esophagitis in children: symptoms, histology and pH probe results. J Pediatr Gastroenterol Nutr 2004;39:373–7.

[24] Noel RJ, Putnam PE, Collins MH, et al. Clinical and immunopathologic effects of swallowed fluticasone for eosinophilic esophagitis. Clin Gastroenterol Hepatol 2004;2:568–75.

[25] Esposito S, Marinello D, Paracchini R, et al. Long-term follow-up of symptoms and peripheral eosinophil counts in seven children with eosinophilic esophagitis. J Pediatr Gastroenterol Nutr 2004;38:452–6.

[26] Baxi S, Gupta SK, Swigonski N, et al. Clinical presentation of patients with eosinophilic inflammation of the esophagus. Gastrointest Endosc 2006;64:473–8.

[27] Kelly K, Lazenby A, Rowe P. Eosinophilic esophagitis attributed to gastroesophageal reflux: improvement with an amino acid-based formula. Gastroenterology 1995;109:1503–12.

[28] Konikoff MR, Blanchard C, Kirby C, et al. Potential of blood eosinophils, eosinophil-derived neurotoxin, and eotaxin-3 as biomarkers of eosinophilic esophagitis. Clin Gastroenterol Hepatol 2006;4:1328–36.

[29] Schwab D, Raithel M, Klein P, et al. Immunoglobulin E and eosinophilic cationic protein in segmental lavage fluid of the small and large bowel identify patients with food allergy. Am J Gastroenterol 2001;96:508–14.

[30] Yu LCH, Montagnac G, Yang PC, et al. Intestinal epithelial CD23 mediates enhanced antigen transport in allergy: evidence for novel spice forms. Am J Physiol 2003;285:G223–4.

[31] Hongxing L, Nowak-Wegrzyn A, Charlop-Powers Z, et al. Transcytosis of IgE-antigen complexes by CD23a in human intestinal epithelial cells and its role in food allergy. Gastroenterology 2006;131:47–58.

[32] Wang FY, Gupta SK, Fitzgerald JF. Is there a seasonal variation in the incidence or intensity of allergic eosinophilic esophagitis in newly diagnosed children? J Clin Gastroenterol 2007; 41:451–3.

[33] Menzies-Gow A, Robinson DS. Eosinophil chemokines and their receptors: an attractive target in asthma? Lancet 2000;355:1741–3.

[34] Hogan SP, Foster PS, Rothenberg ME. Experimental analysis of eosinophil-associated gastrointestinal diseases. Curr Opin Allergy Clin Immunol 2002;2:239–48.

[35] Blanchard C, Wang N, Stringer KF, et al. Eotaxin-3 and a uniquely conserved gene expression profile in eosinophilic esophagitis. J Clin Invest 2006;116:536–47.

[36] Gupta SK, Fitzgerald JF, Kondratyuk T, et al. Cytokine expression in normal and inflamed esophageal mucosa: a study into the pathogenesis of allergic eosinophilic esophagitis (AEE). J Pediatr Gastroenterol Nutr 2006;42:22–6.

[37] Straumann A, Bauer M, Fischer B, et al. Idiopathic eosinophilic esophagitis is associated with a T_H2-type allergic inflammatory response. J Allergy Clin Immunol 2001;108:954–61.

[38] Yang D, Chen Q, Rosenberg H, et al. Human ribonuclease A superfamily members, eosinophil-derived neurotoxin, and pancreatic ribonuclease induce dendritic cell maturation and activation. J Immunol 2004;173:6134–42.

[39] Saitoh O, Kojima K, Sugi K, et al. Fecal eosinophil granule-derived proteins reflect disease activity in inflammatory bowel disease. Am J Gastroenterol 1999;94:3513–20.

[40] Rao GS, Mitchell L, Ohnuki L, et al. Can eosinophil-derived neurotoxin (EDN) act as a surrogate marker of disease activity in children with allergic eosinophilic esophagitis (AEE)? Gastrointest Endosc 2004;59:AB103.

[41] Chehade M, Yershov O, Sampson HA. Serum eosinophil cationic protein and eosinophil-derived neurotoxin are potential non-invasive biomarkers for eosinophilic esophagitis. Gastroenterology 2007;132:A-6.

[42] Jenerowicz D, Czarnecka-Operacz M, Silny W. Selected eosinophil proteins as markers of inflammation in atopic dermatitis patients. Acta Dermatovenerol Croat 2006;14:73–80.

ELSEVIER
SAUNDERS

Gastrointest Endoscopy Clin N Am
18 (2008) 169–178

GASTROINTESTINAL
ENDOSCOPY CLINICS
OF NORTH AMERICA

Pharmacologic Treatment of Eosinophilic Esophagitis

Chris A. Liacouras, MD[a,b,*]

[a]University of Pennsylvania School of Medicine, 34th and Civic Center Boulevard,
Philadelphia, PA 19104, USA
[b]The Children's Hospital of Philadelphia, Division of Gastroenterology, Hepatology
and Nutrition, 34th and Civic Center Boulevard, Philadelphia, PA 19104, USA

There are several treatment options available for patients who have eosinophilic esophagitis (EE) [1–5]. These options include dilatation for mechanical esophageal abnormalities, pharmacologic therapy, and dietary management. Providing the appropriate therapy depends on the significance of clinical symptoms, association of abnormal anatomy, and histologic involvement of underlying the esophageal tissue. When considering therapy for EE, it is important to understand its clinico–pathologic diagnosis [6]. EE is defined histologically by an isolated esophageal eosinophilia of greater then 15 eosinophils in the most densely involved 400 power microscopic field. The histology of the remainder of the gastrointestinal (GI) tract is normal and all other causes of esophageal eosinophila such as gastroesophageal reflux disease, parasitic disease, and inflammatory bowel disease must be ruled out. In general, the exclusion of gastroesophageal reflux disease is determined by ongoing severe esophageal eosinophila despite the use of proton pump inhibitor (PPI) therapy or with a normal pH monitoring of the distal esophagus.

Proton pump inhibitors

Acid blockade has been used in patients with esophageal eosinophilia since the disease originally was described in the late 1990s [7]. Initially, it was thought that severe gastroesophageal reflux led to significant esophageal eosinophilia and thus treatment with a PPI would provide symptomatic and

* The Children's Hospital of Philadelphia, Division of Gastroenterology, Hepatology and
Nutrition, 34th and Civic Center Boulevard, Philadelphia, PA 19104.
  E-mail address: liacouras@email.chop.edu

1052-5157/08/$ - see front matter © 2008 Elsevier Inc. All rights reserved.
doi:10.1016/j.giec.2007.09.012   *giendo.theclinics.com*

histologic relief. As now is known, however, EE is defined by the lack of response to PPI therapy [6].

Currently, PPIs play two important roles for managing patients who have EE. First, as mentioned previously, because it is important to exclude acid reflux disease as a cause for esophageal eosinophila, patients should be treated with PPIs to suppress gastric acid and alleviate any symptoms and mucosal disease associated with acid reflux. Ngo reported three cases of patients who had severe esophageal eosinophilia (greater then 30 eosinophils per higher power field) who were treated with a PPI [8]. In these three cases, both the clinical symptoms and the esophageal eosinophilia resolved. These patients were diagnosed with gastroesophageal reflux disease (GERD) and not EE.

Diagnosis of EE should be made by endoscopy and biopsy only after a patient has been treated with a PPI for at least 4 weeks. Despite the fact that EE is not caused by gastroesophageal reflux, the concomitant use of a PPI is important in many patients who have EE. Because EE may involve the mucosal, submucosal, and muscular layers of the esophagus, esophageal dysmotility is likely to occur which may lead to secondary GERD. The use of PPI therapy, during the initial diagnosis and management phase of patients with EE, often provides symptomatic relief of any symptoms caused by GERD.

There have been no significant pediatric studies demonstrating the effect of PPI therapy on EE. Desai, however, evaluated PPI therapy in 17 adult patients with EE (defined as esophageal eosinophilia of greater then 20 eosinophils per higher power field) [9]. He reported that eight patients clinically improved with the administration of a PPI. unfortunately, these patients did not have histologic follow-up, so it was unknown whether histologic improvement also occurred. Eight additional patients demonstrated no improvement with PPI therapy but later did demonstrate improvement with other medical modalities that treat EE (steroids). One patient was lost to follow-up.

PPI therapy (maximum of 2 mg/kg divided twice daily; maximum of 80 mg/d) is recommended in any patient in whom EE is considered. The lack of histologic response to PPI therapy in patients who have an isolated esophageal eosinophila is virtually diagnostic of EE. Once EE has been treated adequately, PPI therapy can be discontinued. It is important to understand that PPI therapy alone is insufficient for EE treatment.

Corticosteroids

Numerous studies have shown that corticosteroids significantly improve esophageal eosinophila in patients who have EE [10,11]. Over the past 10 years, several methods of steroid administration have been used. These include oral prednisone, topical, swallowed fluticasone, and swallowed budesonide mixed in a sucralose suspension. All of these methods of steroid administration have been shown to successfully improve both the clinical symptoms and abnormal esophageal histology depending upon the dose used.

Systemic corticosteroids

Several decades ago, oral prednisone was administered to patients with eosinophilic GI disease and shown to have an effect on both abnormal mucosal eosinophilia and clinical symptoms [12]. In 1998, Liacouras and colleagues [13] evaluated 20 patients who had EE and demonstrated that the oral administration of 1.5 mg/kg of methylprednisolone significantly improved esophageal inflammation. Clinically, symptoms resolved in 19 of 20 patients, with initial symptom resolution within 8 days of initiating therapy. In addition, in most cases, when steroids were discontinued, the patient's symptoms and abnormal histology recurred.

Oral corticosteroids are an effective therapy for the treatment of EE. Prednisone should be reserved for patients who present emergently with severe dysphagia, small-caliber esophagus, acute weight loss, or the inability to sustain oral intake. Prednisone should be thought of as a short-term therapy used as a bridge until another more acceptable therapy can be initiated. Typically, doses of 1 to 2 mg/kg (maximum of 60 mg/d) of prednisone are used. Symptomatic improvement should occur within 7 to 10 days, and histologic improvement can be seen within 1 month. Without other treatment, EE almost always recurs when oral steroids are discontinued. Additionally, the long-term use of this medication is associated with significant adverse effects (poor growth, adrenal suppression, bone abnormalities, etc.) and is not recommended for maintenance in patients who have EE.

Topical corticosteroids

In 1999, Faubion and colleagues [14] reported four patients with EE who responded to administration of topical, swallowed fluticasone spray. These patients were provided with up to 880 μg of swallowed fluticasone twice daily. All four patients demonstrated significant clinical improvement; furthermore, two patients had normal biopsy specimens upon repeat endoscopy 6 weeks after the initiation of therapy Since that time, there have been other studies that have reported the effectiveness of topical steroids for EE [15].

Teitelbaum and colleagues [16] conducted a prospective trial examining the use of swallowed fluticasone proprionate on children who had EE. Nineteen subjects were identified, of whom, 11 patients were treated with fluticasone and completed the full study. Swallowed fluticasone was administered at a dose of 88 μg twice daily to children 2 to 4 years of age, 220 μg twice daily to children 5 to 10 years of age, and 440 μg twice daily to children greater than 11 years of age. Patients were instructed not to inhale the medication, not to use a spacer, and not to drink or eat for 30 minutes. Clinically, all 11 patients improved. Endoscopically, the visual appearance of the esophagus continued to suggest inflammatory changes in nine patients; however, microscopically, all patients demonstrated significant improvement. In addition, immunohistopathologic studies were performed and revealed a significant reduction of CD3+ and CD8+ lymphocytes, after treatment. Two patients developed esophageal candidiasis.

Noel and colleagues [17] conducted a retrospective analysis of 20 pediatric patients with EE who received swallowed fluticasone. In addition to observing the clinical and histologic effect of fluticasone, they studied the CD8+ lymphocyte infiltration, papillary lengthening and basal layer hyperplasia of the esophageal tissue specimens. Skin prick testing identified allergic and nonallergic patients. All of the nonallergic patients responded clinically and histologically to swallowed fluticasone. In contrast, 20% of the allergic patients demonstrated no response, while another 20% only exhibited a partial response to swallowed fluticasone.

Remedios and colleagues [18] performed a prospective study on 19 adult patients identified as having EE (mean age 36 years). Subjects received 500 μg twice daily of fluticasone proprionate. All 19 patients developed a significant clinical improvement after 4 weeks of therapy; 11 became completely asymptomatic. Esophageal histology also improved in all patients, with a mean reduction of proximal esophageal eosinophils from 25 eosinophils per high-power field (HPF) to less than 5 per HPF and distal esophageal eosinophils from 39 to less than 4.Three patients developed mild esophageal candidiasis.

In 2006, Konikoff and colleagues [19] completed the first placebo-controlled trial using fluticasone proprionate in pediatric patients with EE. They randomly assigned 36 patients to receive either placebo (15 patients) or swallowed fluticasone (440 μg twice daily).Clinical symptoms and histologic changes were evaluated. After treatment, 50% of patients treated with fluticasone achieved full histologic remission compared with one patient who received placebo. Of the remaining 11 patients who received fluticasone, three achieved a significant response, while the remainder had no significant improvement. The clinical response was comparable. Other factors studied included higher responsiveness of fluticasone in younger and nonallergic patients. In addition, fluticasone was found to lower esophageal CD8 + T cell levels and the level of esophageal mastocytosis.

Recently, Aceves and colleagues [20,21] reported the successful treatment of EE by using an oral viscous suspension of budesonide instead of a swallowed fluticasone aerosolized spray. A retrospective review was conducted in 20 EE patients (mean age 5.5 years) who were treated with oral budesonide (1 mg/d, younger than10 years of age; 2 mg/d, older than 10 years of age) mixed with 5 g of sucralose. Sixteen patients responded to therapy. One patient demonstrated a partial response, while three failed treatment. Both clinical symptoms and esophageal histology significantly improved in those who responded to therapy. No significant adverse effects occurred, and morning cortisol levels remained within normal limits.

Overall, through September 2006, 47 adult patients were treated with swallowed fluticasone, in doses ranging from 220 to 500 µg twice a day for 4 to 6 weeks. Symptoms improved in all but one patient, and histologic resolution occurred in 75% of patients. When the medication was discontinued, however, EE recurred in 17 of 37 patients ranging from 3 to 18 months at the time of follow-up. No studies documented follow-up past 18 months. During the same time, 33 pediatric patients were studied and provided doses of fluticasone ranging from 220 to 440 µg twice a day for 8 weeks. Clinical and histologic improvement occurred in 31 of 33 patients; however, long term follow-up were not reported.

Currently, topical, swallowed corticosteroids are the best pharmacologic option for patients who have EE. When used in effective doses, these medications improved both clinical symptoms and the underlying abnormal esophageal inflammation similar to results gained with systemic steroids. Topical steroids have minimal short-term and long term-side effects. While epistaxis and dry mouth occur, up to 20% of patients have developed esophageal candidiasis. Unfortunately, long-term maintenance studies have not been performed.

Cromolyn sodium and leukotriene receptor antagonists

Cromolyn prevents the release of inflammatory mediators from mast cells, inhibits the influx of neutrophils, and inhibits the assembly of an active NADPH oxidase in the neutrophil, thereby preventing oxygen radical-induced tissue damage. Although some investigators have hypothesized that enteric cromolyn may be an effective therapy for EE, Liacouras and colleagues [11] used cromolyn sodium as a treatment for EE without success.

Alternatively, leukotrienes attract eosinophils; thus, by blocking the leukotriene receptor, one could decrease the effects of leukotrienes and prevent clinical symptoms [22,23]. Attwood and colleagues [24] used montelukast in high dosages in patients who had EE. They demonstrated decreased symptoms, but because no follow-up endoscopies were performed, no change in endoscopy was noted. An interesting report from Gupta and colleagues [25] compared cysteinyl leukotriene levels in 12 children who had EE, 10 healthy controls, and five children who had eosinophilic gastroenteritis. They found that the levels did not correlate with the degree of eosinophilic inflammation and that there was no statistical difference between levels from patients who had EE and normal controls. Interestingly, increased levels were found in patients with eosinophilic gastroenteritis and reached statistical significance.

Biologic compounds

A large group of substances, cytokines (interleukins), is produced primarily by leukocytes and have various functions. Each interleukin (IL) acts on a specific, limited group of cells that express the receptor for that interleukin. IL-5 is a cytokine that has been demonstrated to regulate various processes associated with eosinophils [26]. These include antigen-induced eosinophilia, bone marrow release of eosinophils, eosinophil tissue survival, and eosinophil activation. Based on these properties, performed in primate and murine models, neutralizing antibodies against murine IL-5 were generated and shown to be safe and effective in lowering eosinophil blood and tissue levels in models of asthma and parasitic infection [27,28]. Notably, IL-5 has been shown to be overproduced in some patients with idiopathic hypereosinophilic syndrome (IHES) and EE [29] and has also been implicated in the pathogenesis of experimental EE in mice [28]. Thus, these findings and observations have led to the use of humanized antibody therapy blocking IL-5 in the treatment of patients who have IHES and EE.

In 2003, Garrett and colleagues [30] treated four patients who had IHES with anti IL-5 antibody. Each patient was treated with 10 mg/kg (maximum 750 mg dose) of mepolizumab with a single intravenous injection for 3 consecutive months. Anti IL-5 significantly reduced peripheral eosinophils and the clinical symptoms in all four patients. One specific patient had severe dysphagia and marked esophageal eosinophilia. After therapy with mepolizumab, not only did the patient's diet significantly improve, but also a striking decrease in esophageal eosinophils and esophageal narrowing occurred. There were no associated adverse effects from the medication.

Recently, Stein and colleagues [31] conducted an open-labeled study using intravenous mepolizumab in four adult patients with EE who had esophageal narrowing and clinical symptoms. Patients received three doses of intravenous anti IL-5 antibody, at monthly intervals, without change in other therapy and then underwent esophageal biopsy at weeks 0, 8, and 20.Blood eosinophils percentages were decreased significantly, as were the number of esophageal eosinophils. Clinically, the medication was tolerated well, and all patients reported a considerable improvement in their clinical symptoms. These results suggest that biologic compounds are a promising new therapy for patients who have EE. Additional studies are in developmental stages. but this treatment is not US Food and Drug Administration (FDA)-approved for use in EE or available outside of research protocol.

Management

Initial management

Initial management for patients identified with esophageal eosinophilia almost always should focus on aggressive acid blockade with a PPI for 4 to 6 weeks. Once the esophageal eosinophilia has been confirmed to persist despite acid blockade, the diagnosis of EE is established. Whenever a patient receives a diagnosis of EE, a decision should be made regarding the best treatment approach: dietary or pharmacological.

Esophageal narrowing or stricture poses a difficult management decision for patients who have EE. Many adult gastroenterologists have reported the use of esophageal dilatation for their patients who present acutely with esophageal strictures. Although esophageal dilatation may relieve dysphagia and improve an esophageal stricture, esophageal tearing during endoscopy and dilatation may occur. Thus, while esophageal dilatation has a role in alleviating severe esophageal strictures in patients who have EE, the results are generally temporary, and both the clinical symptoms and esophageal narrowing often recur. Gastroenterologists should be extremely careful whenever performing endoscopy or dilatation, as perforation is a distinct possibility. Whenever possible, a diagnostic endoscopy should be performed, and medical or dietary therapy instituted. Esophageal dilatation is discussed in greater detail in articles by Straumann, Fox, and Aceves and colleagues, elsewhere in this issue.

Systemic corticosteroids should be considered, and these are an effective short-term therapy, especially for those patients who present with aggressive symptoms including severe dysphagia, the inability to eat solids, significant weight loss, failure to thrive, or intractable vomiting. Occasionally, a brief hospitalization may be required in cases of food impaction or dehydration. Typically, within a few days, the esophageal inflammation decreases such that a normal diet can be initiated. Unfortunately, upon withdrawal of steroid treatment, EE almost always recurs. In addition, given the extensive adverse effect profile, corticosteroids are not considered a good long-term treatment option for EE. Therefore, whenever systemic steroids are used, an alternate treatment approach needs to be considered.

The use of swallowed aerosolized fluticasone or viscous budesonide has been shown to be an effective initial therapy for treating clinical symptoms and eliminating esophageal eosinophils. Unlike systemic steroids, these medications also have been shown to be effective for maintenance therapy. Again, without other treatment, when topical steroids are discontinued, EE generally recurs. Moreover, although minimal adverse effects have been reported, specific adverse effects, including the development of esophageal candidiasis, dry mouth, and epistaxis may occur.

Several other therapies also have been used in an attempt to initially treat EE. Oral cromolyn sodium has not been shown to be an effective option, as it does not improve either the patient's symptoms or the underlying abnormal histology. In contrast, leukotriene receptor antagonists have been reported to improve the symptoms associated with EE; however, there is no evidence that histologic improvement occurs. These two medications have not been accepted generally for routine use for treating patients who have EE. Finally, the use of anti IL-5 antibody is under investigation.

Patients given medical therapy almost always require prolonged therapy, while those prescribed a special diet must remain off the foods that cause EE for an extended period of time. In most cases, a repeat upper endoscopy with biopsy should be performed after initiating treatment to assess for evidence of histological remission. A small number of patients who have EE may be asymptomatic despite an ongoing aggressive eosinophilic inflammation. In these patients, the argument has been made that they do not require treatment, because they have minimal clinical symptoms. The no treatment approach has been suggested because of the potential adverse effects of medication, the difficult social aspects of being on a limited diet, and the lack of information regarding the effects of chronic eosinophilic inflammation on the esophagus. In contrast, other physicians argue that by not treating this disease, patients eventually will have increased mucosal disease, contributing to dysphagia and the development of esophageal strictures. In addition, one of the histologic features of EE is severe hyperplasia of the basic cell layer. In general, significant cell turnover may be a prelude to tissue dysplasia, although this has not been documented in patients with EE. If the decision is made to withhold therapy, close follow-up and repeat endoscopy are suggested.

Long-term management

The focus of long-term management of EE should be to provide symptom relief along with maintaining histologic healing. At this point, clinical experience and small studies suggest that topical corticosteroids and dietary restriction are successful in the long-term treatment of EE. Several reports have demonstrated esophageal healing and symptom resolution with dietary therapy ranging from the removal of a few foods to the use of a total elemental diet strictly using an amino acid-based formula. Dietary management is discussed in greater detail in the article by Spergel and Shuker, elsewhere in this issue.

With regard to medical therapy, because of the possibility of secondary gastroesophageal reflux caused by chronic esophageal inflammation, acid blockade can be an effective concomitant therapy in improving symptoms. The exact incidence of concomitant GERD affecting patients who have EE is unknown. Although the long-term use of topical steroids appears safe, several adverse effects have been reported, including esophageal candidiasis, epistaxis, and dry mouth. In addition, long-term effects on growth, bone health, and esophageal fibrosis are not known. Finally, in the future, biologic therapy using monoclonal antibodies such as anti IL-5 antibody show promising results for initial and maintenance therapy for patients with moderate to severe EE.

At times, combination therapy may be effective. Pentiuk and colleagues [32] studied 15 pediatric patients with EE referred to a feeding team and documented responses to treatment (1/2000 through 6/2003). All received therapy with PPI, swallowed fluticasone, and dietary restriction (when allergy testing was performed and was positive).With this approach, all endoscopies improved, with 93% resolution with therapy, and 87% had clinical improvement. Ferguson and colleagues [33] suggested that 25% to 40% patients with EE relapse. In this study, pediatric patients were treated with dietary management, while adults received swallowed fluticasone for 6 weeks;

if symptoms recurred, they extended the fluticasone treatment for 12 weeks or changed to oral steroid therapy.

Summary

EE is a chronic disease that generally requires long-term maintenance therapy. There is no single specific therapy that should be used in every patient (pediatric or adult) diagnosed with EE. Several therapies, including dilatation, pharmacologic therapy, and dietary therapy have been shown to provide successful treatment; these therapies should be tailored to each patient. Regardless of the therapy instituted, it is recommended that continued follow-up and repeat evaluation should be performed to assess the effectiveness of treatment and the severity of disease. Presently, endoscopy with biopsy is the only reliable method for evaluation. Because symptoms may be sporadic and intermittent. With all treatments, EGD with biopsy should be performed to assess histologic disease. Future research should focus on clarifying the prevalence and natural history (eg, the potential development of strictures) and optimizing the diagnostic approach and treatment options of EE.

References

[1] Liacouras CA. Eosinophilic esophagitis: treatment in 2005. Curr Opin Gastroenterol 2006; 22(2):147–52.

[2] De Angelis P, Markowitz J, Torroni F, et al. Paediatric eosinophilic oesophagitis: towards early diagnosis and best treatment. Dig Liver Dis 2006;38:245–51.

[3] Ngo P, Furuta GT. Treatment of eosinophilic esophagitis in children. Curr Treat Options Gastroenterol 2005;8(5):397–403.

[4] Khan S, Henderson WA. Treatment of eosinophilic esophagitis in children. Curr Treat Options Gastroenterol 2002;5(5):367–76.

[5] Furuta GT, Straumann A. Review article: the pathogenesis and management of eosinophilic esophagitis. Aliment Pharmacol Ther 2006;24:173–82.

[6] Furuta G, Liacouras C, Collins M, et al. Eosinophilic esophagitis in children and adults: a systematic review and consensus recommendations for diagnosis and treatment. Gastroenterology 2007;133:1342–63.

[7] Ruchelli E, Wenner W, Voytek T, et al. Severity of esophageal eosinophilia predicts response to conventional gastroesophageal reflux therapy. Pediatr Dev Pathol 1999;2(1):15–8.

[8] Ngo P, Furuta GT, Antonioli DA, et al. Eosinophils in the esophagus–peptic or allergic eosinophilic esophagitis? Case series of three patients with esophageal eosinophilia. Am J Gastroenterol 2006;101(7):1666–70.

[9] Desai TK, Stecevic V, Chang CH, et al. Association of eosinophilic inflammation with esophageal food impaction in adults. Gastrointest Endosc 2005;61(7):795–801.

[10] Vitellas KM, Bennett WF, Bova JG, et al. Radiographic manifestations oeosinophilicgastroenteritis. Abdom Imaging 1995;20(5):406–13.

[11] Liacouras CA, Spergel JM, Richelli E, et al. Eosinophilic esophagitis: a 10-year experience in 381 children. Clin Gastroenterol Hepatol 2005;3(12):1198–206.

[12] Kravis LP, South MA, Rosenlund ML. Eosinophilic gastroenteritis in the pediatric patient. Clin Pediatr 1982;21(12):713–7.

[13] Liacouras CA, Wenner W, Voytek T, et al. Primary eosinophilic esophagitis in children: successful treatment with oral corticosteroids. J Pediatr Gastroenterol Nutr 1998;26(4):380–5.

[14] Faubion W Jr, Perrault J, Burgart LJ, et al. Treatment of eosinophilic esophagitis with inhaled corticosteroids. J Pediatr Gastroenterol Nutr 1998;27(1):90–3.

[15] Arora AS, Perrault J, Smyrk TC, et al. Topical corticosteroid treatment of dysphagia due to eosinophilic esophagitis in adults. Mayo Clin Proc 2003;78(7):830–5.

[16] Teitelbaum JE, Fox VL, Twarog FJ, et al. Eosinophilic esophagitis in children: immunopathological analysis and response to fluticasone propionate. Gastroenterology 2002; 122(5):1216–25.

[17] Noel RJ, Putnam PE, Collins MH, et al. Clinical and immunopathologic effects of swallowed fluticasone for eosinophilic esophagitis. Clin Gastroenterol Hepatol 2004;2(7):568–75.

[18] Remedios M, Campbell C, Jones DM, et al. Eosinophilic esophagitis in adults: clinical, endoscopic, histologic findings, and response to treatment with fluticasone propionate. Gastrointest Endosc 2006;63(1):3–12.

[19] Konikoff MR, Noel RJ, Blanchard C, et al. A randomized, double-blind, placebo-controlled trial of fluticasone proprionate for pediatric eosinophilic esophagitis. Gastroenterology 2006;131(5):1381–91.

[20] Aceves SS, Bastian JF, Newbury RO, et al. Oral viscous budesonide: a potential new therapy for eosinophilic esophagitis in children. Am J Gastroenterol 2007;102:2271–9.

[21] Aceves SS, Dahil R, Newbury RO, et al. Topical viscous budesonide suspension for treatment of eosinophilic esophagitis. J Allergy Clin Immunol 2005;116(3):705–6.

[22] Gawrieh S, Shaker R. Treatment options for eosinophilic esophagitis: montelukast. Curr Gastroenterol Rep 2004;6(3):190.

[23] Sinharay R. Eosinophilic oesophagitis: treatment using montelukast. Gut 2003;52(8): 1228–9.

[24] Attwood SE, Lewis CJ, Bronder CS, et al. Eosinophilic oesophagitis: a novel treatment using montelukast. Gut 2003;52(2):181–5.

[25] Gupta SK, Peters-Golden M, Fitzgerald JF, et al. Cysteinyl leukotriene levels in esophageal mucosal biopsies of children with eosinophilic esophageal inflammation: are they all the same? Am J Gastroenterol 2006;101(5):1125–8.

[26] Simon D, Braathen LR, Simon HU. Anti-interleukin-5 antibody therapy in eosinophilic diseases. Pathobiology 2005;72(6):287–92.

[27] Hart TK, Cook RM, Zia-Amirhosseini P, et al. Preclinical efficacy and safety of mepolizumab (SB-240563), a humanized monoclonal antibody to IL-5, in cynomologus monkeys. J Allergy Clin Immunol 2001;108:250–7.

[28] Mishra A, Hogan SP, Brandt EB, et al. An etiological role for aeroallergens and eosinophils in experimental esophagitis. J Clin Invest 2001;107:83–90.

[29] Owen WF, Rothenberg ME, Petersen J, et al. Interleukin 5 and phenotypically altered eosinophils in the blood of patients with the idiopathic hypereosinophilic syndrome. J Exp Med 1989;170:343–8.

[30] Garrett JK, Jameson SC, Thomson B, et al. Anti-interleukin-5 (mepolizumab) therapy for hypereosinophilic syndromes. J Allergy Clin Immunol 2004;113(1):115–9, Epub 2003 Dec 12.

[31] Stein ML, Collins MH, Villanueva JM, et al. Anti-IL 5 (mepolizumab) therapy for eosinophilic esophagitis. J Allergy Clin Immunol 2006;118:1312–9.

[32] Pentiuk SP, Miller CK, Kaul A. Eosinophilic esophagitis in infants and toddlers. Dysphagia 2007;22(1):44–8.

[33] Ferguson DD, Foxx-Orenstein AE. Eosinophilic esophagitis: an update. Dis Esophagus 2007;20(1):2–8.

ELSEVIER
SAUNDERS
Gastrointest Endoscopy Clin N Am
18 (2008) 179–194

Nutritional Management
of Eosinophilic Esophagitis

Jonathan M. Spergel, MD, PhD[a,b,c,*],
Michele Shuker, MS, RD, CSP, LDN[b]

[a]Division of Allergy and Immunology, Wood Building 5314, The Children's Hospital
of Philadelphia, 34th and Civic Center Boulevard, Philadelphia, PA 19104, USA
[b]Center for Pediatric Eosinophilic Disorders, The Children's Hospital of Philadelphia,
34th and Civic Center Boulevard, Philadelphia, PA 19104, USA
[c]Department of Pediatrics, University of Pennsylvania School of Medicine,
34th and Civic Center Boulevard, Philadelphia, PA 19104, USA

Eosinophilic esophagitis (EE) is characterized by infiltration of the esophagus with eosinophils without infiltration in other parts of the gastrointestinal tract. EE has become increasingly prevalent based on studies in the United States and Australia [1–3]. The authors have seen a 35-fold increase, from 2 cases in 1994 to 72 cases in 2003, at The Children's Hospital of Philadelphia [4]. Patients who have EE typically are male (by a 2:1 ratio) [3,5], and the majority of patients have associated allergies (asthma, allergic rhinitis, or atopic dermatitis).

The symptoms of EE are similar to the symptoms of gastroesophageal reflux but do not respond to medications for gastroesophageal reflux disease (GERD). Other symptoms of EE include dysphagia in older children and failure to thrive in infants [3,4,6]. Because of these diverse symptoms, EE can be diagnosed only by esophageal biopsy (after aggressive treatment with gastroesophageal reflux medications) with the finding of 15 or more eosinophils per high-power field (HPF) [3,4].

Foods have been shown to be the cause of EE through the use of elimination diets or elemental formulas [7,8]. The critical evidence that foods play a role in EE came from work done by Kevin Kelly and Hugh Sampson in 1996 [9]. They examined 10 children (aged 8 months to 12.5 years) who had persistent symptoms of reflux and who had not responded to GERD medications, including 6 who had prior Nissen fundoplications. All 10 patients

---

* Corresponding author. Division of Allergy and Immunology, Wood Building 5314, Children's Hospital of Philadelphia, 34th and Civic Center Boulevard, Philadelphia, PA 19104.
E-mail address: spergel@email.chop.edu (J.M. Spergel).

1052-5157/08/$ - see front matter © 2008 Elsevier Inc. All rights reserved.
doi:10.1016/j.giec.2007.09.008 *giendo.theclinics.com*

improved on elemental formula, with 8 patients reaching completely normal levels and the remaining 2 patients reaching nearly normal levels [9]. Symptoms returned when food was reintroduced into the diet, with milk causing symptoms in 7 patients, soy in 4 patients, wheat and peanut in 2 patients, and egg in 1 patient. In larger studies with over 160 patients at The Children's Hospital of Philadelphia, more than 98% of the patients have demonstrated resolution of symptoms and normalization of biopsies with elemental diets [4,7], indicating that food allergies can cause EE. Because of the poor palatability of elemental formulas, patients often refuse this difficult diet. Therefore, elimination diets based on skin prick testing (SPT) and atopy patch testing (APT) [5,8,10] or on the removal of the most common food allergens [11] have been tried with similar rates of improvement (75%).

Therefore, three nutritional or dietary approaches exist for EE. This article examines these approaches with emphasis on the nutritional risks, advantages, and disadvantages of each method.

Overall nutrition assessment of the patient who has eosinophilic esophagitis

Each of the three proposed methods for dietary treatment of EE presents potential nutritional risks. A thorough nutrition assessment by a registered dietitian experienced in food allergy therefore is advisable for all patients after diagnosis. The challenge to the registered dietitian is in educating the patient and family on which foods need to be avoided and also teaching them how to replace nutrients lost when major allergens are removed.

A complete diet history should be obtained and should include food preferences, brand names of food, amounts consumed at meals, eating behaviors, number of caregivers involved in food shopping and preparation, and methods of food preparation. All these factors can affect adherence to the prescribed diet, and a careful review can help identify potential barriers to successful nutrition therapy.

Estimating nutritional requirements

Estimated nutritional requirements are determined using established methods for the pediatric population: Recommended Dietary Allowances and Dietary Reference Intakes [12,13]. Nutritional requirements for children who have EE generally are the same as for healthy children who do not have allergies. Additional calories, protein, and/or micronutrients may be required in certain situations (eg, history of poor weight gain and/or growth, atopic dermatitis).

Carbohydrate intake should provide 45% to 55% of total calories, with an emphasis on whole grains, fruits, and vegetables for nutrients and fiber. Wheat often is removed from the diet of children who have EE, necessitating the use of alternate grain sources, as discussed later.

High-quality sources of protein should comprise 15% to 20% of the diet, with fat providing the remaining 30% to 35% of total calories. Adequate dietary fat helps ensure appropriate energy intake and prevents essential fatty acid deficiency. A variety of dietary fat is encouraged so that appropriate amounts of monounsaturated, polyunsaturated, and saturated fats are consumed.

Micronutrient intake will vary according to the severity of diet restrictions. Salman and colleagues [14] noted that the intake of children who have food allergies was low in calcium, iron, vitamin D, vitamin E, and zinc. The need for supplementation should be assessed continually when diet modifications change throughout treatment.

Elimination diets pose significant challenges to patients and families. Some foods are easier to omit from the diet than others, but the removal of even one dietary staple can make for a difficult adjustment. Milk and wheat proteins generally are the most difficult allergens to remove, because they are present in the diets of so many children. Their removal also results in the greatest nutritional impact. Christie and colleagues [15] found that children who have milk allergy or children with two or more food allergies were shorter, based on height-for-age percentiles, than those who had only one food allergy. As might be expected, children who had cow's milk allergy or multiple food allergies consumed less dietary calcium than children who did not have cow's milk allergy and/or had only one food allergy.

Elemental diets

Markowitz and colleagues [7] confirmed the causative role of foods in EE in a study in 346 children who had chronic GERD symptoms, of whom 51 eventually received the diagnosis of EE. The 51 patients who had EE then were given an elemental formula; 49 of the 51 patients improved symptomatically within 8 days, and the number of eosinophils in the distal esophagus decreased significantly, to normal levels, within 1 month. This finding was confirmed in the authors' larger study at The Children's Hospital Philadelphia, in which biopsies of 158 of 160 patients normalized after treatment with an elemental diet [4]. In a review of all of their nearly 500 patients, the authors found only 5 patients ($<2\%$) who did not respond to an elemental diet. The rest showed complete resolution of symptoms and normalization of biopsies to an average of 1.1 eosinophils per HPF. Kagalwalla and colleagues [11] found similar results at Northwestern Medical Center, where 25 children were treated with an elemental diet and 35 children were treated with selective diet elimination of six common allergens. The biopsies of all the children treated with the elemental diet normalized; counts improved from 58.8 ± 31.9 eosinophils to 3.6 ± 6.5 eosinophils per HPF ($P<.001$). The dramatic improvement with the elemental diet within 6 weeks shows that food allergies cause EE in pediatric patients. This causation has not been studied in adult patients, however. Eighty percent of the patients requiring elemental diets used nasogastric tubes to receive sufficient calories.

An important part of therapy is the addition of foods back into the diet. The rationale and scheme for adding foods back into the diet is discussed later.

Nutritional concerns of elemental diet

An elemental diet requires the replacement of all solid foods with a nutritionally complete elemental formula, in which the protein source is comprised entirely of synthetic amino acids. Hydrolyzed protein or semi-elemental formulas are not acceptable for use, because they contain small amounts of milk proteins.

Flavors/palatability

One of the most frequently encountered barriers to success with an elemental diet is the acceptance of the formulas by patients. The use of amino acids as the main protein source renders the formulas significantly less palatable than their intact protein counterparts. Flavors of these formulas have improved in recent years, although their palatability remains, as expected, largely a matter of opinion. The prospect of drinking at least a liter of these formulas per day can indeed be overwhelming. The two major manufacturers of formulas approved for use in these populations produce both flavored and unflavored formulas. Different strategies can be used to enhance palatability, such as using the sugar-based flavor packets provided by the manufacturer or adding protein-free flavorings of the patient's choice (eg, chocolate syrup, powdered drink mixes). Any flavorings should be discussed with the allergist before use to ensure their safety, although the use of sugar-based or artificially sweetened products that do not contain protein are likely to pose little allergenic risk.

If a patient is unable or unwilling to consume the required volume of elemental formula, the use of a nasogastric tube may be necessary. This concept is foreign to most patients and families, but with proper training the feedings can be provided successfully in almost all cases. The advice of an experienced registered dietician is essential in managing enteral tube feedings.

Other nutrients/vitamins/protein/fat

Micronutrient supplementation may be required, depending on the volume of formula consumed. Most additional needs can be met using over-the-counter supplements that are free of major allergens. Product ingredients should be reviewed on a regular basis to ensure safety.

Elemental formulas do not contain dietary fiber, which can be problematic for some children. Fiber supplements are useful for children who develop or are prone to constipation and for those who remain dependent on elemental formula for longer periods of time if solid foods cannot be re-introduced. Supplements should be free of known allergens (eg, wheat starch). The authors have used guar gum–based fiber supplements without difficulty in patients at the Children's Hospital of Philadelphia.

Elimination diets

An alternative dietary approach is to remove specific foods. There are two ways to remove individual foods, based either on testing or on the removal of common foods. Kagalwalla and colleagues [11] removed the eight most common food groups (milk, soy, egg, wheat, shellfish, fish, tree nuts, and peanut) in 35 pediatric patients. The children treated with this elimination diet showed clinicopathologic improvement (80.2 ± 44.0 eosinophils per HPF before elimination versus 13.6 ± 23.8 after elimination). The nutritional issues of this diet are discussed later.

The other approach to remove selective foods is based on testing to foods. There are two methods to test for IgE-mediated food allergies: in vitro (radioallergosorbent testing or fluoroenzyme immunoassay) and SPT. These tests have been standardized and validated for many IgE-mediated allergies. IgE-mediated allergies are classic food allergies, with symptoms such as urticaria and anaphylaxis that occur immediately (within seconds to 1 hour) after eating the food. Classic IgE-mediated symptoms or reactions usually are not seen in EE, however. Therefore most studies have had limited or no success with using only in vitro specific IgE testing or SPT.

The method for SPT involves placing the allergen on the forearm or back, pricking the skin with a device, and measuring the wheal and flare reaction. If the wheal diameter is greater than 3 mm, the test is considered positive. The authors examined the positive predictive (PPV) and negative predictive values (NPV) for SPT in 104 children who had EE to determine if removal of an individual food led to normalization of esophageal biopsies or if the addition of the individual foods led to greater than 20 eosinophils per HPF in the esophagus. The NPV for the SPT for EE ranged from 58% for milk, 6% to 75% for wheat, soy, egg, corn, and beef, and 85% to 95% for rice, peanut, and oat. (NPV values of SPT for "classic" IgE-mediated food reactions typically are greater than 95% for all foods [16]). In EE, the PPV for the SPT for milk, egg, beef, and peanut was greater than 75%, but the PPV for SPT for oat, rice, potato, peanut, chicken, and barley ranged from 33% to 43% [10]. Similarly, the PPV for the SPT for the classic IgE-mediated reactions (urticaria, anaphylaxis) with a standard positive of wheal greater than 3 mm ranged from 30% for soy and wheat to 70% for egg [16]. Using a large wheal size, a 95% PPV for the major allergens causing IgE-mediated reactions can be determined [17,18], but the authors could not determine a 95% PPV for EE with SPT.

The other method for determining specific IgE reaction to foods is in vitro testing. The standard commercial tests are antibodies against IgE to specific foods. The original radioallergosorbent assays involved detection by radioisotope. The problem with the original assay was a high background and a significant number of false-positive results. The newer assay, which has been in existence for the last 5 years is fluoroenzyme immunoassay. It has a lower background and is supposed to be more specific for true IgE reactions. Sampson and colleagues [19,20] and other laboratories have developed 95% PPVs for milk, egg, and peanut. The specific IgE varied for each food, being 32 kU/L for milk, 6 kU/L for egg, and 14 kU/L for peanut. The investigators could not determine a 95% PPV for other foods they studies (soy and wheat). Also, there was a higher false-negative rate (NPV) for peanut and egg than seen with standard skin tests. There are no reliable studies examining the use of these assays for the diagnosis of food allergies in EE, and anecdotal reports suggest that these assays are not helpful in making the diagnosis of EE.

The IgG reaction to foods has not been studied in EE. The IgG reaction to foods is a normal reaction to foods. There are no well-designed study has found a relationship between the IgG reaction to foods and any type of food allergy.

Because many patients who had EE did not present the clinical picture of IgE-mediated reactions, the authors used APT to look for non–IgE-mediated food reactions. APT was first described for irritants in the early 1900s and later was described for pollen and dust mite in 1950s. The first use of APT for foods was a study by Erika Isoulari [21] to detect milk allergy in atopic dermatitis. APT now is common in Europe for examining non–IgE-mediated food allergies. Like the delayed hypersensitivity test, the APT is thought to provide evidence for a T-cell–mediated reaction. APT is performed by using the food in its native state (ie, fresh milk, plain wheat flour) and placed in an occlusion aluminum Finn Chamber for 48 hours on a patients back. The chamber then is removed, and the reaction is measured for induration and papules 24 hours later (ie, 72 hours after placement). A true-positive reaction is seen not when the patch is removed at 48 hours, but 24 hours later. Although the type of Finn Chamber and recording time have been standardized for other atopic diseases, the quality or quantity of food examined is not standardized. For example, some groups use fresh milk, and others use dried milk.

The authors have developed PPVs and NPVs for SPT in EE using the criteria used for SPT in other diseases. In this analysis, all patients first received an SPT that was followed by APT. If an SPT was positive for a specific food, no APT was completed, because the authors' previous experience demonstrated that APT to SPT-positive foods caused too great an irritant reaction. As in SPT, the PPVs for APT varied from food to food. The PPVs for APT ranged from 94% for beef, to 83% for milk, 60% to 70% for most foods, and 48% for oats [10]. The NPV was more consistent and generally was the mid-80% to the high-90% range for all foods except for milk, which was 59%. This finding suggests if a food is negative on skin test and patch test, it probably is not responsible for EE. The specificity for APT ranged from 43% to 89%, lower than the reported 91% for APT in atopic dermatitis [22]. Interestingly, the sensitivity of APT was better for EE (78%–99%) than for atopic dermatitis (30%–33%) [23].

The authors also examined the combination of skin test and patch test to identify foods causing EE. In this scenario, if either test was positive, the food was eliminated from the diet. If the patient developed clinicopathologic remission and/or developed signs and symptoms of the disease with re-introduction of the food, the specific food was identified as a cause of the patient's EE. The PPV varied from 92% for milk to 50% for oat (Table 1). The NPV ranged from 88% to 100% for all foods except for milk. The high NPV indicates that if a food (other than milk) is negative on skin test or patch test, it is unlikely to cause EE. This finding is problematical, because milk is the most common food causing EE in the authors' pediatric population.

Nutritional needs and evaluation

The risk of dietary inadequacy increases with the number and type of foods removed from the diet and also is influenced by the child's nutritional status on diagnosis and the presence of additional risk factors (refusal of foods/selective eating/texture aversion). The removal of some food groups (dairy, meat, grains) poses more substantial nutritional challenges than the removal of others. Careful attention should be paid to the calories, protein, and micronutrients remaining in the diet. Vitamin and mineral supplements may be necessary.

For example, those on a dairy-free diet may need to replace calcium and protein. Fiber supplements may be needed if grains are removed and intake of fruits and vegetables is suboptimal. The family can keep a 3-day diet

Table 1
Predictive values for skin prick test and atopy patch test for eosinophilic esophagitis

Food	Combined skin prick test and atopy patch test			
	PPV (%)	NPV (%)	Specificity (%)	Sensitivity (%)
Milk	92.0	40.9	63.9	81.8
Egg	84.8	87.5	86.7	85.7
Soy	73.7	92.9	87.5	83.9
Wheat	76.5	90.0	81.3	87.1
Corn	63.4	92.5	86.7	76.6
Beef	85.2	92.5	82.1	93.9
Chicken	62.5	98.6	93.8	88.5
Apple	57.1	97.7	66.7	96.6
Rice	60.9	100.0	100.0	88.8
Potato	61.1	97.4	84.6	91.4
Peanut	71.4	100.0	100.0	95.2

Abbreviations: NPV, negative predictive value; PPV, positive predictive value.

record once the patient has transitioned to the restricted diet. Analysis of the recorded intake is useful in determining nutritional adequacy and the need for nutritional supplementation. Supplementation with an elemental formula may be necessary at the outset of treatment if numerous diet restrictions are required or if intake of solid foods eventually proves inadequate.

Additional calories, when needed, can be provided from a variety of sources. The most efficient way to add calories is with dietary fats (vegetable oils), which generally not are restricted for most patients.

Removal of foods most commonly responsible for eosinophilic esophagitis

Another approach to nutritional management is to remove the foods that most commonly cause EE. In the authors' patient population, the most common foods that they have found responsible for EE are milk, egg, wheat, corn, soy, beef, and chicken. Kagalwalla and colleagues [11] performed a retrospective review of their experience with this method. The investigators removed these six food groups from the diet in patients who had EE (defined as 20 eosinophils per HPF isolated in the esophagus without eosinophils in the stomach or duodenum). Thirty-five children were treated with a 6-week course of selective food elimination from October 2003 to June 2005 with removal of milk, egg, wheat, soy, peanut, tree nuts, and seafood. The children treated with the six-food elimination diet had significant improvement in the number of esophageal eosinophils, but the results were not as dramatic as that seen with the elemental diet. These investigators also examined treatment failures and improvement rates based on counts of fewer than 10 eosinophils per HPF, 10 to 20 eosinophils per HPF, and more than 20 eosinophils per HPF. Eighty-eight percent of the patients on the elemental diet had improvement to less than 10 eosinophils per HPF, and 74% of the patients on the six-food elimination diet had similar improvement.

Nutritional needs and evaluation

The nutritional considerations for this dietary approach are similar to those encountered with the elimination diets. The potential deficits in calories and protein may be more or less significant, depending on the degree to which these foods were consumed previously. The diet of the average child in authors' population probably would not be altered severely by the removal of soy, peanut, and seafood (assuming they were on an open diet before diagnosis). The restriction of dairy and wheat can create numerous nutritional deficiencies, however, and adherence to such restrictions can be difficult. As noted in the previous section, a 3-day diet record is useful in evaluating dietary adequacy. These patients also may require dietary supplementation with an elemental formula (orally or by tube).

Milk avoidance

Milk is a leading dietary source of protein, calcium, phosphorus, vitamin D, riboflavin, pantothenic acid, and vitamin B_{12}. Enriched soymilk can substitute for cow's milk, because it proves protein, calcium, vitamin D, and riboflavin [24]. If soy is also restricted from the diet, enriched rice milk can be used. Rice milk is not a significant source of protein, however, and a registered dietitian should review the remainder of the diet to ensure that protein needs can be met by solid foods. Rice milk is also low in fat, and other sources of dietary fats such as vegetable oils may need to be added to the diet [24]. The same concerns hold true for beverages derived from oat and potato, but these beverages, if accepted, can be used a significant source of calories in an otherwise balanced diet. Again, careful analysis of the diet is required.

Wheat avoidance

Wheat and enriched wheat products provide iron, niacin, riboflavin, thiamin, folate, and fiber. The removal of wheat and other grains can affect dietary fiber intake significantly. Patients should be encouraged to increase their intake of fruits and vegetables, if allowed in the diet. Wheat alternatives such as amaranth, arrowroot, barley, corn, oat, potato, rice, soybean, tapioca, and quinoa flour may be used if allowed in the diet and tolerated by the patient. Many wheat- and gluten-free products are available today, and families should receive information on how to use them or alternative grains in recipes.

Egg avoidance

Eggs provide protein, choline, vitamin A, riboflavin, pantothenic acid, biotin, and selenium. Most of these nutrients usually can provided by other foods, depending on what remains in the diet. Both egg whites and egg yolks must be avoided. Eggs also are an important ingredient in baked goods, providing leavening and structure. Instructions on how to substitute for eggs in baking can be found at The Food Allergy and Anaphylaxis Network (www. foodallergy.org). Cholesterol-free egg substitutes contain egg whites and are not appropriate for use. There is an egg replacement that is safe for almost all restricted diets available from commercial hypoallergenic companies.

Soy avoidance

Soy provides protein, thiamin, riboflavin, pyridoxine, folate, calcium, phosphorus, magnesium, iron, and zinc. Its removal from the diet may not present a significant nutritional risk unless it already is in use as a replacement for dairy products. As mentioned previously, fortified rice milks or other grain- and/or nut-based beverages can replace the calories and some of the nutrients that soy products provide. Soy is a significant source of protein, however, and care must be taken to ensure that protein requirements can be met by the remainder of the diet.

The elimination of soy, egg, peanut, and seafood from an already open diet does not usually present major nutrient losses, because these foods typically do not represent as significant a part of the diet as milk and/or wheat. If the diet is already restricted, however, the removal of these foods can result in significant challenges in ensuring adequate intake. Micronutrient supplementation probably will be needed, and elemental formula or modular supplementation with vegetable oils may be required to provide optimal intake of calories, protein, and fat.

How to reintroduce foods

An important part of nutritional management is the reintroduction of foods into the diet. After the authors have obtained a normal biopsy in a patient on a diet plan, they add foods back into the patient's diet to minimize the foods being avoided. Based on history and testing, the authors have found that fruits and vegetables are unlikely to be the cause of EE. Therefore, these foods typically are the first to be reintroduced. Reintroduction is classified into general food families ranging from group A (the least allergic) to group D (the most allergic) (Table 2). The authors start with foods in column A and then move to column B. The authors recommend a repeat endoscopy 4 to 6 weeks after the introduction of four or five new foods, to ensure that the addition of these foods is not associated with histologic inflammation. If a patient develops symptoms, the authors eliminate the last food reintroduced and wait until symptoms return to baseline before continuing to reintroduce foods. They continue on this approach until esophageal eosinophilia occurs. They then assume the most recently reintroduced foods—or one of them—are causing EE. They eliminate these foods, wait 2 weeks and try a new set of foods.

Nutritional needs and evaluation

Nutritional risks should decrease as foods are successfully reintroduced and the dietary variety expands. Periodic reassessment of the diet using a 3-day food record can be helpful in adjusting micronutrient supplementation.

Patient education

All caregivers should be educated about the need for allergen avoidance to ensure the selection of safe products and food preparation. The registered dietitian should emphasize to all caregivers the need to focus on what children can eat rather than on what they cannot. All the dietary treatments discussed here will affect the family's daily life, and this circumstance should be acknowledged. Families should be referred to appropriate resources for

Table 2
Food reintroduction table for eosinophilic esophagitis

A	B	C	D
Vegetables (non-legume):	Tropical fruits: Bananas	Allergenic fruit and vegetables:	Most commonly allergenic foods:
Carrots	Kiwi	Apples	Corn
Squash	Pineapples	Potatoes	Chicken
Sweet potato	Mangoes	Peas	Wheat
String beans	Papayas		Beef
Broccoli	Guavas		Soy
Lettuce	Avocadoes		Eggs
			Milk
Fruit (non-citrus, non-tropical):	Melons: Honeydews	Grains: Rice	
Pears	Cantaloupes	Oats	
Peaches	Watermelons	Barley	
Plums		Rye	
Apricots			
Citrus fruits:	Berries:	Meat (progress	
Oranges	Strawberries	from well-	
Grapefruit	Blueberries	cooked to	
Lemons	Raspberries	rarer):	
Limes	Cherries	Lamb	
		Chicken	
		Turkey	
		Pork	
	Legumes:	Fish/shellfish:	
	Lima beans	Peanut and tree	
	Chickpeas	nuts:	
	White/black/red beans	Peanuts	
		Almonds	
		Walnuts	
		Hazelnuts	
		Brazil nuts	
		Pecans	

additional information and encouraged to investigate local support groups. The American Partnership for Eosinophilic Disorders (www.apfed.org) is a valuable resource for many families and provides useful information that the families of newly diagnosed patients will find especially helpful.

Label reading

Label reading will become a crucial skill for all involved in food selection and preparation during an elimination diet. New legislation has been passed to assist patients and families with this task. The Food Allergen Labeling and Consumer Protection Act of 2004 (FALCPA) was implemented in January 2006 [25]. An overview of the law is given here, and complete details can be found with the Food Allergy and Anaphylaxis Network (FAAN) at www.foodallergy.org. The FALCPA mandates that any food product manufactured for sale in the Unites States must have on the package label a clear listing of ingredients derived from commonly allergenic foods (milk, egg, soybean, wheat, peanut, tree nut, fish, crustacean shellfish). The law applies to conventional food products, dietary supplements, infant formulas, and medical foods; raw agricultural commodities are not affected. Manufacturers also must list the specific tree nut, fish, or crustacean shellfish used as an ingredient (mollusks are not considered major food allergens under the FALCPA [25]).

Major food allergens must be listed on the product label in one of the following ways [25]:

- In the ingredient list: "milk, egg, or soy"
- Parenthetically following the food protein derivative: "casein (milk)"
- Immediately below the ingredient list in a "contains" statement: "contains milk"

Only one of these methods is required. Patients and families should be taught to avoid looking only for "contains" statements and continue to read ingredient lists as needed. Major food allergens also must be declared in spices, flavorings, colorings or additives, or if used to aid in processing [25,26]. These regulations apply only to ingredients derived from the eight foods listed previously. Individuals who need to avoid ingredients not covered under the FALCPA must contact the manufacturer to confirm product safety.

Some ingredients may be derived from an allergenic source but contain such insignificant amounts of the allergenic protein that they usually are well tolerated. Examples are lecithin (derived from soy) and kosher gelatin (derived from fish) [27,28]. Highly refined vegetable oils derived from major food allergens are exempt from labeling requirements, because they contain very little protein and are not thought to pose a risk of allergic reaction [25–29].

Ingredients and manufacturing processes can change over time, and labels should be read each time a food is purchased or consumed, even if the food has been used safely in the past. The FAAN has available for purchase a Grocery Manufacturer's Directory and small pocket-sized laminated cards listing ingredients to avoid on specific allergen-free diets [30].

Educational materials

Educational materials and instructions should be thorough, up-dated, and easily understood. Allergen-free sample menus can be used to help plan meals and snacks. Some families find it helpful for all family members to follow the prescribed diet restrictions, depending on the number of foods removed. This strategy can assist with dietary adherence in some cases, provided each family member's nutritional requirements are met. Families should be given information about where they can purchase allergen-free foods, either locally or online.

The family also should receive guidance on how to manage diet restrictions when eating outside the home and/or on special occasions. It usually is best to contact restaurants ahead of time and visit during nonbusy hours. Caregivers should ask questions about ingredients and food preparation or storage, so that the risk of cross-contamination can be avoided.

The FAAN has developed excellent educational materials for use in schools. Parents should be encouraged to familiarize themselves and their child's school with these materials [30].

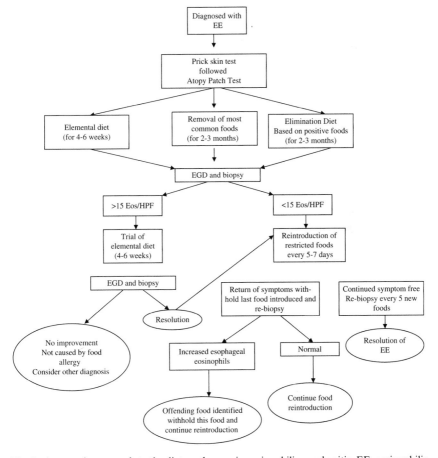

Fig. 1. A systemic approach to the dietary therapy in eosinophilic esophagitis. EE, eosinophilic esophagitis; EGD, esophagogastroduodenoscopy; Eos, eosinophils; HPF, high-powered field. (*Adapted from* Spergel JM, Andrews T, Brown-Whitehorn TF, et al. Treatment of eosinophilic esophagitis with specific food elimination diet directed by a combination of skin prick and patch tests. Ann Allergy Asthma Immunol 2005;95:342.)

Summary

The use of elemental diets leads to dramatic and complete healing of EE in almost all patients who have EE. The reintroduction of foods into the diet leads to the return of symptoms and eosinophil esophageal inflammation, fulfilling Koch's postulate that foods can cause EE. This result has been confirmed in pediatric patients in multiple academic centers, but it has not been studied in adults. Although this form of treatment is extremely effective, compliance can be difficult.

Removal of the most common foods is effective in approximately 70% of patients who have EE. The use of skin test and patch testing, with the additional removal of milk (which is often missed on skin and patch tests), can lead to success rates of up to 80%. Therefore, the authors have developed a systemic approach to dietary therapy in EE (Fig. 1).

After patients receive the diagnosis of EE (GERD having been ruled out with a trial of proton-pump inhibitor or normal pH monitoring of the distal esophagus), the authors look for foods that may be causing EE, using both skin tests and patch tests. After testing is complete, the authors discuss with the family the three options: (1) removal of foods based on testing, (2) removal of the most commonly responsible foods, or (3) an elemental diet. The patients then are started on the diet for a minimum of 2 months, and a repeat endoscopy with biopsy is performed. If the biopsy is normal, removed foods can be reintroduced. If the biopsy is still abnormal, the use of an elemental diet is recommended. If the patient does not respond to an elemental diet, an alternative diagnosis or noncompliance is considered.

Food reintroduction begins with the least allergic foods and progresses slowly to the most allergic foods (see Table 2). Foods typically are reintroduced every week. The authors typically repeat the endoscopy and biopsy after three to five new foods have been reintroduced to make sure those foods are being tolerated clinically and histologically. If the food is associated with symptoms on reintroduction, that food is avoided.

The authors find that with this systematic approach more than 70% of their patients return to a socially acceptable diet. As in all medicine, it is important that physician–family–patient cooperation takes place, because the time from the initial diagnosis and diet therapy to "happy" diet can take months to years.

References

[1] Noel RJ, Putnam PE, Rothenberg ME. Eosinophilic esophagitis. N Engl J Med 2004;351:
    940–1.
[2] Cherian S, Smith NM, Forbes DA. Rapidly increasing prevalence of eosinophilic oesopha-
    gitis in Western Australia. Arch Dis Child 2006;91:1000–4.
[3] Furuta GT, Liacouras CA, Collins MH, et al. Rothenberg ME and the FIGERS subcommit-
    tees. Eosinophilic esophagitis in children and adults: a systematic review and consensus
    recommendations for diagnosis and treatment. Gastroenterology 2007;133(4):1342–63.

[4] Liacouras CA, Spergel JM, Ruchelli E, et al. Eosinophilic esophagitis: a 10-year experience in 381 children. Clin Gastroenterol Hepatol 2005;3:1198–206.

[5] Spergel JM, Andrews T, Brown-Whitehorn TF, et al. Treatment of eosinophilic esophagitis with specific food elimination diet directed by a combination of skin prick and patch tests. Ann Allergy Asthma Immunol 2005;95:336–43.

[6] Orenstein SR, Shalaby TM, Di Lorenzo C, et al. The spectrum of pediatric eosinophilic esophagitis beyond infancy: a clinical series of 30 children. Am J Gastroenterol 2000;95: 1422–30.

[7] Markowitz JE, Spergel JM, Ruchelli E, et al. Elemental diet is an effective treatment for eosinophilic esophagitis in children and adolescents. Am J Gastroenterol 2003;98:777–82.

[8] Spergel JM, Beausoleil JL, Mascarenhas M, et al. The use of skin prick tests and patch tests to identify causative foods in eosinophilic esophagitis. J Allergy Clin Immunol 2002;109: 363–8.

[9] Kelly K, Lazenby A, Rowe P, et al. Eosinophilic esophagitis attributed to gastroesophageal reflux: improvement with an amino acid-based formula. Gastroenterology 1995;109: 1503–12.

[10] Spergel JM, Brown-Whitehorn T, Beausoleil JL, et al. Predictive values for skin prick test and atopy patch test for eosinophilic esophagitis. J Allergy Clin Immunol 2007;119: 509–11.

[11] Kagalwalla AF, Sentongo TA, Ritz S, et al. Effect of six-food elimination diet on clinical and histologic outcomes in eosinophilic esophagitis. Clin Gastroenterol Hepatol 2006;4(9): 1097–102.

[12] Food and Nutrition Board Institute of Medicine. Dietary reference intakes—applications in dietary assessment. A report of the subcommittee on interpretation and uses of dietary reference intakes and the standing committee on the scientific evaluation of dietary reference intakes. Washington, DC: National Academy Press; 2000.

[13] Food and Nutrition Board NRC. Recommended dietary allowances. 10th edition. Washington, DC: National Academy Press; 1989.

[14] Salman S, Christie L, Burks A, et al. Dietary intakes of children with food allergies: comparison of the Food Guide Pyramid and the Recommended Dietary Allowances. J Allergy Clin Immunol 2002;109:S21.

[15] Christie L, Hine RJ, Parker JG, et al. Food allergies in children affect nutrient intake and growth. J Am Diet Assoc 2002;102:1648–51.

[16] Eigenmann PA, Sampson HA. Interpreting skin prick tests in the evaluation of food allergy in children. Pediatr Allergy Immunol 1998;9:186–91.

[17] Sporik R, Hill DJ, Hosking CS. Specificity of allergen skin testing in predicting positive open food challenges to milk, egg and peanut in children. Clin Exp Allergy 2000;30:1540–6.

[18] Hill DJ, Heine RG, Hosking CS. The diagnostic value of skin prick testing in children with food allergy. Pediatr Allergy Immunol 2004;15:435–41.

[19] Sampson HA. Utility of food-specific IgE concentrations in predicting symptomatic food allergy. J Allergy Clin Immunol 2001;107:891–6.

[20] Sampson HA, Ho DG. Relationship between food-specific IgE concentrations and the risk of positive food challenges in children and adolescents. J Allergy Clin Immunol 1997;100: 444–51.

[21] Isolauri E, Turjanmaa K. Combined skin prick and patch testing enhances identification of food allergy in infants with atopic dermatitis. J Allergy Clin Immunol 1996;97L9-15.

[22] Darsow U, Laifaoui J, Kerschenlohr K, et al. The prevalence of positive reactions in the atopy patch test with aeroallergens and food allergens in subjects with atopic eczema: a European multicenter study. Allergy 2004;59:1318–25.

[23] Verstege A, Mehl A, Rolinck-Werninghaus C, et al. The predictive value of the skin prick test weal size for the outcome of oral food challenges. Clin Exp Allergy 2005;35:1220–6.

[24] Mofidi S. Nutritional management of pediatric food hypersensitivity. Pediatrics 2003;111: 1645–53.

[25] Food Allergen Labeling and Consumer Protection Act of 2004. (Title II of Public Law 108-282), USC 343, 303.

[26] US Food and Drug Administration. Questions and answers regarding food allergens including The Food Allergen Consumer Protection Act of 2004, edition 4, 2004. Available at: http://www.cfsan.fda.gov/~dms/alrguid4.html. Accessed April 11, 2007.

[27] Hefle SL, Taylor SL. How much food is too much? Threshold doses for allergenic foods. Curr Allergy Asthma Rep 2002;2:63–6.

[28] Taylor SL, Hefle SL. Food allergen labeling in the USA and Europe. Curr Opin Allergy Clin Immunol 2006;6:186–90.

[29] Crevel RW, Kerkhoff MA, Koning MM. Allergenicity of refined vegetable oils. Food Chem Toxicol 2000;38:385–93.

[30] Munoz-Furlong A. Daily coping strategies for patients and their families. Pediatrics 2003; 111:1654–61.

GASTROINTESTINAL
ENDOSCOPY CLINICS
OF NORTH AMERICA

Gastrointest Endoscopy Clin N Am
18 (2008) 195–217

Integrated Approach to Treatment of Children and Adults With Eosinophilic Esophagitis

Seema S. Aceves, MD, PhD[a], Glenn T. Furuta, MD[b],*,
Stuart Jon Spechler, MD[c]

[a]Division of Allergy, Immunology, Rady Children's Hospital,
San Diego, Pediatrics University of California, 3020 Childrens Way,
San Diego, CA 92123, USA
[b]Section of Pediatric Gastroenterology, Hepatology and Nutrition, The Children's Hospital,
Denver, University of Colorado Medical School, 13123 East 16th Avenue,
Aurora, CO 80045, USA
[c]Department of Medicine, Dallas Department of Veterans Affairs Medical Center,
The University of Texas Southwestern Medical Center at Dallas, Texas,
5323 Harry Hines Boulevard, Dallas, TX 75390, USA

Other articles in this issue provide unique viewpoints on clinical and basic elements of eosinophilic esophagitis (EE) from experts hailing from various disciplines. In this article, a pediatric gastroenterologist, an adult gastroenterologist, and a pediatric allergist combine efforts to provide an approach to the evaluation and treatment of patients who have EE. First, we present our collective clinical experiences, literature interpretations, and unique speculations as they pertain to the treatment of EE. Second, a practical approach to patient management is provided. Because EE is a relatively new disease with diagnostic criteria only recently established [1], this approach represents a best effort to guide clinicians and will likely change as more data accumulate in this dynamic field.

Mucosal esophageal eosinophilia

Esophageal eosinophilia in gastroesophageal reflux disease and eosinophilic esophagitis

Dr. Collin's article clearly elaborated the complexities of interpreting the histologic finding of esophageal eosinophilia. It is worth re-emphasizing

---

* Corresponding author.
E-mail address: furuta.glenn@tchden.org (G.T. Furuta).

doi:10.1016/j.giec.2007.09.003   *giendo.theclinics.com*

here that esophageal eosinophilia alone does not define any disease definitively. The differential diagnosis for esophageal eosinophilia is broad; clinical correlation is required to identify the correct diagnosis associated with the histologic findings. For instance, it has been known since 1982 that gastroesophageal reflux disease (GERD) can be associated with a mild eosinophilic infiltration of the squamous epithelium in the distal esophagus, usually with fewer than seven eosinophils per high-power field [2,3]. Although GERD and EE may share common symptoms, such as heartburn and dysphagia, occasionally it can be difficult to distinguish between the two disorders in children and adults whose esophageal biopsy specimens show mild eosinophilic infiltration.

Several reports have focused on the issue of how to distinguish GERD from EE [4–11]. In children, small studies have suggested that the two disorders might be distinguished by the results of gene expression profiling or by the density of activated mucosal mast cells and IgE-bearing cells in esophageal biopsy specimens [12,13]. Those findings need confirmation in larger studies and in adults.

Some reports suggest that the interaction between GERD and EE can be complex, and that the notion of establishing a clear distinction between the two disorders may be too simplistic [14]. There are at least four situations in which GERD might be associated with esophageal eosinophils: (1) GERD causes esophageal injury that results in a mild eosinophilic infiltration, (2) GERD and EE coexist but are unrelated, (3) EE contributes to or causes GERD, or (4) GERD contributes to or causes EE.

Gastroesophageal reflux disease causes esophageal injury with mild eosinophilic infiltration

Recent studies suggest potential mechanisms whereby GERD might cause eosinophils to be recruited to the esophageal mucosa. In cultures of human esophageal microvascular endothelial cells, for example, acid exposure induces the expression of VCAM-1, an adhesion molecule that is recognized by ligands on the eosinophil cell surface [15]. Acid exposure also induces the release of platelet-activating factor (PAF) in the human esophageal mucosa, and PAF is known to attract and activate eosinophils [16]. Furthermore, acid exposure can increase esophageal blood flow, which can enhance the delivery of eosinophils to the epithelium [17]. It is not clear which, if any, of these potential mechanisms causes the mild eosinophilic infiltration of the esophageal squamous epithelium that can be seen in patients who have GERD.

Gastroesophageal reflux disease and eosinophilic esophagitis coexist but are unrelated

Surveys have shown that approximately 20% of adults in Western countries regularly experience heartburn, the cardinal symptom of

GERD [18,19]. It seems unlikely that EE would protect against GERD and, therefore, a substantial number of adult patients who have EE should have unrelated GERD. In series of adult patients who have EE, 20% to 30% of patients complain of heartburn [8,20]. Although this is approximately the frequency of heartburn that would be anticipated in the general adult population, it is not clear that heartburn is indeed a symptom of EE in adults.

In children who have EE, esophageal pH monitoring studies infrequently show abnormal acid exposure [9,10,21]. In contrast, the few available studies on this issue in adult patients who have EE suggest that pathologic acid reflux is common [20,22]. For example, Remedios found abnormal acid reflux by 24-hour esophageal pH monitoring in 10 (38%) of 26 adults who had EE [22]. If future, well-controlled studies confirm that this high frequency of pathologic acid reflux occurs in the face of a well-documented diagnosis of EE, then that would suggest that there is more than a chance association between adult EE and GERD.

Eosinophilic esophagitis contributes to or causes gastroesophageal reflux disease

Eosinophils secrete several biologically active substances that could contribute to GERD by affecting the function of esophageal smooth muscles and nerves [23]. Some eosinophil secretory products, such as vasoactive intestinal peptide and PAF, can induce relaxation of the lower esophageal sphincter (LES) muscle, which might predispose to gastroesophageal reflux [23,24]. Eosinophils also secrete interleukin (IL)-6, which has been shown to decrease the amplitude of esophageal muscle contractions. Decreased esophageal muscle contractions could contribute to GERD by interfering with esophageal peristalsis and acid clearance [25,26]. EE also can be associated with structural changes in the esophagus that might affect LES function and peristalsis [27,28]. Irrespective of the underlying mechanisms, esophageal motility abnormalities are found in approximately 40% of adults who have EE [27].

Some eosinophil secretory products (eg, major basic protein, eosinophil cationic protein, eosinophil peroxidase) have cytotoxic effects that might render the esophageal epithelium more susceptible to injury by refluxed gastric juice [29–31]. Major basic protein has been shown to down-regulate a cellular tight junction protein (occludin) and to impair barrier function in monolayers of human colonic carcinoma cells [32]. Eosinophilic infiltration of the bronchial mucosa in asthma is known to be associated with damage to tight junctions and dilation of the intercellular spaces similar to that seen in the esophagus of patients who have GERD [33–35]. Eosinophilic infiltration of the esophageal epithelium thus might cause damage to the squamous epithelial cells and their tight junctions, thereby increasing mucosal permeability and rendering the mucosa more susceptible to injury by refluxed gastric juice.

Gastroesophageal reflux disease contributes
to or causes eosinophilic esophagitis

Recent reports document patients who had symptoms and endoscopic and histologic abnormalities typical of EE, all of which resolved during treatment with a proton pump inhibitor (PPI) [6,36]. One conclusion that might be gleaned from this observation is that large numbers of eosinophils can be seen in peptic esophagitis because of GERD. An alternative conclusion is that, in some patients, GERD causes EE.

It is possible that GERD could cause epithelial changes that predispose to the development of an allergic esophagitis. The normal esophageal epithelium is highly impermeable to large molecules like peptides, which might function as allergens if they could penetrate the epithelium. With acid-peptic damage to the tight junctions between esophageal epithelial cells, however, the mucosa becomes leaky and permeable to peptides [37]. This GERD-induced increase in mucosal permeability could expose the deep layers of the esophageal squamous epithelium to antigens that ordinarily would pass by without penetrating the mucosa. GERD-induced esophageal damage also might recruit immune cells that could contribute to the local development of allergies. Such allergic reactions might resolve when the initiating, GERD-induced injury heals with the administration of PPIs.

Although PPIs are highly effective for reducing gastric acid secretion and healing reflux esophagitis, there is one potentially harmful effect of PPIs that clinicians should consider when prescribing these agents for patients who have EE: recent studies suggest that gastric acid suppression could contribute to the development of food allergies [38]. Normally, the digestion of dietary proteins begins when they are exposed to acid and pepsin in the stomach. Acid-peptic digestion of dietary proteins produces oligopeptides that can be ignored by the immune system or that can induce immunologic tolerance to the parent protein. Conversely, it has been shown that dietary proteins that escape gastric digestion can induce immunologic sensitization [39]. By raising the gastric pH to levels at which pepsin loses much of its proteolytic activity, antisecretory medications like PPIs theoretically could contribute to the development of food sensitization and potentially food allergies. Recent studies have shown that the administration of antisecretory medicines is associated with the development of food-allergic reactions in mice and with the formation of IgE antibodies to food allergens in humans [40–42]. This association may be an especially important consideration when treating EE, which seems to be a manifestation of food allergy. Presently, there are no reports of PPIs exacerbating EE, but the potential contribution of PPIs to food allergy is not widely appreciated and this issue needs further investigation. Clinicians should be aware of the intriguing possibility that the treatment of GERD with antisecretory agents might contribute to the development of EE.

Diagnosis of eosinophilic esophagitis

In light of these possibilities, the evaluation of patients who have esophageal eosinophilia requires careful clinicopathologic considerations. The diagnosis of EE is based on the finding of 15 or more eosinophils per high-power field in the clinical context of a patient in whom GERD and other rarer causes of esophageal eosinophilia have been ruled out (2 months of high-dose PPI or normal pH monitoring of the distal esophagus) [1]. (See the article by Gonsalves, elsewhere in this issue.) There may be considerable overlap in the clinical and histologic features of GERD and EE in adults that precludes a clear distinction between the two disorders. In addition, gastric and duodenal mucosal biopsies should be normal in patients who have EE. If a patient suspected of having EE has received treatment for asthma or allergic rhinitis with topical corticosteroids before their mucosal biopsy, anticipated histologic findings also may be diminished. Because the treatment of these diseases is quite diverse, it is imperative that the diagnosis of EE be definitively established before proceeding to further evaluations and treatments.

Considerations for the evaluation of suspected patients

Allergy

Role of allergy
Studies to date suggest that the rates of allergic sensitization in patients who have EE exceed those found in the general population. (See the article by Assa'ad, elsewhere in this issue.) When allergy is defined as the presence of either (1) another atopic diathesis (allergic rhinitis, atopic dermatitis, or asthma) or (2) the presence of antigen-specific IgE for food or aeroallergens by skin prick or plasma-specific IgE testing (RAST), the majority of EE patients (50%–80%) are atopic [43]. Available estimates of the frequency of allergy in children and adults who have EE may be spuriously low, because early studies defining the association between allergy and EE were performed only by gastroenterologists who had no specialized training in recognizing allergic disorders. For instance, it is likely that the gastroenterologists did not take a complete allergic history and thus they may not have uncovered a potentially associated allergic disease. Recent multidisciplinary studies have begun to address this issue more clearly and thus true rates will become better defined.

Food antigens are implicated instigators of EE based primarily on the results of food elimination trials in pediatric patients. (See the article by Spergel and Shuker, elsewhere in this issue.) More than 90% of children treated with complete food antigen elimination by way of elemental formula and 74% of children treated with specific food antigen elimination diets that exclude milk, soy, egg, wheat, peanuts, and fish/shellfish develop histologic, symptomatic, and endoscopic disease resolution [44–47]. Despite the success of empiric elimination diets, however, detecting the inciting food antigens in

EE can be a challenge and elimination diets based on allergy testing have varying success rates [48–50]. This challenge lies in several factors, including inexperience with the disease, sparse data regarding the pathogenesis of disease (IgE versus non IgE), and lack of testing for non–IgE-mediated food allergic diseases. (See the article by Chehade, elsewhere in this issue.) Currently available standardized testing for food allergy is limited to the detection of food-specific IgE using either skin prick testing (SPT) or serum food IgE levels. When detecting food IgE, the presence of specific IgE does not definitively diagnose a clinical reactivity to the food. In the absence of a clinical history consistent with a food-driven process (eg, anaphylaxis) the false-positive rates for food IgE can be as high as 50%. RAST documents the presence of specific IgE to allergens. SPT demonstrates the presence and ability of the antigen-specific IgE to cause mast cell degranulation [13]. RAST-based elimination diets are largely unsuccessful and not recommended [50]. Spergel and colleagues [51] have recently developed predictive values for SPT-based elimination diets in pediatric EE. (See the artilce by Spergel and Shuker, elsewhere in this issue.) Similar to the data for anaphylaxis, negative predictive values are generally greater (ranging from 58% to 98%) than positive predictive values, which range from 33% to 96% depending on the food [51].

It is unlikely that EE pathogenesis relies exclusively on IgE [43]. (See the articles by Blanchard and Rothenberg, and Chehade, elsewhere in this issue.) A definition of allergy that relies solely on antigen-specific IgE is therefore likely inappropriate in EE. To evaluate food triggers that may use a T cell–mediated, delayed-type hypersensitivity mechanism, Spergel and colleagues [51] developed, used, and generated predictive values for food atopy patch tests (APT) in pediatric patients who had EE. (See the article by Spergel and Shuker, elsewhere in this issue.) Their studies show that the most common foods triggering EE are milk and egg, in agreement with the success of empiric diets that exclude these foods [45,48,49,51]. Although the sensitivity of APT for milk and egg were 90% and 92%, respectively, the specificities were significantly lower (44% and 62%, respectively). It is important to remember that APT has been best used and validated for occupational antigens in allergic disorders, such as contact dermatitis; food APT has not been rigorously validated for EE, has been used exclusively in children, and currently remains a research tool. In vitro studies demonstrate that peripheral blood mononuclear cells from adult patients can produce IL-5 when stimulated with milk protein [52]. The presence of food-specific T cells and their pathogenic role in EE continues to be an area for future research.

The institution of elimination diets or elemental formula, especially if done empirically, warrants a detailed discussion with patients and families and careful consideration of the clinical consequences of the interventions. Elemental diets are often unpalatable and patients frequently require nasogastric or gastrostomy tube placement to receive the recommended caloric and nutritional intake [47]. There is speculation that prolonged elimination of solid oral intake in children may contribute to oral aversions and failure to thrive. Elimination diets can lead to nutritional deficits and the incorporation of a trained nutritionist into the care team is essential [53]. Elemental formulas are expensive and may not be paid for by health insurance, resulting in financial burdens for patients. Clinical trials to address whether empiric food avoidance can predispose to IgE-mediated food allergy are currently ongoing. In addition, the length of time that a food needs to be avoided before reintroduction and whether or not mucosal tolerance is ever obtained for the inciting food remain to be determined in EE. In contrast to medical managements with systemic corticosteroids, few if any toxic side effects have been identified with nutritional management, especially when a dietician is a part of the patient's care.

It has been suggested that EE is a form of oral allergy syndrome, an immunologic phenomenon that provokes a localized response attributable to shared antigenic features of pollens and foods. Simon and colleagues [54,55] demonstrated that most adult patients who had EE with wheat or rye allergy also had allergy to grasses. The elimination of these grains did not lead to symptomatic, histologic, or endoscopic resolution in adult patients who had EE. However, because grain allergy was determined by RAST (4 of 6 patients had negative SPT to grains), the lack of resolution with elimination diet may be partially explained by the use of a sub-ideal test for diagnosing true food sensitization in EE [55].

Role of aeroallergens in eosinophilic esophagitis

Human case reports and murine models demonstrate that aeroallergens increase esophageal eosinophilia [56,57]. In humans, spontaneous EE resolution can occur when the pollen season subsides [56]. There seems to be an intimate immunologic connection between the airway and esophagus, and patients who have allergic rhinitis have a positive correlation between the number of blood and esophageal eosinophils [57,58]. Mice develop esophageal eosinophilia after sensitization and intranasal challenge with the mold *Aspergillus fumigatus* in an IL-5– and IL-13–dependent manner [59,60]. Antigen-specific T cells to aeroallergens are also implicated in EE pathogenesis. For instance, peripheral blood mononuclear cells from adult patients who have EE produce IL-13 on stimulation with house dust mite extract, and mice that are unable to recombine the T-cell receptor are protected from aeroallergen-driven, experimental EE [52,61].

Role of surrogate allergy markers in eosinophilic esophagitis

There is a critical need to ascertain surrogate disease markers for EE. (See the article by Gupta, elsewhere in this issue.) Cross-sectional and small retrospective studies demonstrate that peripheral eosinophil levels or eosinophil products can correlate with disease severity, persistence, and response to treatment [21,28,50,62,63]. Because of the high rates of concurrent atopic diatheses in patients who have EE, however, peripheral eosinophil counts likely do not exclusively reflect esophageal eosinophilia. Consistent with this, there is no difference in the number of peripheral CCR3+ cells in the blood of active EE and atopic children who do not have EE [64]. Used together, serum eosinophil-derived neurotoxin (EDN) and blood eosinophils have positive and negative predictive values of 83% and 79%, respectively, in pediatric patients who have EE [63]. The definition of "peripheral eosinophilia" varies between groups of investigators and large, prospective studies that clearly define the relationship between blood and esophageal disease state are necessary. The most signifi-cant esophageal marker associated with EE is eotaxin-3, which increases 53-fold in pediatric patients who have EE as compared with normal children and children who have non–EE-associated esophageal eosinophils [12]. (See the article by Blanchard and Rothenberg, elsewhere in this issue.) A recent cross-sectional comparison study demonstrated that there was a correlation between the number of CCR3+ and CD4+-IL-5+ cells in the blood and the number of esophageal eosinophils and eotaxin-3 in pediatric patients who had EE [64]. These intriguing findings need to be repeated in larger cohort studies that follow patients who have EE over time.

Clinical evaluations

The present-day evaluation of the patient who has EE is complicated by the existence of limited data regarding the pathogenesis and natural history of the disease. As such, plans for the exact testing that each patient undergoes in clinical research programs and by primary care providers (internist/pediatrician, allergist, gastroenterologist) may differ.

In routine care, it is reasonable for the affected patient, who considers the use of allergen avoidance as a primary treatment, to complete a thorough evaluation by an experienced allergist. SPT is the best currently available standardized test to evaluate food allergy in EE.

Given the airway-esophagus immunologic link, it is reasonable and may be important to evaluate the presence of aeroallergen sensitivity by SPT, to insti-tute aeroallergen avoidance measures, and to assess pulmonary function in patients who have EE; this has yet to be validated by clinical studies demon-strating improved outcomes, but may be especially important in patients whose disease is recalcitrant to nutritional or medical management. Together, gastroenterologists and allergists should note the pollen season and degree of aeroallergen avoidance undertaken by the patient at each endoscopic, histo-logic, and symptom evaluation. If a patient has a known seasonal aeroallergen sensitization and definitive EE, it may be reasonable to perform endoscopic evaluation out of the pollen season to check for spontaneous disease remis-sion before instituting more aggressive dietary or medical management.

Detailed recording of the mucosal changes observed at endoscopy and procurement of multiple biopsies of the proximal and distal esophagus are critical in monitoring the long-term outcome for affected patients.

As a part of research protocols, patients may undergo further testing aimed at identifying noninvasive markers of disease activity, determination of genetic phenotypes, or validation of improved methods to specify etiologic allergens. Genetic susceptibility to EE in children has been associated with a single nucleotide polymorphism in the 3-prime untranslated region of the eotaxin-3 gene [12]. Eotaxin-3 is an eosinophil chemokine synthesized and secreted by lymphocytes and the esophageal squamous epithelium. In the future, for those pediatric patients in whom the diagnosis of EE is unclear, evaluation of esophageal transcriptosome profile or eotaxin-3 levels may represent a distinguishing factor.

Allergist's role

Current evidence supports the notion that, in EE, the esophagus becomes a target organ for a new atopic disease of increasing prevalence, and suggests that EE is the newest addition to the allergic march. The production of Th2 cytokines, such as IL-5 and -13, reliance on the presence of a functional TCR, and tissue remodeling analogous to asthmatic airway remodeling have been demonstrated in animal models and humans who have EE. Because there seems to be an intimate immunologic connection between the respiratory tract and esophagus, it is important to adequately evaluate and treat concurrent allergic rhinitis and asthma. In addition, the preponderance of food allergy and the removal of esophageal eosinophilia by dietary manipulations, especially in pediatric patients who have EE, underscores the importance of allergic evaluation by skin prick testing and possibly patch testing, but not RAST testing.

Gastroenterologist's role

The role of the gastrointestinal endoscopist in the diagnosis and management of EE is paramount. Often they are first to encounter affected patients who present with dysphagia or food impaction. Gastroenterologists performing the endoscopies should make careful observations regarding mucosal findings, procure multiple endoscopic biopsy specimens at each evaluation, and note the patient's concurrent atopic diatheses, the pollen season as applicable, and the level of control of other allergic conditions.

Differences in treatment approaches between children and adult patients

The treatment of children and adults who have EE differs in several ways. Because children are often more tolerant of dietary changes, nutritional management may be used with greater compliance in children than adults. Although esophageal strictures have been documented in children, they seem to occur more commonly in adults, making esophageal dilation a more commonly used procedure in affected adults. Finally, the use of corticosteroids must be carefully monitored in all patients, but especially in children whose bodies are still in the developmental stages.

Goals of treatment

There are at least two undisputed goals for the treatment of EE: the complete relief of symptoms and the prevention of complications. Known complications of EE include esophageal strictures (either in the form of esophageal rings or diffuse esophageal narrowing) and consequences of increased esophageal fragility, such as esophageal mucosal tears and esophageal perforations. Tears and perforations in EE may occur spontaneously or as a complication of esophageal intubation and dilation procedures [65,66]. The cause of this increased fragility is not clear, but may be related to the tissue remodeling that has been observed in EE [67]. Chronic inflammation is strongly associated with neoplasia in several gastrointestinal organs (eg, chronic inflammatory bowel disease and colon cancer, chronic gastritis and stomach cancer, chronic pancreatitis and pancreatic cancer), but esophageal neoplasia has not yet been recognized as a complication of EE. Other disease states involving chronic eosinophilic inflammation, such as asthma and the hypereosinophilic syndrome, are associated with target tissue fibrosis, a mechanism that is likely at play in patients who have EE who have stricture formation.

Several treatments have been shown to relieve symptoms of EE, but it remains unclear whether any treatment can prevent the complications of the disease. In this regard, therapeutic endpoints for clinicians to judge treatment adequacy are unclear. Proposed endpoints include complete resolution of symptoms (symptomatic remission), elimination of esophageal eosinophilia (histologic remission), and resolution of endoscopic abnormalities (endoscopic remission). One major issue of significant contention, even among the authors of this article, is whether symptomatic remission alone is an adequate endpoint, or whether clinicians should always strive to achieve histologic and endoscopic remissions for their patients who have EE. It is likely that a composite index that evaluates and accounts for all three components of the disease (symptoms, histology, and endoscopy) would provide the best clinical tool for EE management. Such validated scores for these measures in EE are currently unavailable, however, and are the topic of ongoing research.

Clinical experience and studies show that the achievement of symptomatic remission in EE does not seem to be a good index for histologic remission. For example, treatment with montelukast has been shown to render some patients asymptomatic without affecting the degree of esophageal eosinophilia [68]. The rationale for pursuing a posttreatment evaluation with endoscopy and biopsy is the premise that the elimination of esophageal eosinophils should prevent the return of symptoms and the development of complications. In this light, endoscopy with biopsy is a common, straightforward procedure that has a low risk for complications in otherwise healthy patients. Symptoms do not always match the macro- or microscopic appearance of the target tissues, emphasizing the importance of mucosal biopsy to provide a full assessment of the disease state. Finally, the impact of long-standing eosinophilic inflammation is concerning to some pediatricians because fibrosis has been associated with other diseases with prominent tissue eosinophilia. Mucosal biopsy following a therapeutic intervention confirms histologic remission or at regular time intervals assesses for esophageal narrowing. Alternatively, a barium esophagram could be performed to assess for this anatomic complication.

Although this rationale seems reasonable, it remains unproved and there are several considerable downsides to the practice of insisting on histologic remission in all cases. Documentation that esophageal eosinophilia has resolved entails the substantial expense and inconvenience of repeated endoscopic examinations, with the attendant risks for procedure-related complications, especially those with allergic diseases (latex allergy, soy/egg allergy and reactions with propofol, difficult-to-control asthma). For a patient who has achieved a symptomatic remission, furthermore, the achievement of a histologic remission might require higher doses of the medications that induced the symptomatic remission, or the prescription of additional drugs. Both of those measures would increase expense and the chances for medication side effects.

In the absence of definitive studies, it thus remains unclear whether the theoretic benefits of achieving a histologic remission outweigh the documented risks and disadvantages of the available treatments and of repeated endoscopic examinations necessary to document histologic remission. Even among experts, there is considerable variation in the opinion of treatment endpoints with some adamantly insisting on endoscopic evaluation to document histologic remission after each therapeutic intervention, whereas others rely on symptomatic resolution alone. Decisions on the use of this invasive method of analysis must be made in conjunction with the patient/family, with the overriding goal of improving the short- and long-term outcomes of this enigmatic disease. Future research studies will provide data that will aid in making this difficult decision. Until then, practitioners should have a frank discussion with their patients to balance the potential risks and benefits of treatment endpoints.

Rationale for treatment options

Nutritional management

Although the cause of EE remains unknown, and studies to date are retrospective and uncontrolled, the dramatic response to elemental diet therapy that has been seen in children who have the disorder indicates that food allergens play a major role. (See the article by Spergel and Shuker, elsewhere in this issue.) For example, Liacouras and colleagues [46] reported that 98% of children who had EE who were treated with an elemental diet experienced symptomatic and histologic remissions. Unfortunately, few data are available on the role of diet therapy in adults. If diet therapy is to be tried, there are three general approaches to consider [69]: (1) *directed elimination diets* that are based on the results of skin prick or atopy patch testing for food allergens (>75% success rates reported in children), (2) *empiric elimination diets* that prohibit the most common food allergens (eg, milk, soy, eggs, wheat, nuts, seafood) without formal allergy testing (>70% success rates reported in children), and (3) *elemental diets* using amino acid–based formulas (>95% success rates reported in children). A prospective, controlled trial of food avoidance in children who have EE is needed.

A small study in adults treated with a combination of directed and empiric elimination diets has had encouraging preliminary results [70]. SPT was positive for food and aeroallergens in all of the nine study patients, and three patients who completed 6 weeks of the elimination diet showed some symptomatic and histologic improvement. More studies are needed to elucidate the role of diet therapy for adults who have EE.

Corticosteroid treatment

Lessons from other allergic disorders in the use of corticosteroids

Noting that systemic corticosteroids induce salutary effects in allergic disorders associated with eosinophilia, such as asthma, several investigators have documented that systemic corticosteroids can induce symptomatic and histologic remissions in patients who have EE. (See the article by Liacouras, elsewhere in this issue.) Available studies on corticosteroid treatment of EE so far have been limited in size and duration, however. Symptomatic and histologic remission of EE has been documented in more than 95% of children treated with systemic corticosteroids for 4 weeks, although symptoms and esophageal eosinophilia return within 6 months of stopping therapy in most cases [46,71].

Despite the apparent high efficacy of systemic corticosteroids for inducing symptomatic and histologic remission, the need for protracted treatment and concerns about serious side effects must limit the usefulness of these agents in EE. Asthma management has long relied on the use of inhaled topical corticosteroid therapy (ICS) for the treatment of allergic inflammation. ICS therapy decreases inflammatory markers, such as sputum eosinophils, and improves surrogate asthma markers with minimal side effects. The dose and persistence of ICS therapy is based on asthma severity classification, which is gauged by a combination of symptoms and pulmonary function testing. Consequently, several studies have focused on the role of topical corticosteroids like fluticasone propionate, which are less frequently associated with adrenal suppression and other serious systemic corticosteroid side effects.

In patients who have asthma, indoor aeroallergen sensitization correlates with persistent wheezing. Retrospective and prospective analyses of fluticasone propionate in pediatric EE demonstrate that sensitization to foods or aeroallergens correlates with decreased histologic response to topical steroid therapy [72,73]. This finding suggests that specific IgE sensitization may correlate with an EE phenotype that is more recalcitrant to topical steroid therapy. Whether this corresponds to a more persistent or stricture-prone clinical phenotype remains to be identified, but underscores the importance of careful allergic evaluation in patients who have EE.

Use of topical corticosteroids for the acute management of patients who have eosinophilic esophagitis

Practitioners caring for patients who have EE have used the available ICS therapies for topical esophageal delivery [22,44,50,72–76]. (See the article by Liacouras, elsewhere in this issue.) There are no studies that document the location, penetration, or retention of topical esophageal corticosteroids. However, because esophageal corticosteroid is presumably subjected to first-pass hepatic metabolism (unlike ICSs, which are directly absorbed into the bloodstream through the pulmonary vascular bed), it is expected that there is minimal systemic corticosteroid absorption.

Pediatric and adult studies have demonstrated that fluticasone propionate (FP) that is swallowed rather than inhaled can remediate histologic and endoscopic findings of EE [22,44,50,72–76]. A swallowed viscous suspension of budesonide and sucralose is also effective in clearing esophageal eosinophils and improving symptoms and endoscopic findings in pediatric patients without causing depression of morning cortisol levels [74,77]. Endoscopic findings that can be improved with topical corticosteroids include concentric rings, furrows, plaques, and pallor [22,72,74,77]. Both treatments can be associated with esophageal candidiasis in a small number of patients. Consistent with its capacity to improve endoscopic EE features, FP treatment also decreases epithelial eosinophils, mast cells, CD8+ T cells, and, inconsistently, CD1a+ dendritic cells in the esophageal epithelium [50,72,73,78].

A recent, randomized, placebo-controlled trial of swallowed fluticasone documented histologic remission of EE after 3 months of treatment in 50% of 21 children who received fluticasone (880 µg/d) compared with 9% of 15 children who received placebo ($P < .05$) [72]. Uncontrolled studies in adults suggest that most experience symptomatic improvement of dysphagia during 4 to 6 weeks of treatment with fluticasone [22,75]. Side effects that have been reported during short-term therapy include esophageal candidiasis and dry mouth. Unfortunately, relapses are the rule when fluticasone treatment is stopped [46], and few data are available on the efficacy and safety of protracted maintenance therapy with fluticasone.

Use of topical corticosteroids for the chronic management of patients who have eosinophilic esophagitis

Similar to asthma, EE may have its origins in early childhood [79,80]. The use of preventative ICS therapy in pediatric patients does not alter progression to wheezing in young children at high risk for developing asthma, and patients who have persistent asthma have increased symptoms and decreased lung function on removal of the treating agent [8,81,82]. Similarly, symptoms and esophageal eosinophilia often recur in pediatric and adult patients once topical esophageal corticosteroid therapy is discontinued [22,46,79]. The features of those patients who have higher rates of disease recurrence need to be carefully studied and future clinical trials of clearance versus maintenance and intermittent versus chronic topical corticosteroid in EE will help guide management strategies.

Whether topical esophageal corticosteroid delivery can reverse strictures or decrease the necessity or frequency of esophageal dilation remains to be evaluated. Pediatric patients who have EE with strictures or long-standing EE demonstrate subepithelial fibrosis, increased numbers of cells expressing TGFβ, and increased vascularity with vascular activation [67]. Adult patients also have subepithelial fibrosis [8,28]. Consistent with these findings, endoscopic ultrasound demonstrates increased thickness of the esophagus, suggestive of a transmural esophageal process in EE [83]. Changes of fixed concentric rings, strictures, and narrow caliber esophagus may be endoscopic features of tissue remodeling but further studies are needed to assess if histologic deep tissue changes occur even in younger patients who have milder EE and if these changes correlate with clinical severity or progression.

Other agents

In addition to nutrition and corticosteroids, case series report the use of cromolyn and montelukast with no or limited success [46]. Montelukast diminishes symptoms but does not impact eosinophilia even at supraphysiologic doses [68]. (See the article by Liacouras, elsewhere in this issue.) The successful use of anti–IL-5 antibody has also been reported in and open label study of four adult patients [84]. (See the article by Liacouras, elsewhere in this issue.)

Esophageal dilation

Available data suggest that dysphagia attributable to EE responds adequately to medical therapy in most patients, even those who have esophageal strictures. Dysphagia persists in some patients despite medical therapy, however. There are no published, controlled trials of dilation therapy to guide the clinician in precisely when and how to perform esophageal dilation for patients who have EE. Consequently, it is not clear how long medical therapy should be administered before resorting to esophageal dilation, nor is it clear what diet, medications, or combinations of medications and diets should be tried before a patient is deemed a failure of medical treatment.

The major complications of esophageal dilation are perforation and bleeding, which have been reported in approximately 0.5% of dilations performed for esophageal strictures due to causes other than EE [85]. In addition, bacteremia accompanies esophageal dilation in 20% to 45% of cases, although clinically recognizable infectious complications, such as endocarditis and brain abscesses, are rare [85]. It has been suggested that the esophageal mucosal fragility and tissue remodeling that can accompany EE predispose to esophageal tears and perforations [65]. If this is so, then series of patients who have EE treated with esophageal dilation would be expected to describe inordinately high rates of esophageal tears, perforations, bleeding, and infectious complications.

Unfortunately, reported series of patients who have EE treated with esophageal dilation are small, and the findings have been contradictory and confusing. In 2001, before EE was well known, Morrow and colleagues [86] described the results of esophageal dilation for 19 patients who had a "ringed esophagus." There were no perforations, but deep mucosal tears after dilation were described as "common." All patients were treated with a PPI, and 15 of 16 patients available for follow-up (mean duration 19 ± 2.4 months) described overall improvement of dysphagia. Only 1 patient had recurrent symptoms requiring repeated dilations. In a systematic review of the medical literature, Sgouros [27] summarized the results of esophageal dilation for 64 patients who had EE collected from 11 published reports. Extensive mucosal tears were observed in "the majority of cases," and 9% experienced severe chest pain treated with analgesics and hospitalization. Dilation was complicated by esophageal perforation in 1 patient (1.5%). A total of 83% of patients experienced immediate symptomatic improvement. Long-term follow-up was available for only 12 patients, all of whom experienced symptomatic recurrences after 3 to 8 months. The largest series to date has been reported only in abstract form. Gonsalves and colleagues [87] described the results of esophageal dilation in 81 patients who had EE. There were no serious complications and only 2 patients had chest pain or odynophagia after dilation. One half of the patients required repeated dilations, and the median response to dilation was 18 months.

There are not yet sufficient published data to provide a meaningful estimate of the frequency of serious complications of esophageal dilation in patients who have EE. Although it is clear that esophageal dilation in some patients has resulted in extensive mucosal tears with severe chest pain and protracted odynophagia, it is not clear that EE causes an inordinate predisposition to more serious complications like perforation, hemorrhage, and infections. Indeed, the small series available do not describe serious bleeding and infections complicating esophageal dilation in patients who have EE. Also unclear is the durability of the response to dilation, especially because patients generally were not on any standardized protocol of medical management either before or after dilation. Future studies should insist on standardized criteria for the type and duration of medical therapy tried before resorting to esophageal dilation, and the type of maintenance medical therapy after dilation that might decrease the need for repeated dilations.

Specific treatment approaches

A general approach to the management of patients who have EE is outlined in Fig. 1. In most patients, either nutritional or medical treatments provide effective acute management for symptoms and histologic abnormalities. Chronic remission of ongoing inflammation is achieved when antigenic stimuli can be identified and removed. The long-term use of topical corticosteroids has not yet been studied. The intervention used should be tailored to patient preference, lifestyle, severity of endoscopic findings, and symptoms, and should involve the appropriate health care team, including a gastroenterologist, allergist, and experienced nutritionist.

Confirmation of eosinophilic esophagitis diagnosis

Given the number of plausible mechanisms whereby GERD might contribute to the accumulation of eosinophils in the esophageal epithelium, it seems prudent to recommend an initial clinical trial of PPI therapy for patients suspected of having EE and those who have esophageal eosinophilia (ie, patients who do not yet have a diagnosis of EE) [1]. Presently, there is no compelling reason to recommend any one of the available

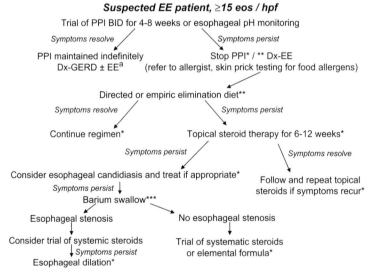

Fig. 1. A general approach to the management of patients who have EE.
[a] There is likely an unmeasured fraction of patients who have a mixed pattern of GERD and EEdpatients who respond symptomatically to PPI therapy but who also have an allergic phenotype; it is likely that the therapeutic response to PPI will not be sustained and symptom recurrence will prompt further investigations [14].
* Consider repeat endoscopy with biopsy to document histologic pattern.
** If patient refuses dietary changes, start topical corticosteroid (TCS) at this step.
*** If esophagogastroduodenoscopy is repeated for continued symptoms TCS and esophageal stenosis is appreciated, may skip barium swallow.

PPIs over another. We recommend a trial of a PPI given twice daily (30 minutes before breakfast and dinner) for at least 4 weeks. If symptoms improve, then PPI therapy can be maintained indefinitely as the patient likely has GERD. The clinician can attempt to decrease the dose of PPI to once a day.

Alternatively, the suspected patient could undergo pH monitoring of the distal esophagus to assess for pathologic acid reflux supporting a diagnosis of GERD.

If PPI treatment is administered and symptoms do not improve, the clinician can consider performing an upper endoscopy and biopsy before stopping PPI therapy to determine if esophageal eosinophilia is persistent, thus providing diagnostic evidence of EE. The validity of this approach to PPI therapy requires formal investigation.

Nutritional management

After the diagnosis is confirmed, we recommend that if nutritional treatment is a viable option for a patient and family, SPT for food allergens should be performed and a directed elimination diet initiated based on the results of that testing. This should be done with the consultation of a nutritionist. An alternative approach that may be similarly effective is to prescribe an empiric elimination diet but, pending further studies, we still prefer the directed elimination diet.

Medical management

If bothersome symptoms/esophageal eosinophilia persist despite nutritional management, or if the patient refuses nutritional management, a trial of topical steroids is appropriate. The optimal, age-adjusted doses of topical corticosteroids for children who have EE are unknown, because these preparations were not designed for esophageal administration. One study extrapolated doses from those used in the treatment of asthma, whereas others have empirically used higher doses without significant side effects. Doses for children range from 44 to 220 μg by mouth twice daily and adolescents/adults 440 to 880 μg by mouth twice daily. Patients should not use a spacer as is used with the metered dose inhaler for asthma. The patient is instructed to spray the steroid into the mouth with lips sealed around the device and should not eat or drink for at least 30 minutes. This regimen is continued for 6 to 12 weeks.

If symptoms and eosinophilia resolve, steroids are weaned and patients are followed with the expectation that repeated courses of steroids will be needed. In children and adults, fluticasone treatment can be continued uninterrupted for patients who have repeated relapses when the steroid is discontinued and patients followed clinically, but the long-term efficacy and safety of this treatment remains unclear. (See the article by Liacouras, elsewhere in this issue.) In children, especially those who are chronologically or developmentally too young to use an MDI puff and swallow technique, a viscous suspension consisting of 1 mg of budesonide mixed with sucralose can be swallowed once daily for the control of symptoms and inflammation without effects on morning cortisol levels.

Persistent symptoms and inflammation

If nutritional or medical treatment with topical steroids is not effective, four considerations should be entertained. First, if patients were using topical corticosteroids, then they could have acquired esophageal candidiasis, which could contribute to the persistent esophageal symptoms. The patient would either undergo an upper endoscopy with biopsy or empiric antifungal treatment. Second, the patient may have a fixed anatomic lesion, such as an isolated stricture or small-caliber esophagus, that may require dilation. A barium esophagram is helpful in assessing this situation. Discussion with the radiologist is critical to clarify the questions that are being addressed. Unless the radiologist is asked specifically to examine for a proximal esophageal stricture or for extensive esophageal narrowing with impaired peristalsis, these findings easily can be missed. If stenoses are identified, we prefer to try a course of systemic steroid therapy before resorting to dilation (eg, prednisone 20 mg every day for 2 to 4 weeks), but there are few data available to either support or refute this approach. Esophageal dilation is used following the same general approach that has been recommended for patients who have benign strictures of the esophagus [14], with careful consideration of the esophageal fragility sometimes associated with EE. (See the articles by Putnam and Fox, elsewhere in this issue.) In addition, it seems prudent to be especially cautious regarding the possibility of esophageal perforation with dilation, and to have a low threshold for ordering prompt radiologic assessment for perforation if there are any clinical features to suggest that possibility. Third, a course of systemic steroid therapy (eg, prednisone 20 mg every day for 2 to 4 weeks) may be used if no anatomic lesion is identified, or if dysphagia persists after esophageal dilation. Finally, a course of an elemental diet or elimination diet may induce remission in refractory cases, but the long-term compliance with this strategy is uncertain.

Unresolved issues

There remain numerous unresolved issues regarding the proper management of patients who have EE (Box 1). Because the natural history and incidence of complications is currently unknown, there is no proof that any treatment can prevent the complications of the disease. The approach recommended above is based on our review of the literature and clinical experience (see Fig. 1). Whether this approach is the optimal one for relieving the symptoms and preventing the complications of EE is yet to be determined, but it represents the authors' best attempt to provide optimal care. Future

---

Box 1. **Future research topics**

Natural history: determination of incidence and severity of
    complications
Scoring tools: symptoms, histology, endoscopy
Prospective treatment trials in adults and children examining
    nutritional and steroid modalities
Usefulness of endoscopic assessment in follow-up of patients
Surrogate markers
Pathogenetic mechanisms
Identification and study of novel therapeutic agents

---

multidisciplinary studies focusing on these issues will improve the care for children and adults affected by EE.

References

[1] Furuta GT, Liacouras C, Collins MH, et al. Eosinophilic esophagitis in children and adults: a systematic review and consensus recommendations for diagnosis and treatment. Gastroenterol 2007;133:1342–63.

[2] Ruchelli E, Wenner W, Voytek T, et al. Severity of esophageal eosinophilia predicts response to conventional gastroesophageal reflux therapy. Pediatr Dev Pathol 1999;2:15.

[3] Winter HS, Madara JL, Stafford RJ, et al. Intraepithelial eosinophils: a new diagnostic criterion for reflux esophagitis. Gastroenterology 1982;83:818.

[4] Aceves SS, Newbury RO, Dohil R, et al. Distinguishing eosinophilic esophagitis in pediatric patients: clinical, endoscopic, and histologic features of an emerging disorder. J Clin Gastroenterol 2007;41:252.

[5] Dahms BB. Reflux esophagitis: sequelae and differential diagnosis in infants and children including eosinophilic esophagitis. Pediatr Dev Pathol 2004;7:5.

[6] Ngo P, Furuta GT, Antonioli DA, et al. Eosinophils in the esophagus—peptic or allergic eosinophilic esophagitis? Case series of three patients with esophageal eosinophilia. Am J Gastroenterol 2006;101:1666.

[7] Noel RJ, Tipnis NA. Eosinophilic esophagitis—a mimic of GERD. Int J Pediatr Otorhinolaryngol 2006;70:1147.

[8] Parfitt JR, Gregor JC, Suskin NG, et al. Eosinophilic esophagitis in adults: distinguishing features from gastroesophageal reflux disease: a study of 41 patients. Mod Pathol 2006;19: 90.

[9] Steiner SJ, Gupta SK, Croffie JM, et al. Correlation between number of eosinophils and reflux index on same day esophageal biopsy and 24 hour esophageal pH monitoring. Am J Gastroenterol 2004;99:801.

[10] Steiner SJ, Kernek KM, Fitzgerald JF. Severity of basal cell hyperplasia differs in reflux versus eosinophilic esophagitis. J Pediatr Gastroenterol Nutr 2006;42:506.

[11] Walsh S, Antonioli D, Goldman H, et al. Allergic esophagitis in children—A clinicopathological entity. Am J Surg Pathol 1999;23:390.

[12] Blanchard C, Wang N, Stringer KF, et al. Eotaxin-3 and a uniquely conserved gene-expression profile in eosinophilic esophagitis. J Clin Invest 2006;116:536.

[13] Kirsch R, Bokhary R, Marcon MA, et al. Activated mucosal mast cells differentiate eosinophilic (allergic) esophagitis from gastroesophageal reflux disease. J Pediatr Gastroenterol Nutr 2007;44:20.

[14] Spechler SJ, Genta RM, Souza RF. Thoughts on the complex relationship between gastroesophageal reflux disease and eosinophilic esophagitis. Am J Gastroenterol 2007; 102:1301.

[15] Rafiee P, Theriot ME, Nelson VM, et al. Human esophageal microvascular endothelial cells respond to acidic pH stress by PI3K/AKT and p38 MAPK-regulated induction of Hsp70 and Hsp27. Am J Physiol Cell Physiol 2006;291:C931.

[16] Cheng L, Cao W, Behar J, et al. Acid-induced release of platelet-activating factor by human esophageal mucosa induces inflammatory mediators in circular smooth muscle. J Pharmacol Exp Ther 2006;319:117.

[17] Hollwarth ME, Smith M, Kvietys PR, et al. Esophageal blood flow in the cat. Normal distribution and effects of acid perfusion. Gastroenterology 1986;90:622.

[18] Locke GR 3rd, Talley NJ, Fett SL, et al. Prevalence and clinical spectrum of gastroesophageal reflux: a population-based study in Olmsted County, Minnesota. Gastroenterology 1997;112:1448.

[19] Shaheen N, Provenzale D. The epidemiology of gastroesophageal reflux disease. Am J Med Sci 2003;326:264.

[20] Gonsalves N, Policarpio-Nicolas M, Zhang Q, et al. Histopathologic variability and endoscopic correlates in adults with eosinophilic esophagitis. Gastrointest Endosc 2006;64: 313.

[21] Sant'Anna AM, Rolland S, Fournet JC, et al. Eosinophilic esophagitis in children: symptoms, histology and pH probe results. J Pediatr Gastroenterol Nutr 2004;39:373.

[22] Remedios M, Campbell C, Jones DM, et al. Eosinophilic esophagitis in adults: clinical, endoscopic, histologic findings, and response to treatment with fluticasone propionate. Gastrointest Endosc 2006;63:3.

[23] Cheng L, Harnett KM, Cao W, et al. Hydrogen peroxide reduces lower esophageal sphincter tone in human esophagitis. Gastroenterology 2005;129:1675.

[24] Farre R, Auli M, Lecea B, et al. Pharmacologic characterization of intrinsic mechanisms controlling tone and relaxation of porcine lower esophageal sphincter. J Pharmacol Exp Ther 2006;316:1238.

[25] Cao W, Cheng L, Behar J, et al. IL-1beta signaling in cat lower esophageal sphincter circular muscle. Am J Physiol Gastrointest Liver Physiol 2006;291:G672.

[26] Cao W, Cheng L, Behar J, et al. Proinflammatory cytokines alter/reduce esophageal circular muscle contraction in experimental cat esophagitis. Am J Physiol Gastrointest Liver Physiol 2004;287:G1131.

[27] Sgouros SN, Bergele C, Mantides A. Eosinophilic esophagitis in adults: a systematic review. Eur J Gastroenterol Hepatol 2006;18:211.

[28] Straumann A, Spichtin HP, Grize L, et al. Natural history of primary eosinophilic esophagitis: a follow-up of 30 adult patients for up to 11.5 years. Gastroenterology 2003;125: 1660.

[29] Motojima S, Frigas E, Loegering DA, et al. Toxicity of eosinophil cationic proteins for guinea pig tracheal epithelium in vitro. Am Rev Respir Dis 1989;139:801.

[30] Tai PC, Hayes DJ, Clark JB, et al. Toxic effects of human eosinophil products on isolated rat heart cells in vitro. Biochem J 1982;204:75.

[31] Young JD, Peterson CG, Venge P, et al. Mechanism of membrane damage mediated by human eosinophil cationic protein. Nature 1986;321:613.

[32] Furuta GT, Nieuwenhuis EE, Karhausen J, et al. Eosinophils alter colonic epithelial barrier function: role for major basic protein. Am J Physiol Gastrointest Liver Physiol 2005;289: G890.

[33] Barlow WJ, Orlando RC. The pathogenesis of heartburn in nonerosive reflux disease: a unifying hypothesis. Gastroenterology 2005;128:771.

[34] Ohashi Y, Motojima S, Fukuda T, et al. [Relationship between bronchial reactivity to inhaled acetylcholine, eosinophil infiltration and a widening of the intercellular space in patients with asthma]. Arerugi 1990;39:1541 [in Japanese].

[35] Tobey NA, Carson JL, Alkiek RA, et al. Dilated intercellular spaces: a morphological feature of acid reflux–damaged human esophageal epithelium. Gastroenterology 1996;111: 1200.
[36] Genta RM, Jon Spechler S, Souza RF. The twentieth eosinophil. Adv Anat Pathol 2007;14: 340.
[37] Tobey NA, Hosseini SS, Argote CM, et al. Dilated intercellular spaces and shunt permeability in nonerosive acid-damaged esophageal epithelium. Am J Gastroenterol 2004;99:13.
[38] Untersmayr E, Jensen-Jarolim E. The effect of gastric digestion on food allergy. Curr Opin Allergy Clin Immunol 2006;6:214.
[39] Astwood JD, Leach JN, Fuchs RL. Stability of food allergens to digestion in vitro. Nat Biotechnol 1996;14:1269.
[40] Scholl I, Ackermann U, Ozdemir C, et al. Anti-ulcer treatment during pregnancy induces food allergy in mouse mothers and a Th2-bias in their offspring. Faseb J 2007;21:1264.
[41] Scholl I, Untersmayr E, Bakos N, et al. Antiulcer drugs promote oral sensitization and hypersensitivity to hazelnut allergens in BALB/c mice and humans. Am J Clin Nutr 2005;81: 154.
[42] Untersmayr E, Bakos N, Scholl I, et al. Anti-ulcer drugs promote IgE formation toward dietary antigens in adult patients. Faseb J 2005;19:656.
[43] Rothenberg ME. Eosinophilic gastrointestinal disorders (EGID). J Allergy Clin Immunol 2004;113:11.
[44] De Angelis P, Markowitz JE, Torroni F, et al. Paediatric eosinophilic oesophagitis: towards early diagnosis and best treatment. Dig Liver Dis 2006;38:245.
[45] Kagalwalla AF, Sentongo TA, Ritz S, et al. Effect of six-food elimination diet on clinical and histologic outcomes in eosinophilic esophagitis. Clin Gastroenterol Hepatol 2006;4: 1097.
[46] Liacouras CA, Spergel JM, Ruchelli E, et al. Eosinophilic esophagitis: a 10-year experience in 381 children. Clin Gastroenterol Hepatol 2005;3:1198.
[47] Markowitz JE, Spergel JM, Ruchelli E, et al. Elemental diet is an effective treatment for eosinophilic esophagitis in children and adolescents. Am J Gastroenterol 2003;98:777.
[48] Spergel JM, Andrews T, Brown-Whitehorn TF, et al. Treatment of eosinophilic esophagitis with specific food elimination diet directed by a combination of skin prick and patch tests. Ann Allergy Asthma Immunol 2005;95:336.
[49] Spergel JM, Beausoleil JL, Mascarenhas M, et al. The use of skin prick tests and patch tests to identify causative foods in eosinophilic esophagitis. J Allergy Clin Immunol 2002;109:363.
[50] Teitelbaum J, Fox V, Twarog F, et al. Eosinophilic esophagitis in children: immunopathological analysis and response to fluticasone propionate. Gastroenterology 2002;122:1216.
[51] Spergel JM, Brown-Whitehorn T, Beausoleil JL, et al. Predictive values for skin prick test and atopy patch test for eosinophilic esophagitis. J Allergy Clin Immunol 2007;119:509.
[52] Yamazaki K, Murray JA, Arora AS, et al. Allergen-specific in vitro cytokine production in adult patients with eosinophilic esophagitis. Dig Dis Sci 2006;51:1934.
[53] Jones M, Campbell KA, Duggan C, et al. Multiple micronutrient deficiencies in a child fed an elemental formula. J Pediatr Gastroenterol Nutr 2001;33:602.
[54] Simon D, Marti H, Heer P, et al. Eosinophilic esophagitis is frequently associated with IgE-mediated allergic airway diseases. J Allergy Clin Immunol 2005;115:1090.
[55] Simon D, Straumann A, Wenk A, et al. Eosinophilic esophagitis in adults—no clinical relevance of wheat and rye sensitizations. Allergy 2006;61:1480.
[56] Fogg MI, Ruchelli E, Spergel JM. Pollen and eosinophilic esophagitis. J Allergy Clin Immunol 2003;112:796.
[57] Mishra A, Hogan SP, Brandt EB, et al. An etiological role for aeroallergens and eosinophils in experimental esophagitis. J Clin Invest 2001;107:83.
[58] Onbasi K, Sin AZ, Doganavsargil B, et al. Eosinophil infiltration of the oesophageal mucosa in patients with pollen allergy during the season. Clin Exp Allergy 2005;35:1423.

[59] Mishra A, Hogan SP, Brandt EB, et al. IL-5 promotes eosinophil trafficking to the esophagus. J Immunol 2002;168:2464.

[60] Mishra A, Rothenberg ME. Intratracheal IL-13 induces eosinophilic esophagitis by an IL-5,
eotaxin-1, and STAT6-dependent mechanism. Gastroenterology 2003;125:1419.

[61] Mishra A, Schlotman J, Wang M, et al. Critical role for adaptive T cell immunity in experimental eosinophilic esophagitis in mice. J Leukoc Biol 2007;81:916.

[62] Esposito S, Marinello D, Paracchini R, et al. Long-term follow-up of symptoms and peripheral eosinophil counts in seven children with eosinophilic esophagitis. J Pediatr Gastroenterol Nutr 2004;38:452.

[63] Konikoff MR, Blanchard C, Kirby C, et al. Potential of blood eosinophils, eosinophil-
derived neurotoxin, and eotaxin-3 as biomarkers of eosinophilic esophagitis. Clin Gastroenterol Hepatol 2006;4:1328.

[64] Bullock JZ, Villanueva JM, Blanchard C, et al. Interplay of adaptive Th2 immunity with
eotaxin-3/c-C chemokine receptor 3 in eosinophilic esophagitis. J Pediatr Gastroenterol
Nutr 2007;45:22.

[65] Lucendo AJ, De Rezende L. Endoscopic dilation in eosinophilic esophagitis: a treatment
strategy associated with a high risk of perforation. Endoscopy 2007;39:376, author reply:
377.

[66] Prasad GA, Arora AS. Spontaneous perforation in the ringed esophagus. Dis Esophagus
2005;18:406.

[67] Aceves SS, Newbury RO, Dohil R, et al. Esophageal remodeling in pediatric eosinophilic
esophagitis. J Allergy Clin Immunol 2007;119:206.

[68] Attwood SE, Lewis CJ, Bronder CS, et al. Eosinophilic oesophagitis: a novel treatment using
Montelukast. Gut 2003;52:181.

[69] Spergel JM. Eosinophilic esophagitis in adults and children: evidence for a food allergy component in many patients. Curr Opin Allergy Clin Immunol 2007;7:274.

[70] Gonsalves N, et al. A prospective clinical trial of allergy testing and food elimination diet in
adults with eosinophilic esophagitis. Gastroenterol 2007;132:A6.

[71] Liacouras CA, Wenner WJ, Brown K, et al. Primary eosinophilic esophagitis in children:
successful treatment with oral corticosteroids. J Pediatr Gastroenterol Nutr 1998;26:380.

[72] Konikoff MR, Noel RJ, Blanchard C, et al. A randomized, double-blind, placebo-controlled
trial of fluticasone propionate for pediatric eosinophilic esophagitis. Gastroenterology 2006;
131:1381.

[73] Noel RJ, Putnam PE, Collins MH, et al. Clinical and immunopathologic effects of swallowed
fluticasone for eosinophilic esophagitis. Clin Gastroenterol Hepatol 2004;2:568.

[74] Aceves SS, Dohil R, Newbury RO, et al. Topical viscous budesonide suspension for treatment of eosinophilic esophagitis. J Allergy Clin Immunol 2005;116:705.

[75] Arora AS, Perrault J, Smyrk TC. Topical corticosteroid treatment of dysphagia due to
eosinophilic esophagitis in adults. Mayo Clin Proc 2003;78:830.

[76] Faubion WA Jr, Perrault J, Burgart LJ, et al. Treatment of eosinophilic esophagitis with
inhaled corticosteroids. J Pediatr Gastroenterol Nutr 1998;27:90.

[77] Aceves SS, Bastian JF, Newbury RO, et al. Oral viscous budesonide: a potential new therapy
for eosinophilic esophagitis in children. Am J Gastroenterol 2007;102:2271-9.

[78] Lucendo AJ, Navarro M, Comas C, et al. Immunophenotypic characterization and quanti-
fication of the epithelial inflammatory infiltrate in eosinophilic esophagitis through stereol-
ogy: an analysis of the cellular mechanisms of the disease and the immunologic capacity of
the esophagus. Am J Surg Pathol 2007;31:598.

[79] Assa'ad AH, Putnam PE, Collins MH, et al. Pediatric patients with eosinophilic esophagitis:
an 8-year follow-up. J Allergy Clin Immunol 2007;119:731-8.

[80] Pentiuk SP, Miller CK, Kaul A. Eosinophilic esophagitis in infants and toddlers. Dysphagia
2007;22:44.

[81] Long-term effects of budesonide or nedocromil in children with asthma. The Childhood
Asthma Management Program Research Group. N Engl J Med 2000;343:1054.

[82] Guilbert TW, Morgan WJ, Zeiger RS, et al. Long-term inhaled corticosteroids in preschool children at high risk for asthma. N Engl J Med 2006;354:1985.

[83] Fox VL, Nurko S, Teitelbaum JE, et al. High-resolution EUS in children with eosinophilic "allergic" esophagitis. Gastrointest Endosc 2003;57:30.

[84] Stein ML, Collins MH, Villanueva JM, et al. Anti-IL-5 (mepolizumab) therapy for eosinophilic esophagitis. J Allergy Clin Immunol 2006;118:1312.

[85] Spechler SJ. American gastroenterological association medical position statement on treatment of patients with dysphagia caused by benign disorders of the distal esophagus. Gastroenterology 1999;117:229.

[86] Morrow JB, Vargo JJ, Goldblum JR, et al. The ringed esophagus: histological features of GERD. Am J Gastroenterol 2001;96:984.

[87] Gonsalves N, Hirano I. Safety and response of esophageal dilation in adults with eosinophilic esophagitis (EE): a single center experience of 81 patients. Gastroenterol 2007;132:A607.

ELSEVIER
SAUNDERS

Gastrointest Endoscopy Clin N Am
18 (2008) 219–224

GASTROINTESTINAL
ENDOSCOPY CLINICS
OF NORTH AMERICA

Index

Note: Page numbers of article titles are in **boldface** type.

Moving?

Make sure your subscription moves with you!

To notify us of your new address, find your **Clinics Account Number** (located on your mailing label above your name), and contact customer service at:

E-mail: elspcs@elsevier.com

800-654-2452 (subscribers in the U.S. & Canada)
407-345-4000 (subscribers outside of the U.S. & Canada)

Fax number: 407-363-9661

Elsevier Periodicals Customer Service
6277 Sea Harbor Drive
Orlando, FL 32887-4800

*To ensure uninterrupted delivery of your subscription, please notify us at least 4 weeks in advance of move.